Clinical Companion to Accompany

Contemporary Medical-Surgical Nursing

Clinical Companion to Accompany

Contemporary Medical-Surgical Nursing

Rick Daniels, RN, PhD
Oregon Health and Science University
Ashland, Oregon

Laura John Nosek, PhD, RN
Frances Payne Bolton School of Nursing
Case Western Reserve University
Cleveland, Ohio
and
Marcella Niehoff School of Nursing
Loyola University Chicago
Chicago, Illinois
and
Excelsior College
Albany, New York

Leslie H. Nicoll, PhD, MBA, RN, BC
Principal and Owner
Maine Desk, LLC
Portland, Maine

Prepared by
Janice Tazbir, RN, MS, CS, CCRN
Associate Professor of Nursing
Purdue University Calumet
Hammond, Indiana

THOMSON

DELMAR LEARNING

Clinical Companion to Accompany Contemporary Medical-Surgical Nursing

by Rick Daniels, Laura John Nosek, and Leslie H. Nicoll

Prepared by Janice Tazbir

Vice President, Health Care Business Unit:
William Brottmiller

Director of Learning Solutions:
Matthew Kane

Acquisitions Editor:
Tamara Caruso

Product Manager:
Patricia Gaworecki

Editorial Assistant:
Tiffiny Adams

Marketing Director:
Jennifer McAvey

Marketing Channel Manager:
Michele McTighe

Marketing Coordinator:
Danielle Pacella

Technology Director:
Laurie Davis

Technology Project Manager:
Mary Colleen Liburdi

Production Director:
Carolyn Miller

Production Manager:
Barbara Bullock

Art Director:
Robert Plante
Jack Pendleton

Content Project Manager:
Stacey Lamodi
Jessica McNavich

Printed in the United States of America
1 2 3 4 5 6 7 8 XXX 09 08 07 06

For more information, contact Thomson Delmar Learning, 5 Maxwell Drive, Clifton Park, NY 12065
Or find us on the World Wide Web at http://www.delmarlearning.com

Library of Congress Cataloging-in-Publication Data
ISBN 1-4018-3721-2

Introduction

The first edition *Clinical Companion to Accompany Contemporary Medical-Surgical Nursing* is designed as a quick reference guide for nursing in the clinical setting. It is also designed to accompany the *Contemporary Medical-Surgical* text with a more clinical approach to diseases and conditions commonly seen in the clinical setting. It is written to give the nurse answers to the questions: What is the condition? What should I look for? What should I do?

The book is divided into two parts. The first section, Diseases and Disorders, focuses on over 200 diseases and disorders, which are alphabetically arranged so that topics can be found quickly. Each topic contains a definition, key assessments, diagnostics, lab tests, points for planning and implementing nursing care, and the nursing diagnosis based on NANDA's *Nursing Diagnoses: Definitions and Classifications.* In addition, discharge planning and special concerns are addressed when appropriate to the topic and include cultural, gender, geriatric, and teaching concerns. The second section, Special Procedures and Treatments, includes special procedures and treatments commonly seen in the acute care setting. Some procedures, such as Pallative Care, are common, general in nature, and affect many types of patients, and others, such as Valve Repair, are more specific.

The appendices incorporate reference materials to assist the nurse with common needs in the health care setting, including common Spanish phrases, a quick head-to-toe assessment guide, a common abbreviations list, and a lab reference list.

As the health care setting becomes more complex, relying on references is necessary. It is not always how smart you are, but how good your references are. My hope is that this *Clinical Companion* will help increase your knowledge base as you provide safe and effective nursing care.

ACKNOWLEDGMENTS

I would like to thank Katherine Kraines for her editorial support and for cheerleading me through this incredible process. To the people who have meant, and continue to mean, the most to me: my father, for giving me the ability to dream; my mother, for making me understand strength and grace; my grandmother, for helping me value service; my husband, for loving me no matter what; and my girls, for making life more precious than I could have ever dreamed.

Janice Tazbir, RN, MS, CS, CCRN
Associate Professor of Nursing

Contents

SECTION 1
Diseases and Disorders

A

B

C

F

G

H

O

P

R

SECTION

1

Diseases and Disorders

Abscess, Hepatic

DEFINITION

- Hepatic abscess is an area of infection in the liver caused by bacteria, amoeba, or protozoa.

KEY ASSESSMENTS

- Right upper quadrant pain
- Chills
- Malaise
- Pleuritic chest pain
- Right shoulder pain
- Anorexia
- Weight loss
- Hepatomegaly
- Jaundice

Diagnostics

- Abdominal X-ray
- Computed tomography (CT) of the abdomen

Lab Tests

- Liver function tests
- Complete blood count (CBC)
- Prothrombin time (PT)
- Blood cultures

PLANNING AND IMPLEMENTATION

- Monitor intake and output (I & O)
- Encourage adequate fluid and nutritional intake
- Daily weight
- Administer antibiotics
- Monitor vital signs
- Administer analgesics for pain
- Administer antipyretic
- Anticipate CT guided draining

A

SPECIAL CONCERNS

Cultural Considerations

- Hepatic abscesses are common in developing countries and are usually caused by amoeba or protozoa.

Gender Considerations

- Men are twice as likely as women to develop a hepatic abscess.

NURSING DIAGNOSIS

- Pain, Acute
- Hyperthermia
- Infection, Risk for

Abscess, Lung

DEFINITION

- A lung abscess is a collection or cavity of cellular debris formed as a result of necrosis. It can be acute or chronic and can develop from pulmonary infections, such as pneumonia, or from aspiration of bacteria from the oral pharynx. Aspiration may be from mental status changes, pharyngeal dysfunction, or periodontal disease.

KEY ASSESSMENTS

- Fever and chills
- Night sweats
- Productive cough
- Dyspnea
- Pleuritic chest pain
- Weight loss
- Percussed localized dullness over involved lung

Lab Tests

- Sputum samples
- Complete blood count (CBC)
- Chest X-ray (CXR)
- Computed tomography (CT) or bronchoscopy (to rule out malignancy)

PLANNING AND IMPLEMENTATION

- Monitor respiratory system
- Administer oxygen therapy
- Elevate head of bed
- Encourage incentive spirometry
- Plan frequent rest periods
- Monitor fluid and nutritional intake
- Treat pleuritic pain
- Administer appropriate antibiotics

Discharge Planning

- Patients need to understand long-term antibiotic therapy is often necessary.
- Make certain the patient has the financial means to continue antibiotic therapy once discharged.

NURSING DIAGNOSIS

- Infection, Risk for
- Breathing pattern, Ineffective
- Tissue perfusion, Ineffective

Abscess, Peritonsillar

DEFINITION

- A peritonsillar abscess, also known as quinsy, is a localized accumulation of pus in the peritonsillar tissue that forms as a complication of acute tonsillitis. The highest incidence is in the 15 to 35 age group. The most common bacterial organism is *Streptococcus pyogenes*.

KEY ASSESSMENTS

- Sore throat
- Painful swallowing
- Fever
- Trismus (difficulty opening the mouth)
- Enlarged tonsil displaced on the side of the abscess
- Uvula displaced to opposite side
- Red, swollen soft palate

PLANNING AND IMPLEMENTATION

- Encourage cool liquids and frequent gargling for pain
- Administer analgesics
- Monitor respiratory status
- Encourage adequate intake by mouth
- Needle aspiration (for culture and sensitivity)
- Appropriate antibiotics (based on culture results)
- Tonsillectomy (for repeated episodes of peritonsillar abscess)

SPECIAL CONCERNS

- Complications of peritonsillar abscess may include airway obstruction. The nurse must quickly identify any signs of airway obstruction, such as stridor, and report to the health care provider immediately.

NURSING DIAGNOSIS

- Infection, Risk for
- Pain, Acute
- Breathing pattern, Ineffective

Achalasia

DEFINITION

- Achalasia is the loss of peristalsis and failure of the lower esophagus to relax with eating, causing pain and dysphagia (swallowing difficulties).

KEY ASSESSMENTS

- Esophageal pain that may radiate to the throat, neck, or back
- Dysphagia
- Weight loss

Diagnostics

- Video esophagram
- Esophageal manometry (measures pressure in the esophagus)
- Endoscopy

PLANNING AND IMPLEMENTATION

- Provide small, frequent, soft meals
- Upright positioning with meals
- Daily weight
- Monitor intake and output (I & O)
- Treat pain
- Administer vasodilator medications including nitroglycerin and calcium channel blockers
- Treatment options: balloon dilation of the esophagus, esophageal myotomy (severing muscle fibers), or esophageal muscle injection with botulism toxin

NURSING DIAGNOSIS

- Pain, Acute
- Swallowing, Impaired
- Nutrition: less than body requirements, Imbalanced

Acromegaly

DEFINITION

- Acromegaly is caused by a hypersecretion of pituitary growth hormone from a tumor over a period of time. The chronic effects of excess growth hormone are cardiovascular, cerebrovascular, and respiratory disease and an increased risk for diabetes mellitus.

KEY ASSESSMENTS

- Large, thick-boned head and hands
- Headaches
- Hypertension
- Decreased libido
- Arthralgias

Diagnostics

- Magnetic resonance imaging (MRI)

Lab Tests

- Serum growth hormone (perform the test in the morning)
- Growth hormone suppression test
- Postprandial plasma glucose

PLANNING AND IMPLEMENTATION

- Monitor for long-term effects of growth hormone on other body systems
- Monitor glucose levels
- Anticipate surgical removal of the tumor or use of a gamma knife

NURSING DIAGNOSIS

- Body image, Disturbed
- Knowledge, Deficient

Acute Respiratory Distress Syndrome (ARDS)

DEFINITION

- ARDS is a noncardiac pulmonary edema with increased permeability of the alveolar-capillary membrane because of injury. Increased permeability allows interstitial edema, which prohibits gas exchange and may cause death. Synonyms include adult respiratory distress syndrome, shock lung, wet lung, capillary leak syndrome, and adult hyaline membrane disease.

Clinical Causes

- Aspiration
- Near drowning
- Smoke inhalation
- Pneumonia
- Chest trauma
- Sepsis
- Acute pancreatitis
- Systemic inflammatory response syndrome (SIRS)
- Disseminated intravascular coagulation (DIC)
- Shock

KEY ASSESSMENTS

- Dyspnea
- Hypoxia
- Cyanosis

Diagnostics

- Chest X-ray ([CXR], ground glass appearance)

Lab Tests

- Arterial blood gases ([ABGs], hypoxia and acidosis)

PLANNING AND IMPLEMENTATION

- Intubation and mechanical ventilation
- Monitor pulse oximetry
- Monitor vital signs
- Monitor neurological status
- Maintain patent intravenous (IV) fluids
- Provide adequate fluid balance with IV therapy
- Monitor intake and output (I & O)
- Turn patient every two hours with head of bed elevated
- Anticipate prone positioning
- Oral care every four hours
- Sedation may be required
- Prevent complications associated with immobility
- Monitor ABGs

NURSING DIAGNOSIS

- Tissue perfusion, Ineffective
- Fluid volume, Risk for imbalanced
- Infection, Risk for
- Breathing pattern, Ineffective
- Mobility, Impaired physical

Acute Myocardial Infarction (AMI)

DEFINITION

- AMI is when an atherosclerotic plaque ruptures, resulting in occlusions of a coronary artery and leading to myocardial tissue anoxia and death.

KEY ASSESSMENTS

- Integumentary: cool, clammy, pale, or ashen skin
- Neurological: altered level of consciousness (LOC) or syncope

- Respiratory: dyspnea, tachypnea, crackles, or shortness of breath
- Cardiovascular: tachycardia, bradycardia, arrhythmias, hypotension, hypertension, S_3, S_4, or murmur
- Gastrointestinal (GI) and genitourinary (GU): vomiting, decreased urine output
- Unrelieved angina

PLANNING AND IMPLEMENTATION

- Obtain electrocardiogram (ECG) (ST depression—acute ischemia, ST elevation—AMI)
- Place patient on cardiac monitor
- Obtain creatine kinase-megabase (CK-MB) and troponin levels
- MONA acronym for chest pain
  - **M**orphine intravenously for pain
  - **O**xygen
  - **N**itroglycerin
  - **A**spirin
- Vital signs with O_2 saturation
- If AMI: fibrinolytic therapy or percutaneous coronary intervention (PCI)

Fibrinolytic Therapy

- The goal of fibrinolytic therapy is to dissolve the thrombus and reperfuse the myocardium before myocardial cellular death occurs.
- It must be initiated within six hours of first symptoms.
- Patient selection is vital because major bleeding is a risk of therapy.
- Many contraindications to fibrinolytic therapy exist, such as known bleeding disorder and active peptic ulcer disease.
- The patient will also receive anticoagulation therapy, such as heparin, low molecular weight heparin, or glycoprotein Ib/IIIa receptor inhibitors.
- Monitor the patient for external and internal bleeding.
- Monitor LOC (cerebrovascular bleeding).
- Monitor coagulation and coronary studies.
- Monitor for resolution of chest pain.
- Monitor for resolution of ST segment abnormalities.

Percutaneous Coronary Interventions (PCI)

- PCI includes percutaneous transluminal coronary angioplasty (PTCA), a procedure performed under fluoroscopy in which a balloon-tipped catheter is inserted through a peripheral artery and guided into the stenotic segment of the coronary vessel. The balloon is inflated, and the plaque is compressed against the wall of the artery, restoring coronary perfusion.

- Monitor coagulation and coronary studies.
- Monitor for resolution of chest pain.
- Monitor for resolution of ST segment abnormalities.
- Monitor puncture site for bleeding or hematoma formation.
- Monitor vital signs for shock related to reaction or hemorrhaging frequently as ordered.
- Do not move the punctured limb for four to six hours or as prescribed by physician.
- Encourage fluids.
- Assess and document pulses frequently as ordered.
- Monitor distal pulses.

Complications of AMI

Arrhythmias

- Eighty percent of patients with AMI experience arrhythmias, including bradycardias, tachycardias, heart blocks, or atrial or ventricular fibrillation.
- Ventricular fibrillation is the most common cause of sudden death in the prehospital setting.
- Continuous ECG monitoring is essential.
- Arrhythmias can be treated with medication.

Cardiogenic shock

- Cardiogenic shock occurs when the contractility of the myocardium is inadequate and may require intra-aortic balloon pump therapy to stabilize the patient.
- Inotropic and vasoactive drugs are used to increase cardiac performance.
- Cardiogenic shock related to AMI has a 70 percent mortality rate.

Dressler's syndrome

- Dressler's syndrome is a pericarditis (inflammation of the pericardium) that develops 2 to 10 weeks after an AMI.
- Pain is mild to severe and is aggravated by coughing, inspiration, and upper body movement.
- It is thought to be an inflammatory response caused by an autoimmune reaction to myocardial neo-antigens.

Sudden cardiac death

- Sudden cardiac death is an unexpected death from cardiac causes.
- Ventricular fibrillation is a common cause of sudden cardiac death.
- Twenty-five percent of people who die of sudden cardiac death have no symptoms of coronary artery disease (CAD).

Congestive heart failure (CHF)

- CHF occurs when there is decreased contracting power of the heart.
- AMI may leave a portion of the heart necrotic, decreasing its contracting power.
- Dyspnea, jugular vein distention, crackles, and the presence of an S_3 heart sound are indications of CHF.

Cardiac Rehabilitation

- Cardiac rehabilitation combines exercise training with coronary risk factor modification in patients with established heart disease.
- The goals of cardiac rehabilitation are to:
  - Improve functional capacity
  - Alleviate or lessen activity related symptoms
  - Reduce disability
  - Identify and modify coronary risk factors
  - Reduce mortality and morbidity because of cardiovascular illness

Four phases of cardiac rehabilitation

- Phase 1—takes place in the hospital after a cardiac event. The emphasis is on light exercise and education regarding cardiac status. Referrals are made at this time for outpatient follow up.
- Phase 2—a transitional phase in which the patient begins to recover at home. The focus is on increasing activity.
- Phase 3—includes supervised exercise restoring physical function and reducing the risk of future heart conditions. There is counseling and education on adhering to prescribed dietary, physical, and medication therapy.
- Phase 4—is often referred to as the maintenance phase of cardiac rehabilitation. It emphasizes long-term lifestyle changes and is tailored to the patient.

SPECIAL CONCERNS

- See Special Procedures and Treatments for information on Coronary Artery Bypass Grafting (CABG).
- See Special Procedures and Treatments for information on Coronary Angioplasty.
- See Special Procedures and Treatments for information on Coronary Angiogram.

Cultural Considerations

- African Americans typically experience longer delays in seeking treatment for AMI and have higher mortality rates than Caucasians.
- African Americans have a greater incidence of dyspnea as an acute symptom of myocardial infarction (MI) rather than classic chest discomfort.

Gender Considerations

- CAD is the number one killer of women.
- Women have a higher mortality rate and reinfarction rate then men.
- Diabetes mellitus is the most powerful predictor of CAD in women.

Geriatric Considerations

- Elderly patients often do not experience chest pain when having an AMI.
- Many elderly present with dyspnea or pulmonary edema when experiencing an AMI.
- Elderly patients may be more sensitive to medications and should be monitored closely for dietary, physical, and medication side effects.

NURSING DIAGNOSIS

- Cardiac output, Decreased
- Tissue perfusion, Impaired
- Fluid volume, Risk for imbalanced
- Pain, Acute
- Knowledge, Deficit

Acute Pulmonary Edema

DEFINITION

- Acute pulmonary edema is an emergent condition in which there is an accumulation of fluid in the lungs resulting from heart failure and fluid overload.

KEY ASSESSMENTS

- Rapid, labored breathing
- Frothy, pink sputum
- Tachycardia and possible arrhythmias
- Decreased oxygen saturation
- Hypotension
- Thready pulse
- Cold, clammy, cyanotic skin
- Anxious with possible confusion

PLANNING AND IMPLEMENTATION

- Place patient in high Fowler's position
- Administer oxygen
- Anticipate diuretic administration
- Anticipate possible endotracheal intubation
- Monitor oxygenation status
- Monitor vital signs

NURSING DIAGNOSIS

- Airway clearance, Ineffective
- Breathing pattern, Ineffective
- Tissue perfusion, Ineffective

Addison's Disease

DEFINITION

- Addison's disease is adrenal insufficiency resulting from the destruction of the cortex of the adrenal gland (primary adrenal insufficiency) or from a deficient adrenocorticotropic hormone (ACTH) secretion due to a dysfunction of the pituitary hypothalamic axis (secondary adrenal insufficiency).

Clinical Causes

- Autoimmune disease
- Adrenal hemorrhage
- Infections (histoplasmosis or mycobacterium tuberculosis)
- Metastatic cancer
- Medications (ketoconazole, metyrapone, or etomidate)
- Rapid withdrawal of glucocorticoid therapy

KEY ASSESSMENTS

- Weakness
- Fatigue
- Hypotension
- Hyperpigmentation (only with primary adrenal insufficiency)
- Nausea

Lab Tests

- Glucose (low)
- Electrolytes (hyperkalemia or hyponatremia)
- Plasma cortisol (low)

PLANNING AND IMPLEMENTATION

- Implement safety measures
- Monitor glucose
- Monitor intake and output (I & O)
- Daily weight
- Cardiac monitoring
- Assist with activities of daily living
- Treat nausea
- Ensure adequate fluid and nutritional intake
- Administer cortisol as requested
- Anticipate increases in cortisol dose with stress or illness
- Monitor for signs of Addison's crisis
  - Shock, profound hypotension, and tachycardia
- Treat with aggressive fluid administration and IV cortisol

Discharge Planning

- Wear a medical alert bracelet at all times
- Teach patient and family members the signs of Addison's crisis
- Explain how to use hydrocortisone self-injection in case of crisis
- Contact the health care provider to adjust cortisol dose with stress or infection
- Never miss a dose of medication
- Keep extra cortisol medication in the home

NURSING DIAGNOSIS

- Activity intolerance
- Knowledge, Deficient
- Injury, Risk for
- Fluid volume, Deficient

Alpha-Antitrypsin Deficiency

DEFINITION

- Alpha-antitrypsin deficiency is a genetic deficiency of alpha trypsin that is normally produced in the liver and then transported to the lungs. Alpha trypsin neutralizes enzymes released by white blood cells (WBCs). Without adequate alpha trypsin, the WBCs attack healthy lung tissue and can lead to cirrhosis of the liver.

KEY ASSESSMENTS

- Shortness of breath
- Productive cough
- Pulse oximetry
- Ascites
- Abdominal pain

Lab Tests

- Alpha-antitrypsin deficiency
- Aspartate transaminase (AST) and alanine aminotransferase (ALT)
- Pulmonary function tests

PLANNING AND IMPLEMENTATION

- Hepatitis B vaccination
- Flu and pneumococcal vaccines
- Avoid alcohol
- Administer oxygen
- Smoking cessation
- Monitor for worsening lung and liver function
- Administer alpha-1 proteinase inhibitor replacement therapy intravenously every week
- Lung and/or liver transplantation may be necessary

NURSING DIAGNOSIS

- Knowledge, Deficient
- Breathing pattern, Ineffective
- Infection, Risk for

Alzheimer's Disease

DEFINITION

- Alzheimer's disease is a progressive degenerative neurological disorder noted clinically with progressive dementia. Pathophysiological findings include neuronal degeneration in the hippocampus and cerebral cortex, neuritic plaques, also called spherical bodies, and neurofibrillary tangles inside the neurons. The cause is unknown, and risk factors include increasing age and family history.

Classifications

Stages of Alzheimer's disease

- Early stage is characterized by forgetfulness and inability to learn new information.
- Middle stage is characterized by disorientation; impaired ability to follow commands; wandering at night; and irritable, anxious behavior.
- Late stage is characterized by weight loss, severe impairment of all cognitive functions, inability to communicate, incontinence, and loss of motor skills leading to becoming bedridden.

KEY ASSESSMENTS

- Assess memory and cognitive skill using the Mini-Mental State Examination (MMSE)
- Dementia
- Behavioral changes
- Changes in communication
- Incontinence
- Motor skill and strength
- Weight loss

Diagnostics

- Diagnostic tests are used to rule out any other cause for the patient's symptoms.
- Dementia workup includes evaluation for delirium, depression, infection, thyroid dysfunction, nutritional deficits, heart failure, chronic obstructive pulmonary disease (COPD), arrhythmias, liver failure, brain lesions, or tumors.
- The only definitive test is brain biopsy confirming the presence of neurofibrillary tangles and neuritic plaques.

PLANNING AND IMPLEMENTATION

- Implement safety measures
- Meticulous skin care
- If restricted to the bed, reposition every two hours
- Monitor bowel and bladder function
- Monitor for motor weakness
- Monitor for progression of dementia
- Assist with activities of daily living
- Reorientate frequently
- Use memory aids, such as notes on items, and put the patient's first name on the door
- Anticipate night wandering
- Anticipate administering cholinesterase inhibitors, selective serotonin reuptake inhibitors (SSRIs), and antipsychotic medications

SPECIAL CONCERNS

Geriatric Considerations

- Alzheimer's disease is the fourth leading cause of death among the elderly. After the age of 65, the risk of Alzheimer's disease doubles every 20 years. Children of a parent diagnosed with Alzheimer's disease have a 50 percent risk of developing the disease.

Teaching Considerations

- Teaching should address the physical, emotional, and social aspects of the disease.
- In the early stages of the disease encourage the patient to address long-term issues, such as advanced directives, estate planning, and care options.
- Encourage the use of door alarms to warn if the patient tries to leave the home.
- Teach memory aids, such as the use of notes on items to improve the patient's ability to perform self-care and simple tasks.

NURSING DIAGNOSIS

- Injury, Risk for
- Thought process, Disturbed
- Sleep pattern, Disturbed
- Anxiety
- Self-care deficit, Bathing/hygiene

Amputation

DEFINITION

- Amputation is the surgical removal of a limb and is most commonly performed to the lower extremities due to peripheral vascular disease associated with diabetes mellitus.

Clinical Causes

- Frostbite
- Electrical burns
- Gangrene
- Trauma
- Cancer
- Peripheral vascular disease
- Diabetes mellitus
- Osteomyelitis

Classifications

- Above the knee amputation (AKA) loses joint function of the extremity
- Below the knee amputation (BKA) perseveres joint function

KEY ASSESSMENTS

- Pain level
- Limb color, temperature
- Evidence of bleeding
- Vital signs
- Oxygenation status
- Neurological status

PLANNING AND IMPLEMENTATION

- Treat phantom pain (pain felt where limb was preoperatively, which may be burning or itching in nature). It is real pain and needs to be treated as such.
- Monitor vital signs.
- Monitor wound for bleeding and infection.
- Residual limb should be monitored for color and temperature.
- Inspect incision for staple intactness and wound approximation.
- Keep residual limb elevated on one pillow for first 24 hours only.
- Prone patient as requested to prevent joint contracture.

- Keep residual limb wrapped to decrease swelling.
- Cleanse stump with sterile saline solution.
- Promote quadriceps exercises.
- Promote crutch use, if appropriate, until fit with a prosthetic.
- Anticipate grieving over loss.
- Institute safety precautions.

SPECIAL CONCERNS

Cultural Considerations

- Disposition of the limb should be discussed preoperatively. Jewish patients bury the limbs.

Teaching Considerations

- Inspect residual limb with mirror daily
- Change positions frequently
- Cleanse residual limb with soap and water
- Change stump sock daily

NURSING DIAGNOSIS

- Grieving, Anticipatory
- Pain, Acute
- Fall, Risk for
- Infection, Risk for

Amyotrophic Lateral Sclerosis (ALS)

DEFINITION

- ALS, also known as Lou Gehrig's disease, is a motor neuron disease causing progressive demyelination of the motor neurons in the anterior horn of the spinal cord, brainstem, and cerebral cortex. The progression of the disease leads to paralysis of all muscles, including those for respiratory function. The cause of ALS is unknown, there is no cure, and death usually occurs within two to six years of the diagnosis.

KEY ASSESSMENTS

- Dyspnea progressing to respiratory failure
- Muscle weakness, spasticity, and wasting

- Deep tendon reflexes
- Dysarthria and dysphasia
- Fatigue

Diagnostics

- There are no specific diagnostic studies to confirm ALS. Computed tomography (CT), magnetic resonance imaging (MRI), and electromyogram (EMG) may be used to rule out other causes for manifestations.

PLANNING AND IMPLEMENTATION

- Monitor airway
- Keep emergency airway equipment near
- Reposition every two hours
- Oral care every four hours
- Inspect skin for breakdown
- Implement safety measures
- Monitor bowel and bladder function
- Monitor gag reflex and ability to swallow
- Offer alternative means of communication
- Assist with activities of daily living
- Monitor fluid and nutritional intake
- Range of motion exercises
- Anticipate administering glutamate inhibitor and benzodiazepine medications

SPECIAL CONCERNS

- The issue of ventilation and long-term ventilatory support should be addressed with the patient early in the disease. Obtain advanced directives and do not intubate orders if the patient does not want mechanical ventilation.
- Patients should understand if the disease progresses and they choose to receive ventilation, they might be considered "locked-in." Locked-in is a term describing a patient who has full cognitive function (alert and orientated) but is unable to move or communicate in any way.

Teaching Considerations

- Teaching should address the physical, emotional, and social aspects of the disease.
- In the early stages of the disease encourage the patient to address long-term issues, such as advanced directives, estate planning, and care options.

NURSING DIAGNOSIS

- Ventilation, Impaired spontaneous
- Breathing pattern, Ineffective
- Fatigue
- Anxiety, Death
- Communication, Impaired verbal
- Mobility, Impaired physical

Anaphylaxis

DEFINITION

- Anaphylaxis is an immediate, life-threatening hypersensitive allergic reaction and may cause death within minutes if not promptly treated. Histamine and other substances are released causing smooth muscle contraction, vascular dilation, edema, and airway obstruction. Anaphylaxis triggers include food (i.e., peanuts), medications (i.e., penicillin), insect venom (i.e., bee stings), and latex products.

KEY ASSESSMENTS

- Dyspnea
- Wheezing
- Airway angioedema
- Tachycardia
- Hypotension
- Chest pain
- Cardiac arrest
- Urticaria
- Angioedema
- Flushing
- Nausea and vomiting
- Headaches
- Seizures
- Severe anxiety

PLANNING AND IMPLEMENTATION

- Recognize symptoms of anaphylaxis
- Administer high-flow oxygen
- Intubation equipment at bedside
- Initiate two large-bore peripheral intravenous (IV) lines

- Maintain blood pressure with isotonic IV fluids
- Administer epinephrine, histamine H_1 and H_2 antagonists, or steroids intravenously as ordered
- Anticipate administering inhaled beta agonists
- Stop offending agent if possible
- Recumbent position
- Cardiac monitoring
- Continuous pulse oximetry
- Vital signs every two to three minutes until resolution
- Prevent future occurrences
- Place allergy band on patient
- Note allergy in the patient's chart and notify pharmacy

SPECIAL CONCERNS

Teaching Considerations

- Causes of anaphylaxis
- Signs and symptoms of anaphylaxis
- Wear medical alert bracelet
- Notify the pharmacist of allergy
- Teach family and patient the use of Epipen

NURSING DIAGNOSIS

- Ventilation, Impaired spontaneous
- Tissue perfusion, Ineffective
- Allergy response, Latex
- Fluid volume, Risk for deficient

Anemia

DEFINITION

- Anemia is a condition in which the hemoglobin concentration is lower than normal. This results in fewer circulating red blood cells (RBCs) and lack of oxygen to the body's cells.

Clinical Causes

- Anemia from blood loss—the loss could be acute or chronic from wounds, trauma, or loss from the gastrointestinal (GI) tract
- Anemia from a decreased production of RBCs—including a lack of erythropoietin from renal disease or deficiency of

coproducers of RBCs, such as vitamin B_{12}, folic acid, or iron deficiency
- Anemia from increased destruction of RBCs—from abnormal RBC structure, such as sickle cell anemia or hypersplenism

Classifications

- Bleeding that results in RBC loss
- Hemolytic anemia caused by RBC destruction
- Hypoproliferative caused by defective RBC production

KEY ASSESSMENTS

- Fatigue, weakness
- Skin pallor
- Tachycardia
- Shortness of breath
- Arrhythmias
- Relate cause of anemia for other key assessments

Diagnostics

- Bone marrow aspiration may be necessary to evaluate malignancy

Lab Tests

- Complete blood count (CBC)
- RBC indices
- Hemoglobin and hematocrit
- Reticulocyte count
- Iron studies
- Serum vitamin B_{12}

PLANNING AND IMPLEMENTATION

- Monitor oxygenation status including pulse oximetry
- Administer oxygen
- Monitor for signs of hypovolemia (poor skin turgor, tachycardia, or decreased urine output)
- Obtain consents for blood
- Type and cross-match for blood products
- Anticipate administering blood
- Implement safety measures
- Space nursing activities
- Allow frequent rest periods
- Monitor skin color, temperature, and capillary refill

Types of Anemia

- Acquired hemolytic anemia may result from burns, radiation, hemodialysis, drugs, toxins, autoimmune diseases, transfusion reactions, and bacterial infections.
  - In addition, the patient may exhibit have an enlarged spleen, an increase in bilirubin, and exhibit jaundice.
- Thalassemia is an inherited disease in which hemoglobin synthesis is missing either the alpha or beta chains of the hemoglobin molecule. This disorder affects Asian, Mediterranean, and African populations.
  - Symptoms range from asymptomatic to moderate anemia to organ failure and ultimately death.
- Glucose-6-phosphate dehydrogenase anemia (G6PD) is a form of anemia caused by a defect in RBC metabolism and may be genetic, caused by an inflammatory disorder, or from medications. G6PD occurs more frequently in males, is more common in African and Mediterranean people, and can be diagnosed by a quantitative assay for G6PD.
- Hereditary spherocytosis is an autosomal dominant disorder that begins in utero, causing the blood cells to develop into a spherical shape and resulting in their premature destruction in the spleen. Removal of the spleen is a treatment for this disorder.
- Iron deficiency anemia develops when there is a loss of iron that becomes inadequate for RBC production. It is the most common type of anemia and is common in the elderly.
  - Common causes include poor dietary intake of iron, upper GI bleeding, prolonged menstrual bleeding, pregnancy hemorrhoids, and cancer.
  - Patients may have brittle nails, cheilosis (small fissures at the corner of the mouth), pica (craving to ingest things other than food, such as dirt or ice), and a smooth, painful tongue.
  - Iron replacements and a diet rich in iron may correct the deficiency.
- Folic acid deficiency anemia is found in the chronically undernourished, such as alcoholics, drug abusers, or elderly, and may occur during pregnancy.
  - Diets high in folic acid or supplements may correct the deficiency.

NURSING DIAGNOSIS

- Fatigue
- Nutrition: less than body requirements, Imbalanced

A

Anemia, Sickle Cell

DEFINITION

- Sickle cell anemia is a hereditary disorder of an autosomal recessive defect causing crescent-shaped red blood cells. Sickle cell anemia is seen predominately in Africans but may be present in people of Mediterranean and Central and South American descent. A sickle solubility test confirms the presence of HbS—the gene responsible for sickle cell disease (presence of hemoglobin S).

Sickle Cell Crisis

- Excessive sickling can precipitate a crisis due to occluded circulation, sequestering of large amount of blood in the liver or spleen, and impaired erythropoiesis.
- Crisis can be precipitated by stress, infection, or dehydration.

KEY ASSESSMENTS

For sickle cell crisis

- Severe extremity pain, joint pain, or abdominal pain
- Extremity swelling and coolness to the touch

PLANNING AND IMPLEMENTATION

For sickle cell crisis

- Treat pain
- Correct fluid and electrolyte imbalances
- Infections are treated with appropriate antibiotic therapy
- Administer oxygen therapy
- Monitor respiratory status
- Monitor extremity temperature and observe for swelling
- Anticipate blood transfusions
- Splenectomy or bone marrow transplant may be required

Anemia, Vitamin B_{12} Deficiency

DEFINITION

- Vitamin B_{12} deficiency anemia is caused by a lack of intake or malabsorption of vitamin B_{12}. Inability to absorb vitamin B_{12} exists with the lack of intrinsic factor as seen in pernicious anemia. Vitamin B_{12} deficiency affects approximately 20 percent of the population in industrialized countries and affects 30–40 percent of the elderly.

KEY ASSESSMENTS

- Hunter's glossitis or atrophied lingual papillae (smooth, shiny tongue)
- Spinal cord degeneration
- Polyneuritis
- Ataxia
- Positive Babinski reflex
- If not treated, symptoms may be irreversible
- Megaloblastic anemia
- Schilling test (radioactive testing for absorption capabilities)
- Intrinsic factor serum test

PLANNING AND IMPLEMENTATION

- Increase dietary intake of foods rich in vitamin B_{12}.
- If the cause is lack of intrinsic factor, intramuscular (IM) injections of vitamin B_{12} are necessary.

SPECIAL CONCERNS

- Many anemias are related to ethnic backgrounds and genetics. While taking health histories, be aware of the genetic and ethnic propensity of certain anemias.
- Diet history is important to see if there are dietary causes of anemia.
- Teach patients about foods that are rich in the deficiency they are experiencing.

NURSING DIAGNOSIS

- Knowledge, Deficient
- Nutrition: less than body requirements, Imbalanced

Aneurysm

DEFINITION

- An aneurysm is a permanent bulging and stretching of an artery. This localized abnormality puts the artery at risk for dissection or tearing. Common sites include aortic arch, thoracic aorta, and abdominal aorta. There are higher risks for aneurysm formation in patients who are smokers or those with cardiovascular disorders, circulatory disorders, or hypertension.

Classifications

Etiology classification

- Congenital (including Marfan's, Turner's, Ehler's-Danlos, and Menkes syndromes)
- Mechanical—related the arterial-venous fistulas and amputations
- Inflammatory—related to an infectious process causing aneurysms
- Traumatic—from blunt or penetrating trauma
- Anastomotic—aneurysms that form at a suture line

Type classification

- False aneurysm—pulsating hematoma on all three layers of the artery
- True aneurysm—involvement of one, two, or all three layers of the artery
- Fusiform aneurysm—symmetrical and diffuse involvement of the entire vessel
- Saccular aneurysm—one-sided protrusion or out pouching of one area of the vessel
- Dissecting aneurysm—splits the layers of the vessel wall and forms a hematoma

KEY ASSESSMENTS

- Medical history
- Nausea and vomiting
- Bruit over aneurysm site
- Cyanosis distal to aneurysm site
- Decreased pulses
- Back pain
- Vital signs
- Dysphasia
- Hypovolemic shock
- Cardiogenic shock

PLANNING AND IMPLEMENTATION

- Computerized tomography (CT)
- Treat pain
- Monitor vital signs
- Monitor kidney function

- Monitor extremity strength
- Monitor distal pulses
- Monitor for dissection
- Monitor level of consciousness (LOC)
- Teach patient to avoid straining during defecation
- Provide smoking cessation materials
- Administer antihypertensive medications
- Obtain consents for blood
- Type and cross-match for blood products

Surgical Aneurysm Repair

Surgical aneurysm repair involves the placement of a Dacron graft above and below the proximal and distal sites of the aneurysm. Postoperative complications include bleeding, hematoma formation, wound infection, paralysis, paralytic ileus, and kidney failure.

Key assessments—Postoperative

- Vital signs
- Urine output
- Distal pulses
- Extremity movement and color
- Bowel sounds
- Respiratory status

Planning and implementation—Postoperative

- Frequent vital signs
- Encourage deep breathing
- Monitor urine output
- Treat pain
- Monitor wound
- Monitor bowel sounds
- Monitor extremity pulse, color, and movement
- Monitor LOC
- Monitor for signs of bleeding
- Monitor hemoglobin
- Monitor intake and output (I & O)

NURSING DIAGNOSIS

- Tissue perfusion, Ineffective
- Cardiac output, Decreased
- Pain, Acute

Ankylosing Spondylitis

DEFINITION

- Ankylosing spondylitis is a chronic, progressive, inflammatory arthritis that affects the synovial joints and the soft tissue of the spine causing fusion of the inflamed spine over time. Symptoms usually begin in the hips, knees, and feet and progress to the spine. The cause is unknown, and it is genetically linked.

KEY ASSESSMENTS

- Back pain (worse in the morning)
- Decrease in spine mobility
- Kyphosis (over time)

Diagnostics

- X-rays

PLANNING AND IMPLEMENTATION

- Administer nonsteroidal anti-inflammatory drugs (NSAIDs), indomethacin, and methotrexate as ordered
- Encourage exercise
- Assist with activities of daily living

SPECIAL CONCERNS

Gender Considerations

- Men are 3 times more likely to develop ankylosing spondylitis with onset occurring between the ages 16 and 35 years.

NURSING DIAGNOSIS

- Mobility, Impaired physical
- Pain, Chronic
- Self-care deficit, Toileting

Anthrax

DEFINITION

- Anthrax infections are caused by the *Bacillus anthracis,* a gram-positive bacterium. Infection occurs in three forms: cutaneous, inhaled, and gastrointestinal (GI). Inhaled anthrax is the greatest concern, because the bacterium is readily available and can be aerosolized and spread over large populations quickly. One hundred percent of patients with inhaled anthrax will die if no treatment is rendered, and 95 percent will die with treatment initiated within 48 hours of symptoms.
- Spread has a low potential for person to person.
- Average incubation period is one to six days.

KEY ASSESSMENTS

Initial

- Headache
- Nonproductive cough

After One to Three Days

- High fever
- Dyspnea
- Stridor
- Cyanosis
- Shock

Diagnostics

- Chest X-ray (CXR)

Lab Tests

- Blood and sputum cultures for *Bacillus anthracis*

PLANNING AND IMPLEMENTATION

- Isolate patient
- Standard precautions
- Wash patient if aerosol transmission is suspected
- Initiate intravenous (IV) ciprofloxacin
- Oral ciprofloxacin for all exposed
- Health care workers exposed immunized (confirmed cases)
- Anticipate intubation and mechanical ventilation

A

- Initiate two large-bore peripheral IVs
- Fluid resuscitation with 0.9% normal saline (NS)
- Monitor vital signs
- Monitor oxygenation status
- Administer antipyretics for fever
- Monitor CXR
- Frequent pulmonary suctioning

NURSING DIAGNOSIS

- Breathing pattern, Ineffective
- Tissue perfusion, Ineffective
- Hyperthermia
- Fluid volume, Risk for deficient

Aortic Regurgitation

DEFINITION

- Aortic regurgitation is a disorder of the aortic valve in which the incompetent valve allows blood back through the left ventricle during diastole. The increased pressure in the left ventricle can cause hypertrophy and an increase in the force necessary to expel blood from the left ventricle into the aorta. Aortic regurgitation may result from an inflammatory disease or congenital conditions.

KEY ASSESSMENTS

- Systolic hypertension
- Diastolic murmur
- Increased intensity of carotid and temporal pulse
- Pulses are intense and then quickly weaken
- Dyspnea on exertion
- Fatigue
- Paroxysmal nocturnal dyspnea

PLANNING AND IMPLEMENTATION

- Echocardiogram
- Teach patients to avoid caffeine, alcohol, and smoking
- Monitor vital signs
- Monitor cardiac status

- Prophylactic antibiotics required before going through dental procedures
- Educate patients and family about treatments
- Surgical valve replacement may be necessary
- If mechanical valve is inserted, lifelong anticoagulation therapy may be necessary

SPECIAL CONCERNS

Gender Considerations

- Three quarters of patients with pure aortic regurgitation are male, and it may be genetically linked.

NURSING DIAGNOSIS

- Cardiac output, Decreased
- Fluid volume, Risk for imbalanced
- Knowledge, Deficient

Aortic Stenosis

DEFINITION

- Aortic stenosis is a narrowing of the diameter of the opening between the left ventricle and the aorta. The left ventricle has to work harder causing hypertrophy.

Clinical Causes

- Congenital valve defects, rheumatic heart disease, cusp calcification, and degenerative changes associated with aging. Aortic stenosis is the most common valvular disorder.

KEY ASSESSMENTS

- Asymptomatic patients
- Systolic murmur
- Thrill along the left sternal border radiating to the neck
- Dyspnea on exertion
- Chest pain
- Dizziness
- Syncope
- Signs of heart failure

PLANNING AND IMPLEMENTATION

- Echocardiogram
- Monitor vital signs
- Monitor cardiac status
- Institute safety precautions
- Educate patient and family about treatments
- Surgical valve replacement may be necessary
- If mechanical valve is inserted, lifelong anticoagulation therapy may be necessary

SPECIAL CONCERNS

- See Special Procedures and Treatments for information on Valve Replacement.

Gender Considerations

- Aortic stenosis occurs three to four times more frequently in men than women with no clear genetic link.

Geriatric Considerations

- Approximately 25 percent of patients over the age or 65 and 35 percent of those over 70 years of age have evidence of aortic stenosis.

NURSING DIAGNOSIS

- Cardiac output, Decreased
- Fluid volume, Risk for imbalanced
- Knowledge, Deficient

Appendicitis

DEFINITION

- Appendicitis is the inflammation of the appendix, located below the ileocecal valve in the bowel, and it is the most common reason for emergency abdominal surgery.

Classifications

- Simple appendicitis—the appendix is inflamed and intact.
- Gangrenous appendicitis—the appendix tissue has infection, necrosis, and microscopic areas of perforation.

- Perforated appendicitis—large perforations of the appendix allow contents to spill in the peritoneal cavity.

KEY ASSESSMENTS

- Periumbilical pain radiating over the lower abdomen
- Right lower quadrant (RLQ) pain
- Fever
- Local tenderness at McBurney's point (pain elicited in the RLQ when pressure is applied)
- Rovsing's sign (when pressure is applied to the left lower quadrant [LLQ] for five seconds and pain is felt in the RLQ)
- Signs of peritonitis (infection of the peritoneal cavity), severe pain drawing knees to the chest, tachycardia, diaphoresis, or high fever

Diagnostics

- Abdominal X-rays (RLQ density)
- Abdominal ultrasound
- Abdominal computed tomography (CT)

Lab Tests

- Complete blood count ([CBC], white blood count will be elevated)

PLANNING AND IMPLEMENTATION

Preoperative

- Insert peripheral IV
- Initiate IV fluids
- Treat pain with narcotics
- Initiate nothing by mouth (NPO) status
- Initiate antibiotic therapy
- Obtain surgical consents

Postoperative

- Frequent vital signs
- Treat pain
- Monitor intake and output (I & O)
- Monitor wound for signs of infection
- Monitor patient for signs of peritonitis
- Encourage deep breathing and coughing
- Administer antibiotics

NURSING DIAGNOSIS

- Pain, Acute
- Infection, Risk for
- Skin integrity, Impaired

Arrhythmias

DEFINITION

- Arrhythmias are a deviation from normal cardiac rhythm. There are many causes of arrhythmias, including cardiac disease, electrolyte disturbances, MI, respiratory disorders, and side effects of medications.

KEY ASSESSMENTS

- Identify and interpret arrhythmias
- Monitor level of consciousness (LOC)
- Apical and peripheral pulses
- Respirations
- Oxygenation status
- Patient's response to the arrhythmia
- Syncope
- Chest pain

PLANNING AND IMPLEMENTATION

(See Tables 1–3)

- Clean skin and remove excess hair prior to attaching electrodes
- To verify rhythm, use 12 lead electrocardiogram (ECG)
- Oxygen
- Initiate peripheral intravenous (IV) line
- Implement appropriate basic life support (BLS) and algorithms from advanced cardiac life support (ACLS)
- Institute safety measures

NURSING DIAGNOSIS

- Tissue perfusion, Ineffective
- Injury, Risk for
- Knowledge, Deficient

TABLE 1

Lead Placement of Standardized Electrocardiogram (ECG)

Lead	Electrode Placement	Axis
Limb lead Lead I	Bipolar lead Positive: Left arm Negative: Right arm	Shoulder-to-shoulder, which reflects the left lateral side of the left ventricle
Limb lead Lead II	Bipolar lead Positive: Left leg Negative: Right arm	Right shoulder to the left leg, which reflects the inferior surface of the left ventricle
Limb lead Lead III	Bipolar lead Positive: Left leg Negative: Left arm	Left shoulder to left leg, which reflects the inferior surface of the left ventricle
Unipolar lead aV_R	Positive electrode: Right arm	Reflects electrical activity on the right side of the heart
Unipolar lead aV_L	Positive electrode: Left arm	Reflects electrical activity on the left side on the heart
Unipolar lead aV_F	Unipolar lead Positive lead: Left leg	Reflects electrical activity on the inferior surface of the left ventricle
Precordial lead V_1	Electrode placement: Fourth intercostal space on the right side of the sternum	Looks at the right ventricle
Precordial Lead V_2	Electrode placement: Fourth intercostal space on the left side of the sternum	Reflects depolarization of the interventricular septum
Precordial Lead V_3	Electrode placement: Halfway between V_2 and V_4	Reflects depolarization of the interventricular septum
Precordial Lead V_4	Electrode placement: Fifth intercostal space, midclavicular line	Electrical activity of the apex of the heart
Precordial Lead V_5	Electrode placement: Fifth intercostal space, anterior axillary line	Left lateral wall of the ventricle
Precordial Lead V_6	Electrode placement: Fifth intercostal space, midaxillary line	Left lateral wall of the ventricle

TABLE 2

Nursing Management for the Patient with Arrhythmias

Nursing Management	Rationale
Provide continuous electrocardiogram (ECG) monitoring.	To detect rapidly the occurrence of arrhythmias.
Maintain heart rate alarms at appropriate limits.	To detect bradycardia or tachycardia promptly.
Administer antiarrhythmic medications per protocol or as ordered.	To maintain therapeutic blood levels of appropriate medications.
Administer cardiopulmonary resuscitation (CPR) or defibrillation as appropriate for life-threatening arrhythmias.	To restore perfusion or terminate ventricular fibrillation promptly.
Maintain SpO_2 levels greater than 90 percent with supplemental O_2 if needed.	To prevent hypoxia-induced arrhythmias.
Monitor electrolyte levels and replace as necessary.	Abnormally high or low potassium and low magnesium levels can precipitate arrhythmias.
Maintain at least one patent IV site.	To be able to administer emergency medications when needed.
Monitor serum levels of antiarrhythmic medications.	To prevent toxicity of medications and to maintain therapeutic blood levels.
Provide information to the patient regarding disease process, procedures, and medications.	To allay patient anxiety and promote compliance with medical and nursing regimes.
Teach patient regarding symptoms of arrhythmias, such as chest pain, syncope, weakness, and fatigue.	So patient can identify arrhythmias and seek early treatment.
Teach patient to take own pulse.	To monitor for side effects of medications or to detect arrhythmias.
Teach patient to avoid proarrhythmic substances.	Patient should avoid caffeine and recreational drugs that may be proarrhythmic.

TABLE 3

Summary of Arrhythmias: Characteristics, Causes, and Treatments

Arrhythmia/ Dysrhythmia	Characteristics	Origin	Possible Causes	Possible Treatments
Sinus Rhythm	Rate: 60–100 Rhythm: Regular P wave: Upright in Lead II PR interval: 0.12–0.20 seconds QRS complex: Less than 0.10 seconds QT interval: 0.40–0.44 (rate of 60) to 0.31–0.34 (rate of 100)	SA node	Expected rhythm	None
Sinus Bradycardia	Rate: Less than 60 Rhythm: Regular P wave: Upright in Lead II PR interval: 0.12–0.20 seconds QRS complex: Less than 0.10 seconds T wave: Upright in Lead II QT interval: 0.40–0.44 (rate of 60)	SA node	Athlete's heart Vagal stimulation Carotid sinus syndrome	Only treated if symptomatic Treatment: atropine, pacemaker, avoid vagal stimulation
Sinus Tachycardia	Rate: 100–180 beats per minute Rhythm: Regular to slightly irregular P wave: Upright in Lead II PR interval: 0.12–0.20 seconds QRS complex: 0.10 seconds or less QT interval: 0.31–0.34 (rate of 100)	SA node	Sympathetic stimulation Exercise Emotion Pain Fever Inflammation Drugs Thyroid Nicotine Caffeine	Treat underlying cause

Sinus Arrhythmia	Rate: Rate varies more that 10 percent (less than 60–100) beats per minute Rhythm: Irregular P wave: Normal sinus P wave PR interval: 0.12–0.20 seconds may vary slightly QRS complex: 0.10 seconds or less QT interval: 0.40–0.44 (rate of 60) to 0.31–0.34 (rate of 100)	SA node	Occurs more often in children Variations due to respirations In older patient, may be due to coronary artery disease	Not treated unless patient is symptomatic during bradycardia
Sinus Block	Rate: Less than 60 beats per minute during block Rhythm: Regular with pauses that do not have a pattern P wave: Normal sinus P waves, may have atrial escape beats PR interval: 0.12–0.20 seconds when present QRS complex: 0.10 seconds or less QT interval: 0.40–0.44 (rate of 60) to 0.31–0.34 (rate of 100)	SA node	Sick sinus syndrome Drugs: cardiac glycosides, beta blockers, calcium channel blockers Increased vagal tone	Not treated unless patient is symptomatic If symptomatic, then a pacemaker is indicated
Premature Atrial Complex (PAC)	Rate: 60–100 if underlying rhythm is SR Rhythm: Irregular because of PAC P wave (P'); P' wave of the PAC usually a different shape from sinus P wave P wave location: Premature, may be in preceding T wave PR interval: P'R may be the same as PR with sinus beat or may be prolonged or P' may not be conducted QRS complex: Usually 0.10 seconds or less QT interval: 0.40–0.44 (rate of 60) to 0.31–0.34 (rate of 100)	Atrial focus	Sympathetic nervous system stimulation Tobacco Alcohol Caffeine Myocardial ischemia Infection Medications Mitral stenosis Atrial septal defect	Treatment of underlying cause; stop precipitating elements

continued

TABLE 3

Summary of Arrhythmias: Characteristics, Causes, and Treatments—cont'd

Arrhythmia/ Dysrhythmia	Characteristics	Origin	Possible Causes	Possible Treatments
Atrial Tachycardia	Rate: 130–180 beats per minute Rhythm: Usually regular P wave: P' shape depends on ectopic site of origin in the atrium PR interval: P'R may be normal or prolonged QRS complex: 0.10 seconds or less unless it is associated with a bundle branch block aberration QT interval: 0.31.	Atrial focus	Digitalis intoxication (especially with hypokalemia) Myocardial ischemia Dilated cardiomyopathy Cardiac tumors Bypass pathways	Radio frequency ablation Evaluation of digitalis levels Correcting underlying electrolyte abnormalities
Atrial Flutter	Atrial rate: 240–340 (type 1) Ventricular rate: Depends on conduction, usually 150–170 if 2:1 conduction Rhythm: Regular with fixed conduction; irregular with variable conduction P wave = F (flutter) wave: sawtooth pattern PR interval: N/A F–R relationship: Fixed with a regular ventricular rhythm QRS complex: 0.10 seconds or less unless there is bundle branch block aberration QT interval: 0.40–0.44 (rate of 60) to 0.31–0.34 (rate of 100)	N/A	Open-heart surgery MI Pulmonary embolism Mitral stenosis Accessory pathway	Rate control with calcium channel blockers and beta blockers Rapid atrial pacing Antiarrhythmic drug therapy Direct current (DC) cardioversion Radio frequency ablation of accessory pathway

Atrial Fibrillation	Atrial rate: greater than 400 beats per minute Ventricular rate: 100 to 180 beats per minute in uncontrolled atrial fibrillation Rhythm: Irregularly irregular P wave: Absent, replaced by fine or coarse fibrillatory lines (F waves) PR interval: Cannot be measured QRS complex: 0.10 seconds or less. QT interval: 0.40–0.44 (rate of 60) to 0.31–0.34 (rate of 100)	Atrial focus	Atrial enlargement Open-heart surgery AMI Pericarditis Heart failure Mitral stenosis Alcohol Hyperthyroidism	Anticoagulation digoxin Rate control with calcium channel blockers Beta blockers Antiarrhythmic medications DC cardioversion Radio frequency ablation
Wandering Atrial Pacemaker	Rate: 60–100 Rhythm: Irregular P wave: Varies in configuration in Lead II PR interval: 0.12–0.20 seconds; may not be constant QRS complex: 0.10 seconds or less QT interval: 0.40–0.44 (rate of 60) to 0.31–0.34 (rate of 100)	SA node to atrium	COPD	Treat underlying cause
Premature Junctional Complexes (PJC)	Rate: Same as underlying rhythm Rhythm: Irregular with the PJC P wave: P' negative in leads II, III, aV_F, or not present, may occur before, during, or after QRS complex PR interval: If P' before the QRS P'R interval is less than 0.12 seconds QRS complex: 0.10 seconds or less QT interval: 0.40–0.44 (rate of 60) to 0.31–0.34 (rate of 100)	AV Junction	Digitalis toxicity	Not usually treated Assess digitalis level

continued

TABLE 3

Summary of Arrhythmias: Characteristics, Causes, and Treatments—cont'd

Arrhythmia/ Dysrhythmia	Characteristics	Origin	Possible Causes	Possible Treatments
Junctional Escape Rhythm	Rate: 35–60 beats per minute Rhythm: Regular P wave P' may not be present PR interval: N/A QRS complex: 0.10 seconds or less QT interval: 0.40–0.44 (rate of 60) to 0.31–0.34 (rate of 100)	AV Junction	Protective mechanism when sinus node does not fire	No treatment unless symptomatic; increase rate of SA node Pacemaker
Junctional Tachycardia	Rate: 70–140 beats per minute Rhythm: Regular P wave: P', may occur before, during, or after QRS complex PR interval: P'R if P' precedes QRS less than 0.12 seconds QRS complex: 0.10 seconds or less QT interval: 0.31–0.34 (rate of 100)	AV Junction	Digitalis toxicity MI Myocarditis Acute rheumatic fever Open-heart surgery	Stop digitalis Digibind if necessary
Atrioventricular Block (Incomplete) First Degree	Rate: 60–100 beats per minute Rhythm: Regular P wave: Normal sinus P wave PR interval: Greater than 0.20 seconds; constant from beat to beat QRS complex: 0.10 seconds or less; normal shape and duration QT interval: 0.40–0.44 (rate of 60) to 0.31–0.34 (rate of 100)	SA node Delayed impulse through the AV junction	AMI (inferior) Digitalis Myocardial ischemia	Usually there is no treatment

Atrioventricular Block (Incomplete) Second Degree Type I	Rate: 60–100 beats per minute Rhythm: Irregular P wave: Normal sinus P wave PR interval: Becomes progressively longer until one P wave is not conducted through the AV node QRS complex: 0.10 seconds or less; normal shape and duration QT interval: 0.40–0.44 (rate of 60) to 0.31–0.34 (rate of 100)	SA node Delayed impulse through the AV junction until impulse is blocked	AMI (inferior) Digitalis Myocardial ischemia Open-heart surgery	Monitor for increasing block Stop digitalis if a contributing cause
Atrioventricular Block (Incomplete) Second Degree Type 2	Atrial rate: 60–100 beats per minute Ventricular rate: variable depending on number of impulses conducted Rhythm: Irregular P wave: Normal sinus P wave PR interval: Constant PR interval: Some P waves not conducted QRS complex: 0.10 seconds or less; normal shape and duration QT interval: 0.40–0.44 (rate of 60) to 0.31–0.34 (rate of 100)	SA node impulse blocked in lower part of system Some impulses get through; some are blocked	AMI	Treatment if symptomatic Pacemaker

continued

TABLE 3

Summary of Arrhythmias: Characteristics, Causes, and Treatments—cont'd

Arrhythmia/ Dysrhythmia	Characteristics	Origin	Possible Causes	Possible Treatments
Atrioventricular Block (Complete) Third Degree	Atrial rate: 60–100 beats per minute Ventricular rate: Depends on escape Junctional pacemaker: 35–60 beats per minute Ventricular pacemaker: 10–40 beats per minute Atrial rhythm: regular; ventricular rhythm: regular P wave: Normal sinus P wave not conducted to ventricles PR interval: Variable QRS complex: 0.10 seconds or less if junctional escape pacemaker; greater than 0.10 if ventricular pacemaker QT interval: 0.40–0.44 (rate of 60) to 0.31–0.34 (rate of 100)	SA node Impulses	Congenital heart block MI	If symptomatic: pacemaker
Premature Ventricular Complexes (PVC)	Rate: Underlying rhythm 60–100 beats per minute Rhythm: Irregular because of PVC P wave: P wave not related to PVC unless there is retrograde conduction PP intervals: Sinus P waves not reset by PVC PR interval: Normal for underlying rhythm QRS complex or PVC: QRS complex greater than 0.12 seconds, QRS, Premature, increased amplitude	Ectopic focus in the ventricle	Myocardial ischemia Bradycardia Decreased volume Infection Increased sympathetic activity Medications Hypokalemia Hypercalcemia Alcohol	No treatment for asymptomatic patient

	T wave of the PVC: opposite direction of the last part of QRS Compensatory pause: Full about 50 percent of time QT interval: 0.40–0.44 (rate of 60) to 0.31–0.34 (rate of 100)			
Ventricular Escape Rhythm	Rate: Less than 40 beats per minute Rhythm: Usually regular P wave: Not associated with QRS PR interval: Cannot be measured QRS complex: Greater than 0.14 seconds QT interval: rate of 0.40–0.44	Ectopic impulse in the ventricle	Occurs when the ventricle is not activated by a higher pacemaker	Advanced cardiac life support (ACLS) protocol Transcutaneous pacing Dopamine Epinephrine Isoproterenol Transvenous pacemaker
Ventricular Tachycardia	Rate: Greater than 100 beats per minute Rhythm: Regular P wave: Dissociated or retrograde PR interval: unknown QRS complex: Greater than 0.14 seconds QT interval: 0.31–0.34 (rate of 100)	Ectopic impulse in the ventricle	MI Cardiomyopathy Valvular heart disease Congenital heart disease Potassium imbalance Drug toxicity Prolonged PT interval	Treatment: ACLS protocol Stable/normal heart: beat blockers, lidocaine, amiodarone, procainamide, sotalol Impaired heart: amiodarone, or lidocaine, then DC cardioversion if persistent

continued

TABLE 3

Summary of Arrhythmias: Characteristics, Causes, and Treatments—cont'd

Arrhythmia/ Dysrhythmia	Characteristics	Origin	Possible Causes	Possible Treatments
Ventricular Fibrillation	Rate: Not identifiable Rhythm: Unknown P wave: Not identifiable PR interval: Not measurable QRS complex: Not identifiable QT interval: Not identifiable	N/A	MI Cardiomyopathy Valvular heart disease Congenital heart disease Potassium imbalance Drug toxicity Prolonged PT interval	ACLS protocol DC Cardioversion if rhythm does not convert after 3 shocks, airway, breathing, circulation Medications: epinephrine, vasopressin, amiodarone, lidocaine, magnesium sulfate, procainamide with alteration of DC cardioversion.
Asystole	Rate: 0 Rhythm: Not measurable P wave: Unknown PR interval: Not measurable QRS complex: Not present QT interval: Not measured			ACLS protocol Airway, breathing, circulation, supplemental oxygen Advanced airway Occasionally transcutaneous pacing IV medications: epinephrine, atropine, or sodium bicarbonate (if associated with lactic acidosis) Rare circumstances: isoproterenol

Torsades de Pointes	Atrial rate: Cannot determine rate Ventricular rate: 150–250 complexes per minute Rhythm: Irregular P wave: Not present PR interval: Not measurable QRS complex: Twisting points of complexes QT interval: QT prolonged onset before tachycardia	N/A	N/A	N/A
Pulseless Electrical Activity (PEA)	Rhythm: Any organized rhythm that does not have a pulse	Varies as to location	Hypovolemia Hypoxia Acidosis Hyperkalemia Hypokalemia Hypothermia Drug overdose Cardiac tamponade Tension	Airway, breathing, circulation, cardiopulmonary resuscitation (CPR).

Asthma

DEFINITION

- Asthma is a chronic inflammatory disease characterized by episodic exacerbations of acute inflammation of the airways. The airways become hyperresponsive to stimuli or triggers, resulting in bronchoconstriction, mucus production, and inflammation.
- Triggers that exacerbate asthma may include allergens, medications, environmental factors (dust or pets), air pollution, occupational exposures, infections, and exercise.

Status Asthmaticus

- Status asthmaticus is a life-threatening acute exacerbation of asthma with severe airway constriction, and it is a medical emergency.

Key assessments for status asthmaticus

- High pitched stridor
- Cyanosis
- Change in level of consciousness (LOC)
- Severe anxiety
- Rapid desaturation of pulse oximetry
- Tachycardia, tachypnea, or hypertension

Planning and implementation for status asthmaticus

- High Fowler's position
- Oxygen to maintain pulse oximetry greater than 90 percent
- Continuous cardiac and pulse oximetry monitoring
- Insert two large-bore intravenous (IV) lines
- Promote a calm environment
- Anticipate administering inhaled $beta_2$ agonist therapy, and IV corticosteroids
- Keep intubation equipment at the bedside

KEY ASSESSMENTS

- Chest tightness
- Wheezing
- Shortness of breath
- Chest tightness
- Tachycardia and tachypnea
- Use of accessory muscles to breath

- Anxiety
- Reported drop in peak flow
- Productive cough

Diagnostics

- Chest X-ray (CXR)
- Pulmonary function testing
- Sputum cultures (if infection suspected)

PLANNING AND IMPLEMENTATION

- High Fowler's position
- Maintain a calm environment
- Monitor peak flows
- Oxygen administration (hypoxia)
- Avoid triggers
- Anticipate administering a combination of leukotriene modifier, mast cell stabilizer, beta$_2$-adrenergic agonist, anticholinergic, and bronchodilator medications

SPECIAL CONCERNS

Cultural Considerations

- Asthma is more common in African American adults and children. The death rate for asthma is highest among African Americans age 15 to 24 years.

Teaching Considerations

- Educate patients with asthma on how to:
  - Assess peak flow and how to interpret findings
  - Properly use inhaler
  - Determine when they need medical attention
  - Assess triggers and how to avoid them

NURSING DIAGNOSIS

- Breathing pattern, Ineffective
- Anxiety
- Knowledge, Deficient

Bacterial Endocarditis

DEFINITION

- Bacterial endocarditis is a bacterial infection of the heart's inner lining or heart valves. People with artificial valves, a history of previous endocarditis or rheumatic fever, heart valve defects, and hypertrophic cardiomyopathy are at higher risk for bacterial endocarditis.

KEY ASSESSMENTS

- Malaise
- Anorexia, weight loss
- Back and joint pain
- Janeway lesions (flat red-bluish spots on the palms and soles)
- Roth's spots (retinal hemorrhages with a central area of clearing)
- Petechiae in the conjunctiva
- Clubbing of fingers
- Transient ischemic attacks due to emboli
- Murmur

PLANNING AND IMPLEMENTATION

- Blood cultures
- Echocardiogram
- Antibiotic therapy
- Monitor vital signs
- Monitor cardiac status
- Monitor for emboli
- Teach patient and family about treatments
- Surgical valve replacement may be necessary

SPECIAL CONCERNS

- See Special Procedures and Treatments for information on Valve Repair.

Bell's Palsy

DEFINITION

- Bell's palsy is a facial neuropathy characterized by pain and paresis of the seventh cranial nerve. It is considered an inflammatory disorder that may be associated with herpes simplex virus, and 90 percent of patients will recover without any residual deficits.

KEY ASSESSMENTS

- Unilateral facial weakness
- Pain and facial stiffness
- Difficulty eating

Diagnostics

- Diagnosis is usually based on examination; other tests may be performed to rule out other etiologies.

PLANNING AND IMPLEMENTATION

- Treat pain
- Monitor fluid and nutritional intake
- Assess eye for closing and dryness
- Anticipate administering steroid

NURSING DIAGNOSIS

- Pain, Acute
- Nutritional: less than body requirements, Imbalanced

Benign Prostatic Hyperplasia (BPH)

DEFINITION

- BPH is the enlargement of the prostate gland due to an overgrowth in the number of cells. The enlargement constricts the urethra causing urinary symptoms. It commonly affects middle age and elderly men.

KEY ASSESSMENTS

- Weak and dribbling urine stream
- Difficulty in initiating urine stream
- Nocturia (urination at night)
- Void small amounts

History and Examination

- History of urinary symptoms
- Digital rectal exam to palpate prostate for enlargement and tenderness

Diagnostics

- Rectal ultrasonography
- Postvoiding bladder scan
- Cystoscopy

Lab Tests

- Prostate-specific antigen (PSA)
- Blood urea nitrogen (BUN) and creatinine (Cr)
- Urinalysis

PLANNING AND IMPLEMENTATION

- Encourage oral fluids. (Many men restrict fluids to alleviate urinary symptoms.)
- Monitor intake and output (I & O).
- Monitor urine for signs of infection (cloudy, malodorous).
- Implement safety measures.
- Ensure a clear path to the bathroom.
- Treatment is aimed to reduce prostate size and decrease urinary symptoms.
- Administer nonselective alpha blockers to relax muscles of the bladder neck and prostate (Hytrin, Uro Xatral, or Cardura).
- Monitor for orthostatic hypotension associated with nonselective alpha blockers.
- Administer antiandrogen agents to shrink hyperplastic cells (finasteride).
- Administer antispasmodics if bladder spasm occur.
- Treat surgical pain.

Surgical Treatment

- Transurethral resection of the prostate (TURP) is the surgical removal of hypertrophied prostate tissue.

B

  - A double lumen urinary catheter is placed to wash out blood oozing from the surgical site.
  - Continuous bladder irrigation (CBI) is performed by instilling 0.9% normal saline (NS) via 5-liter bags to prevent blood from clotting and obstructing urine flow.
  - Postoperatively the outflow will be bright red (looks like fruit punch) and will lighten with time.
  - If there is no outflow, contact the health care provider and stop the irrigation (to prevent bladder distention).
  - Manually irrigate and attempt to withdraw clots with sterile Toomey syringe and sterile saline.
- Transurethral microwave procedure (TUMP) is an outpatient procedure in which a transurethral catheter is heated to reduce urinary symptoms.
- Transurethral needle ablation (TUNA) is an outpatient procedure that emits low-level radio frequency via needles in the urethra that burn away the enlarged prostate tissue impeding the urethral flow.

SPECIAL CONCERNS

Cultural Considerations

- Men of southern European descent are at higher risk for developing BPH, and Asian and Scandinavian men are at lower risk for developing BPH.

Geriatric Considerations

- Ninety percent of men over 70 have BPH symptoms.

NURSING DIAGNOSIS

- Urinary elimination, Impaired
- Pain, Acute
- Infection, Risk for
- Sleep pattern, Disturbed

Brain Injury

DEFINITION

- Brain injury is a neurological injury resulting from any type of trauma. Primary brain injury is the initial brain injury. Secondary brain injury is an effect of the initial injury and includes increased intracranial pressure (ICP).

Classifications

Open

- Basilar skull fracture results from a fracture of the basilar skull. Battle sign (bruising behind the ear) and Raccoon sign (bilateral black eyes) are common indicators of this injury.
- Depressed skull fracture results from a fracture that depresses bone into the brain. There is a high chance of infection with this type of injury.
- Penetrating wounds result from an object piercing the skull and lodging in the brain tissue. Gunshot wounds and arrow injuries are examples.

Closed

- Coup-contracoup injuries occur commonly in motor vehicle accidents in which the forehead strikes the windshield (coup injury), and then the head snaps back forcing the brain against the rear of the skull and injuring the opposite side (contracoup).
- Contusions are brain bruises. Severity depends on the size and location.
- Concussions are a loss of consciousness, a period of memory loss before or after an injury, or a change in level of consciousness (LOC) associated with the accident.
- Diffuse axonal injury is caused from rapid acceleration and deceleration of the head in which the brain moves and shears the axons of the nerve cells.
- Subdural hematoma occurs when there is bleeding into the subdural space. The bleed is venous, onset is typically slower, and treatment involves surgical evacuation of the hematoma.
- Epidural hematoma occurs when there is bleeding in the epidural space. The bleed is arterial with a rapid onset, and prompt surgical evacuation of the hematoma is necessary.
- Subarachnoid hemorrhage is bleeding into the subarachnoid space and is associated with cerebral aneurysm rupture. The patient usually complains of photosensitivity, neck stiffness, and the worst headache of his or her life.

KEY ASSESSMENTS

- Airway, breathing, and signs of circulation
- Frequent vital signs

- Pulse oximetry and cardiac monitoring
- Insert two large-bore peripheral intravenous (IV) lines
- Observe for cerebral spinal fluid leak from ears and nose
- Change in LOC
- Determine if consciousness was lost
- Determine mechanism or cause of injury
- Assess neurological function using the Glasgow Coma Scale
- Assess for other injuries (especially neck injuries)

Diagnostics

- Computed tomography (CT) scan of the head
- Magnetic resonance imaging (MRI)

Lab Tests

- Complete blood count (CBC)
- Electrolytes and glucose
- Coagulation studies
- Toxicology

PLANNING AND IMPLEMENTATION

- Administer oxygen
- Frequent neurological exams
- Call health care provider for any neurological changes
- Implement safety precautions
- Seizure precautions
- Maintain adequate blood pressure
- Prevent hypercarbia
- Prevent increased ICP
- Head of bed elevated
- Maintain a calm environment
- Prevent gagging, vomiting, and straining for defecation
- Monitor for Cushing's response (bradycardia, bradypnea, and systolic hypertension)
- Maintain normothermia
- ICP monitoring device care
- Monitor cerebral perfusion pressure with ICP monitor (mean arterial pressure [MAP] − ICP = cerebral perfusion pressure [CPP]) and maintain above 70 mm Hg
- Provide adequate nutritional intake
- Provide adequate hydration
- Anticipate administering osmotic diuretics
- Prevent all complications of immobility

Discharge Planning

- Depending on the severity of the injury, the patient may require long-term care and extensive rehabilitation.

SPECIAL CONCERNS

- See Special Procedures and Treatments for information on Craniotomy.
- Forty-four percent of traumatic brain injuries result from motor vehicle accidents in which people did not wear seatbelts or drove while intoxicated.
- Thirteen percent of traumatic brain injuries result from sports injuries. Encourage the use of appropriate headgear.

Geriatric Considerations

- Falls are more common in the geriatric population. Falls with subsequent brain injury account for 26 percent of traumatic brain injuries.

NURSING DIAGNOSIS

- Intracranial adaptive capacity, Decreased
- Mobility, Impaired physical
- Thought process, Disturbed
- Caregiver role strain, Risk for

Brain Tumors

DEFINITION

- Brain tumors are an abnormal growth of cells within the brain tissue.

Classifications

- Benign brain tumors are noncancerous, usually grow slowly, and are confined to one area of the brain.
  - Meningiomas are slow growing, account for 25 percent of all brain tumors, and may reoccur if excised.
  - Adenomas or pituitary tumors are tumors that originate in the pituitary gland.

- Schwannomas form around nerve fibers and commonly affect the eighth cranial nerve, affecting balance and hearing (acoustic neuroma).
- Vascular tumors are rare and involve the blood vessels of the brain. The most common is a hemangioblastoma.

- Malignant brain tumors are cancerous, usually grow quickly, and may be considered primary (the cancer originated in the brain) or, more commonly, secondary (the cancer originated in another location and spread to the brain). Secondary brain tumors occur in 20–40 percent of all oncology patients.
  - Gliomas are tumors that arise from the glial cells (see Table 4).
  - Central nervous system (CNS) lymphomas develop from lymphocyte cells and disseminate throughout the brain and in the cerebrospinal fluid.

KEY ASSESSMENTS

- Headache (experienced by 50 percent of patients with brain tumors)
- New onset of seizures
- Nausea and vomiting
- Visual disturbances
- Balance disturbances
- Hemiplegia
- Hearing loss
- Aphasia
- Change in level of consciousness (LOC)
- Personality change

Diagnostics

- Computed tomography (CT)
- Magnetic resonance imaging (MRI)
- Spinal tap
- Electroencephalogram (EEG)
- Cerebral angiography
- Brain biopsy

PLANNING AND IMPLEMENTATION

- Complete and frequent neurological assessments
- Institute seizure precautions
- Institute safety measures
- Monitor and treat headaches, nausea, and vomiting

TABLE 4

Types of Gliomas

Type	Incidence	Treatment

Astrocytomas	Most common
	Three types:
	▪ Pilocytic Astrocytoma (Grade I)
	  ▪ Least malignant
	  ▪ Grows slowly
	▪ Astrocytoma (Grade II)
	▪ Astrocytoma (Grade III)
	▪ Glioblastoma multiforme (Grade IV)
	  ▪ Rapidly grows
	  ▪ Invades tissue nearby
	  ▪ Extremely malignant
	  ▪ Most common in adults
		Surgery
		Surgery, radiation, chemotherapy
		Surgery, radiation, chemotherapy

Ependymomas	Mostly in children Usually benign	Surgery with radiation Chemotherapy if tumors reoccur
Oligodendrogliomas	Five percent of all gliomas Usually in young adults Occurs in cerebral hemispheres	Surgery with radiation
Ganglioneuromas	Rarest form Develops from glial cells and mature neurons Grows slowly	Surgery
Mixed Gliomas	Develops from more than one type of glial cell	Focuses on treatment of the most malignant cell type
Brainstem Gliomas	Located at base of brain Most common in children and young adults	Radiation No surgery due to location near vital brain centers
Optic Nerve Gliomas	Tumor develops on or near nerves between the brain visual center and the eye Common in people with neurofibromatosis	Surgery or radiation

(Adapted from National Institute for Neurological Disorders and Stroke-Hope through Research, 2001; Brain Tumor Association, 2004.)

- Assist with activities of daily living if hemiplegia is present
- Encourage adequate nutritional intake
- Report any neurological change immediately to the health care provider
- Discuss and educate patient about main treatments for brain tumors, including surgery, radiation, and chemotherapy

Discharge Planning

- Many brain tumor patients receive outpatient treatments and need to know when to contact their health care provider.
- If the patient has cognitive or motor impairment, home safety should be addressed before discharge.

SPECIAL CONCERNS

- See Special Procedures and Treatments for information on Craniotomy and Cancer.

NURSING DIAGNOSIS

- Intracranial adaptive capacity, Decreased
- Mobility, Impaired physical
- Thought process, Disturbed
- Caregiver role strain, Risk for

Buerger's Disease

DEFINITION

- Buerger's disease, also known as thromboangiitis obliterans, is an occlusive disease usually located in small- to medium-sized arteries and rarely in veins. Inflammation of vessels occurs, and over time scarring and fibrosis cause tissue hypoxia and decreased peripheral pulses. Weakened vessels are at risk for spasm induced by extreme temperatures.

KEY ASSESSMENTS

- Extreme sensitivity to heat and cold
- Pain in the digits
- Decreased peripheral pulses
- Reports of intermittent claudication (leg cramping with walking)

- Thick nail beds
- Cyanotic extremities
- Presence of blackish ulcerations

PLANNING AND IMPLEMENTATION

- Offer smoking cessation materials
- Monitor peripheral extremity for pain, pallor, pulse, paresthesia, and paralysis
- Treat pain
- Wound care

SPECIAL CONCERNS

Gender Considerations

- Buerger's disease occurs more frequently in young males who smoke, and it has a genetic predisposition.

Teaching Considerations

- Instruct patient to do the following exercises several times a day.
    - Lie flat on a bed with both legs elevated above the heart for two to three minutes.
    - Sit on the edge of the bed with legs dependent for three minutes.
    - Move the feet and toes up, down, inward, and outward.
    - Return to the first position and hold for five minutes.

Burns

DEFINITION

- A burn is an injury to the skin and underlying tissues caused by heat, chemicals, or electricity. Classifications are based on the degree of destruction. Systemic changes develop when more than 25 percent of the total body surface area is burned. The inflammatory response causes massive fluid shifts and burn shock. Hypovolemic and cellular shock may also occur.

Classifications

- Superficial burns, or first-degree burns, involve the epidermal layer, or outer layer, of the skin and are painful.

- Partial thickness and deep partial thickness burns, or second-degree burns, involve the destruction of the epidermal layer and varying depths of the dermis, the layer below the epidermal layer, and are painful.
- Full thickness burns, or third-degree burns, include destruction of the epidermis, the entire dermis, and damage to structures below the dermis, including subcutaneous tissue, muscle, and bone. Nerve endings are destroyed, and the burn is painless.

Causes

- Scald burns are caused by steam or hot fluid, are most common in children, and cause superficial or partial thickness burns.
- Flame and flash burns occur from fires or ignited gasoline and cause partial to full thickness burns. Inhalation injuries are common with this type of burn.
- Chemical burns occur from accidental exposure to a hazardous chemical. The severity of the injury depends on the chemical involved, the concentration of the chemical, and the length of exposure.
- Electrical burns result from accidental contact with an exposed object that conducts electricity. The area burned is not always apparent and often is internal. Arrhythmias and neurological dysfunction are common with this type of burn.

KEY ASSESSMENTS

Emergent Phase: First 24–48 Hours after a Burn Injury

- Airway
- Presence of inhalation injury (singed nasal hairs, inhaled flames, steam or smoke, laryngeal edema, or stridor)
- Breathing
- Circulation
- Signs of burn shock (hypotension or decreased urine output)
- Temperature (hypothermia)
- Pain
- Edema
- Presence of neurological deficit
- Medical history
- Classify and identify type of burn injury
- Use rule of nines to estimate percentage of total body surface burned
    - Head and arms are each considered 9 percent of the total body surface.

- Legs, chest, and back are each considered 18 percent of the total body surface.
- Perineum is remaining 1 percent of the total body surface area.

Acute Phase: From 48 Hours to Weeks after Burn Injury

- Assess for hypothermia
- Hourly urine output
- Oxygenation status
- Neurological status
- Hematemesis
- Bowel sounds (ileus may form)
- Presence of infection
- Signs of organ dysfunction
- Wound appearance
- Pain

Rehabilitation Phase: Days to Years after Injury

- Level of functioning
- Psychological adjustment to injury
- Resumption of preburn activities (work and social function)

PLANNING AND IMPLEMENTATION

Emergent Phase

- Stop the burning process by separating the patient from the causative agent.
- Secure the airway.
- Administer 100 percent oxygen.
- Intubate if signs of inhalation injury present.
- Insert two large-bore peripheral intravenous (IV) lines.
- Initiate fluid resuscitation with lactated Ringer's solution.
- Remove the patient from a hazardous environment.
- Remove all clothing.
- Irrigate eyes for ocular chemical burns.
- Cover burns with sterile dressings dampened with NS.
- Wrap body to prevent heat loss.
- Provide analgesic pain relief.
- Initiate nothing by mouth (NPO) status.
- Insert indwelling urinary catheter.
- Administer tetanus prophylaxis if the patient has not received tetanus toxoid in the preceding five years.
- Type and cross-match for blood products.
- Replace fluids using Parkland Formula: 2–4 mL of lactated Ringer's solution times body weight in kilograms times percent

B

burn = fluid requirement for the first 24 hours. Half of the total amount calculated is given the first 8 hours after the injury; the second half is given over the subsequent 16 hours.

- Monitor arterial blood gases (ABGs) and O_2 saturation.
- Monitor vital signs for shock and cardiac arrhythmias.
- Insert nasogastric tube and apply to low intermittent suction.
- Anticipate administering ulcer prophylaxis medications.
- Initial wound care needed to remove dirt, debris, and dead tissue.
- Obtain baseline wound cultures.
- Photograph wounds to provide a record of the appearance of the wound on admission.
- Monitor distal pulses.
- Escharotomy (linear surgical incision that releases the constriction of the affected part) should be performed for circumferential burns (burns encompassing a body part such as a leg).
- Provide emotional support.

Acute Phase

- Maintain fluid volume noted by adequate urine output of at least 30 mL/hr
- Oxygenate to maintain O_2 saturation above 90 percent
- Monitor vital signs frequently for arrhythmias and hypotension
- Monitor neurological status frequently
- Monitor temperature and prevent hypothermia
- Monitor ABGs
- Monitor and treat electrolyte imbalance
- Observe for organ dysfunction
- Monitor serum creatinine, aspartate transaminase (AST), alanine aminotransferase (ALT), electrolytes, protein, albumin, red blood cells (RBCs), and white blood cells (WBCs)
- Anticipate administering blood
- Administer pain medication prior to wound care
- Daily weight
- Provide adequate nutritional intake
- Sterile wound care as appropriate for location of burn, the size, and depth
- Emotional support
- Alleviate anxiety
- Incentive inspirometry every hour while awake
- Anticipate skin grafting for full thickness wounds
- Anticipate hydrotherapy (immersion of patient in water to help remove debris)
- Routine wound cultures to monitor microorganisms

- Wound cultures if temperature is elevated or the wound appearance changes
- Anticipate administering antibiotics for infection
- Range of motion
- Prevent contractures with use of orthotics and splints as ordered
- Monitor for infection (fever, tachycardia, or tachypnea)

Rehabilitation Phase

- Offer emotional support
- Correct positioning using orthotic devices and elastic pressure garments
- Teach family to perform daily wound care
- Teach family to assess limbs for signs of adequate circulation and when to contact the health care provider
- Promote daily exercise
- Occupational therapy to gain optimal function
- Discuss body image disturbance
- Anticipate corrective surgery if deformities or contractures have formed

SPECIAL CONCERNS

- See Special Procedures and Treatments for information on Pain.
  - Burn injury is the second leading cause of accidental death.
  - Eighty percent of burns occur in the home.
  - Respect a Jehovah's Witness patient's choice if they refuse blood.

NURSING DIAGNOSIS

- Skin integrity, Impaired
- Infection, Risk for
- Pain, Acute
- Knowledge, Deficient
- Nutrition: less than body requirements, Imbalanced

Cancer, Bladder

DEFINITION

- Bladder cancer is cancer originating in the bladder. Cigarette smoking is the single greatest risk factor.

KEY ASSESSMENTS

- Painless, gross hematuria (80–90 percent of patients have this.)
- Dysuria
- Urgency
- Frequency

Diagnostics

- Intravenous pyelogram (IVP)
- Computed tomography (CT)

Lab Tests

- BladderChek (urine test to levels of tumor markers)

PLANNING AND IMPLEMENTATION

- Monitor urine output
- Smoking cessation
- Chemotherapy, radiation, or surgical excision (depends on stage of cancer)

SPECIAL CONCERNS

- See Special Procedures and Treatments for information on Cancer, Pain, and Palliative Care.

NURSING DIAGNOSIS

- Urinary elimination, Impaired
- Knowledge, Deficient

Cancer, Breast

DEFINITION

- Breast cancer is malignancy of the breast. It is the most common type of cancer in women, and one in eight women are expected to be diagnosed with breast cancer.
- Risk factors include female gender, age greater than 50, first-degree relative with breast cancer, inheriting BRAC1 or BRAC2 genes (breast cancer susceptibility genes), Caucasian, early menarche, late menopause, age greater than 30 with first

pregnancy, hormone replacement therapy, obesity, high fat diet, excessive alcohol consumption, and smoking.

KEY ASSESSMENTS

- Palpable lump
- Skin retraction
- Orange peel appearance of breast skin
- Inverted or nipple changes

History and Examination

- Family history of breast cancer

Diagnostics

- Mammography
- Breast ultrasound
- Surgical biopsy
- Fine needle aspiration biopsy
- Image guided core needle biopsy
- Ductal lavage (microcatheter inserted in breast ducts)
- Ductoscopy (microcatheter visualizes breast ducts)

Lab Tests

- Testing for breast cancer susceptibility genes (BRAC1, BRAC2)

PLANNING AND IMPLEMENTATION

- Anticipate treatment depending on size and extent of cancer, including hormonal, biological, and chemotherapies, radiation, and surgical excision.
- Cryotherapy, laser ablation, and radio frequency ablation may be used for small tumors.

Surgical Options

- Lumpectomy—local excision of the tumor and immediately surrounding tissue.
- Mastectomy—removal of breast tissue and lymph nodes located in the breast tissue.
- Modified radical mastectomy—excision of the breast tissue and some of the chains of axillary lymph nodes (most common surgery).

- Radical mastectomy—excision of breast tissue axillary, supraclavicular, internal mammary lymph nodes, and chest wall muscles under the breast (rarely performed).
- Breast reconstruction may be performed at the time of the mastectomy or later. Implants or autologous tissue may be used.

Postsurgical Care

- Monitor vital signs frequently.
- Encourage deep breathing.
- Monitor level of consciousness (LOC).
- Elevate arm on operative site.
- Do not ever perform venipuncture or blood pressures on operative site arm if any type of mastectomy has been performed.
- Monitor site for hemorrhage and infection.
- If drains are present, monitor color and quantity of drainage.
- Encourage early ambulation.
- Deep venous thrombosis (DVT) prophylaxis.
- Administer prophylactic antibiotics.
- Treat pain.
- Change dressing per request.
- Monitor intake and output (I & O).
- Encourage physical therapy for arm strengthening exercises.

SPECIAL CONCERNS

- See Special Procedures and Treatments for information on Cancer, Pain, and Palliative Care.
- Women will experience body image disturbances postsurgery and need support when viewing surgical site for the first time.
- Encourage the patient to discuss fears or questions related to sexuality.

NURSING DIAGNOSIS

- Pain, Acute
- Body image, Disturbed
- Skin integrity, Impaired
- Infection, Risk for
- Sexual dysfunction

Cancer, Cervical

DEFINITION

- Cervical cancer is cancer of the cervix. Squamous cell carcinomas account for 80–90 percent of cervical cancers; the rest are adenocarcinomas.
- Risk factors include human papillomavirus (HPV) infection (chances of HPV infection increase with early onset of sexual intercourse, multiple sexual partners, and having sex with uncircumcised men), smoking, human immunodeficiency virus (HIV) infection, chlamydia infection, obesity, multiple pregnancies, diethylstilbestrol (DES) exposure, and family history of cervical cancer.

KEY ASSESSMENTS

- Asymptomatic (most cancers)
- Abnormal discharge
- Vaginal bleeding
- Dyspareunia (painful intercourse)

Diagnostics

- Ultrasound
- Cervical biopsy
- Ultrasound
- Computed tomography (CT)
- Colposcopy

Lab Tests

- Human chorionic gonadotropin (HCG)
- Cancer antigen 125 (CA 125)
- Alpha-fetoprotein (AFP)

PLANNING AND IMPLEMENTATION

- Treatment is based on cancer extent and may include local laser excision, cryosurgery, hysterectomy, or pelvic exenteration (removal of the uterus, lymph nodes, bladder, vagina, and rectum) in combination with radiation and chemotherapy.
- Monitor for complications of surgery, including hemorrhage, infection, and deep venous thrombosis (DVT) formation.
- Monitor intake and output (I & O).

- Promote adequate nutritional and fluid intake by mouth.
- Monitor for complications of radiation therapy and chemotherapy, if indicated.
- Monitor complete blood count (CBC) and electrolytes.
- Monitor vital signs.
- Promote early ambulation.
- Encourage deep breathing.
- Encourage discussing body image and sexuality changes.

SPECIAL CONCERNS

- See Special Procedures and Treatments for information on Cancer, Pain, and Palliative Care.
- Surgery alters the appearance of the vaginal opening and may result in scar tissue that causes painful intercourse and difficulties attaining orgasm.
- Discuss sexual concerns with the patient and significant other.

NURSING DIAGNOSIS

- Body image, Disturbed
- Sexual dysfunction
- Anxiety
- Knowledge, Deficient

Cancer, Colorectal (CRC)

DEFINITION

- CRC is the presence of adenoma or adenocarcinoma tumors in the colon or rectum. Risk factors for developing CRC include being older than 50; a diet high in animal protein intake; obesity; cigarette smoking; a history of adenomatous polyps, Crohn's disease, CRC, or irritable bowel syndrome; genetic disposition with a family history of CRC, familial adenomatous polyposis (FAP), or hereditary, nonpolyposis colon cancer (HNPCC).

KEY ASSESSMENTS

- Family history
- Fatigue
- Unintended weight loss
- Anorexia

- Change in bowel habits
- Hematochezia (bloody stools)
- Tenesmus (urge to evacuate rectum)
- Narrow stools
- Alternating constipations and diarrhea

Postsurgical

- Vital signs
- Pulse oximetry
- Surgical site
- Stoma site (pink, moist, warm)
- Monitor intake and output (I & O)
- Pain

Diagnostics

- Fecal occult blood test (recommended annually for patients over 50)
- Flexible sigmoidoscopy (recommended every 5 years for patients over 50)
- Colonoscopy (recommended every 10 years for patients over 50)

PLANNING AND IMPLEMENTATION

- Surgery, chemotherapy, radiation, or palliative care (depends on size and stage of cancer)
- Monitor I & O
- Daily weight
- Administer preoperative or preprocedure antibiotics
- Calorie counts

Endoscopic Procedures

- Curative polypectomy (removal of polyps)
- Endoscopic mucosal resection (remove lesions through deep submucosa)

Surgical Resection

- Abdominal-perineal resection (APR) with permanent sigmoid colostomy with an ostomy (a surgically created opening between the intestine and the abdominal wall)

Postsurgical Resection

- Assess and treat pain
- Frequent vital signs

- Infection surveillance
- Monitor I & O
- Monitor electrolytes
- Encourage deep breathing
- Deep venous thrombosis (DVT) prophylaxis (antiembolism stockings, early ambulation)
- Maintain intravenous (IV) fluids to prevent dehydration
- Nasogastric tube to low intermittent suction (LIS)
- Assess incision site
- Wound care
- Observe stoma site for complications (narrowing of stoma opening, stoma separation from the abdominal wall, intestine bulging out of the stoma, dry stoma with no stool output, unusual drainage, rash around stoma site, and dark or purplish stoma color); if any, notify the health care provider
- Monitor for development of peritonitis (infection of the peritoneal cavity), severe pain drawing knees to the chest, tachycardia, diaphoresis, or high fever
- Apply ostomy appliances in collaboration with the enterostomal nurse
- Administer antibiotics

Discharge Planning

- The patient and the family require education and support regarding ostomy care prior to discharge.

SPECIAL CONCERNS

- See Special Procedures and Treatments for information on Cancer, Pain, and Palliative Care.
- Colorectal cancer is the third most common cancer and the third leading cause of cancer deaths.
- Five-year survival rate for CRC is 90 percent when diagnosed early.

NURSING DIAGNOSIS

- Pain, Acute
- Infection, Risk for
- Fluid volume, Risk for deficient
- Body image, Disturbed
- Skin integrity, Risk for impaired

Cancer, Endometrial

DEFINITION

- Endometrial cancer is malignancy of the endometrium and is the most common cancer of the female reproductive system.
- Risk factors include early age at menarche, late menopause, infertility, obesity, use of tamoxifen, ovarian tumors, a diet high in animal fat, age greater than 40, and family history of colon, breast, or ovarian cancer.

KEY ASSESSMENTS

- Irregular vaginal bleeding
- Weight loss
- Pelvic pain

Diagnostics

- Ultrasound
- Endometrial biopsy
- Ultrasound
- Computed tomography (CT)
- Colposcopy

Lab Tests

- Human chorionic gonadotropin (HCG)
- Cancer antigen 125(CA 125)
- Alpha-fetoprotein (AFP)

PLANNING AND IMPLEMENTATION

- Treatment involves hysterectomy and possible removal of the ovaries, and it may include radiation or chemotherapy.
- Monitor for complications of surgery including hemorrhage, infection, and deep venous thrombosis (DVT) formation.
- Monitor intake and output (I & O).
- Promote adequate fluid and nutritional intake by mouth.
- Monitor for complications of radiation therapy and chemotherapy, if indicated.
- Monitor complete blood count (CBC) and electrolytes.
- Monitor vital signs.
- Promote early ambulation.
- Encourage deep breathing.
- Encourage discussing body image and sexuality changes.

SPECIAL CONCERNS

- See Special Procedures and Treatments for information on Cancer, Pain, and Palliative Care.

NURSING DIAGNOSIS

- Body image, Disturbed
- Sexual dysfunction
- Anxiety
- Knowledge, Deficient

Cancer, Esophageal

DEFINITION

- Esophageal cancer is cancer of the esophagus and has a five-year survival rate of only 15 percent.

Classifications

- Risks for adenocarcinoma esophageal cancer include smoking, gastroesophageal reflux disease (GERD), and Barrett's esophagus.
- Risks for squamous cell carcinoma esophageal cancer include smoking, alcohol ingestion, achalasia, exposure to nitrosamines, ingestion of lye, Plummer-Vincent webs, and tylosis.

KEY ASSESSMENTS

- Dysphagia
- Pyrosis
- Anorexia
- Weight loss
- Hoarseness
- Recurrent upper respiratory infections
- Cough

History and Examination

- Smoking history
- GERD
- Alcohol consumption
- Exposure to nitrosamines
- Ingestion of lye

Diagnostics

- Endoscopy with esophageal biopsy
- Barium swallow

PLANNING AND IMPLEMENTATION

- Provide small meals
- Upright position while eating and for one hour after meals
- Encourage weight loss if obese
- Avoid hot and cold beverages
- Avoid alcohol, caffeine, and tobacco
- Avoid eating before bedtime
- Administer antacids, H_2 blockers, and proton pump inhibitors as ordered
- Chemotherapy, surgical resection, or palliative care (depends on size and stage of tumor)

SPECIAL CONCERNS

- See Special Procedures and Treatments for information on Cancer, Pain, and Palliative Care.

Gender Considerations

- Esophageal cancer is most common in white males from 65 to 74 years of age.

NURSING DIAGNOSIS

- Pain, Acute
- Anxiety
- Nutrition: less than body requirements, Imbalanced

Cancer, Gallbladder

DEFINITION

- Cancer of the gallbladder is a rare malignancy occurring more commonly in the elderly, the obese, and in patients with bile duct abnormalities.

KEY ASSESSMENTS

- Abdominal pain (upper right quadrant)
- Anorexia
- Weight loss
- Nausea and vomiting
- Jaundice
- Pruritus

Diagnostics

- Ultrasound
- Computed tomography (CT)
- Endoscopic retrograde cholangiopancreatography (ERCP)

PLANNING AND IMPLEMENTATION

- Monitor intake and output (I & O)
- Daily weight
- Promote adequate fluid and nutritional intake by mouth
- Cool baths for pruritus
- Treat pain
- Surgical resection or palliative treatments (depends on stage of cancer)

SPECIAL CONCERNS

- See Special Procedures and Treatments for information on Cancer, Pain, and Palliative Care.

NURSING DIAGNOSIS

- Pain, Acute
- Nutrition: less than body requirements, Imbalanced
- Knowledge, Deficient

Cancer, Larynx

DEFINITION

- Cancer of the larynx is a malignancy rising from the supraglottic, glottic, or subglottic area of the larynx with 95 percent of cases occurring in the glottic area, which includes the vocal cords. A clear association between smoking, excess alcohol ingestion, and laryngeal cancer exists. Other carcinogens associated with higher risk include exposure to wood dust, paint fumes, tar products, and asbestos. Other factors that increase risk are human papillomavirus (HPV), nutritional deficiencies, and gastroesophageal reflux disease (GERD).

KEY ASSESSMENTS

- Sore throat
- Pain with swallowing
- Cough
- Weight loss
- Hoarseness
- Hemoptysis
- Pain in ears
- Difficulty swallowing
- History of smoking, excessive alcohol consumption, GERD, or exposure to carcinogenic agents

Diagnostics

- Laryngoscopy and biopsy
- Computed tomography (CT)
- Magnetic resonance imaging (MRI)
- Diagnostics will stage and locate the cancer

PLANNING AND IMPLEMENTATION

- Radiation or endoscopic transoral laser surgery (depends on stage and area of cancer)
- Surgical intervention may include:
  - Partial laryngectomy—only one vocal cord is removed, and the voice is preserved.
  - Supraglottic laryngectomy—removal of the hyoid bone, glottis, and false cords.
  - Hemilaryngectomy—removes one true vocal cord, one false vocal cord, and part of the thyroid. Postoperatively the patient will have a tracheostomy.
  - Total laryngectomy—the entire larynx and surrounding tissues are removed. The patient will have a permanent tracheal stoma, and the airway is permanently altered.

- Radical neck dissection—in addition to a total laryngectomy the sternocleidomastoid muscle and surrounding tissue will be removed.

Postoperative Care for a Tracheostomy

- Monitor and maintain a patent airway
- Oxygen administration with humidified air
- Elevate head of bed
- Tracheostomy care
- Provide a means of communication
- Pain relief
- Adequate nutritional and fluid intake
- Monitor for signs of infection
- Frequent vital signs
- Monitor for signs of hemorrhage

SPECIAL CONCERNS

- See Special Procedures and Treatments for information on Cancer, Pain, Palliative Care.
- A nurse caring for a patient with a total laryngectomy must realize that the tracheal stoma is the only communication with the lungs. If the tracheostomy becomes obstructed or dislodged, the nurse must reestablish the tracheostomy to ventilate the patient. The mouth no longer communicates with the lungs because of the surgical alteration.

Cultural Considerations

- Cancer of the larynx has a higher incidence in African Americans in the United States.
- There is a higher incidence of the disease in Spain, Poland, France, and Italy.

Gender Considerations

- Cancer of the larynx occurs four times more frequently in men than in women.

NURSING DIAGNOSIS

- Pain, Acute
- Swallowing, Impaired
- Communication, Impaired verbal

Cancer, Liver

DEFINITION

- Liver cancer is malignant tumors in the liver.

Clinical Causes

- There is an increased incidence of liver cancer in many conditions, including hepatitis B, hepatitis C, cirrhosis, hemochromatosis, smoking, obesity, Wilson's disease, and alpha-antitrypsin deficiency.

Classifications

- Primary liver cancer originates in the hepatocytes of the liver.
- Secondary liver cancer is metastatic liver cancer from cancer originating in another body part, such as breast or colon.

KEY ASSESSMENTS

- Epigastric pain
- Fatigue
- Anorexia
- Weight loss
- Right upper quadrant pain

Diagnostics

- Computed tomography (CT) of liver
- Needle biopsy

Lab Tests

- Complete blood count (CBC)
- Prothrombin time (PT), partial thromboplastin time (PTT), international normalized ratio (INR)
- Liver panel

PLANNING AND IMPLEMENTATION

- Monitor and treat pain
- Monitor intake and output (I & O)
- Daily weight
- Encourage adequate fluid and nutritional intake
- Treat nausea
- Monitor liver panel

- Monitor for signs of worsening liver function (confusion, ascites, or coagulopathies)
- Anticipate treatment consisting or one or more of the following:
  - Surgical resection
  - Radio frequency ablation (high energy radio waves to destroy cancer cells)
  - Chemoembolization (impregnating chemotherapy drugs next to the tumor)
  - Radiation
  - Chemotherapy
  - Palliative care
- Monitor and care for effects of treatments

SPECIAL CONCERNS

- See Special Procedures and Treatments for information on Cancer, Pain, and Palliative Care.

NURSING DIAGNOSIS

- Pain, Acute
- Anxiety
- Tissue perfusion, Ineffective

Cancer, Lung

DEFINITION

- Lung cancer is malignancy of the lungs caused by a malignant neoplasm in which cells mutate and invade the tissue, and it can travel via the lymphatic system and blood vessels to other sites. The expected five-year survival rate for all people diagnosed with lung cancer is 16 percent because it is usually metastasized to other sites by the time it is initially diagnosed. Cigarette smoking and asbestos exposure are the biggest risk factors for developing lung cancer.

KEY ASSESSMENTS

- Cough, blood sputum
- Wheezing
- Shortness of breath (SOB)
- Anorexia

- Weakness
- Weight loss
- Difficulty swallowing
- Change in voice

Diagnostics

- Chest X-ray (CXR)
- Sputum cytology
- Computed tomography (CT) of lung
- Bronchoscopy, needle, or open biopsy (classify by the tumor-nodes-metastasis [TNM] classification)
- Brain, liver, and bone scans to look for metastasis

PLANNING AND IMPLEMENTATION

- Oxygen administration
- Frequent vital signs including pulse oximetry
- Assess mental status frequently
- Treat pain around the clock
- Encourage expression of emotions about cancer and death
- Administer antianxiety medications if necessary
- Administer medications to treat nausea
- Encourage frequent oral care
- Provide frequent rest periods
- Prevent infections
- Encourage adequate fluid and nutritional intake
- Monitor complete blood count (CBC) and platelets
- Implement safety precautions
- Meticulous skin care
- Chemotherapy, radiation therapy, or surgical intervention
- Surgical interventions include:
  - Lobectomy removal of a lobe or section of the lung
  - Pneumonectomy removal of an entire lung

Postoperative Care

- Frequent vital signs
- Continuous pulse oximetry
- Oxygen administration
- Maintain fluid volume status
- Monitor for hemorrhage
- Pain control
- Managing chest tubes
- Encourage incentive spirometry

SPECIAL CONCERNS

- See Special Procedures and Treatments for information on Cancer, Pain, and Palliative Care.
- People caring for patients with lung cancer at home are at risk for caregiver strain.
- Encourage caregivers to attend support groups, and ask family members to stay with the patient so caregivers can have time to themselves.

NURSING DIAGNOSIS

- Activity intolerance, Risk for
- Breathing pattern, Ineffective
- Infection, Risk for

Cancer, Musculoskeletal

DEFINITION

- Musculoskeletal cancers include carcinoma of the bone, muscle, and associated soft tissue (see Table 5).

TABLE 5

Soft Tissue Sarcomas

Name	Origin	Characteristics
Osteosarcoma	Highly malignant bone sarcoma in which malignant cells produce osteoid	Most common type of primary bone tumor. Occurs in the growth plate region of long bones and pelvis. Of all cases, 75 percent occur between ages 10 and 25.
Ewing's sarcoma	Primitive small round cell	Primary bone tumor that can present in soft tissues, but more commonly found in the diaphysis of the femur and the flat bones of the pelvic girdle.

(American Cancer Society, 2005c)

continued

TABLE 5

Soft Tissue Sarcomas—cont'd

Name	Origin	Characteristics
Chondrosarcoma	Malignant cells produce cartilage instead of osteoid	Primary bone tumor, most commonly seen in the knees, shoulders, and pelvis. It can either arise from within the bone or from the surface. It can also be classified as either primary or secondary (from a benign lesion).
Fibrosarcoma	Originates from intermuscular or intramuscular fibrous tissue, fascia, or tendons	A rare primary bone tumor. Point of origin is the medullary cavity and primarily affects the metaphyseal portions of the femur and tibia.
Malignant fibrous histiocytoma	Tumors contain a mixture of fibroblast-like and histiocyte-like cells	Can be a primary bone tumor, but most commonly seen as soft tissue tumor. Most often found in the deep fascia and skeletal muscles, but can be found in almost any soft tissue. Occurs most often (70–75 percent) in the extremities.
Liposarcoma	Adipose tissue	Soft tissue tumor found in the deep tissues of the thigh and retroperitoneal space of the abdomen.
Leiomyosarcoma	Smooth muscle	Soft tissue tumor, mostly found in the gastrointestinal tract, retroperitoneum, and skin.
Neurofibrosarcoma	Ectodermal embryologic origin	A soft tissue tumor that is also called malignant peripheral nerve sheath tumor (MPNST). Found in nerve sheaths in the proximal extremity and trunk.
Synovial sarcoma	Epithelial and spindle cells that resemble cells found in synovial fluid in joints	Soft tissue tumor that can be found anywhere in the body. The most common location is in and around the knee joint.
Angiosarcoma	Vascular endothelium	Soft tissue tumor that resembles blood or lymph vessels. Often seen in the skin, soft tissues, and organs.
Rhabdomyosarcoma	Skeletal muscle	Soft tissue tumors resembling developing striated muscle. Most often seen in the extremities, head, neck, urinary tract, or reproductive organs.

KEY ASSESSMENTS

- Dull aching pain that worsens at night
- Swelling, localized enlargement of extremity
- Fever
- Night sweats
- Pathologic fracture (fracture without injury or trauma)
- Limp
- Limited range of motion to affected limb

Diagnostics

- X-ray
- Biopsy
- Computed tomography (CT)
- Bone marrow aspirate

Lab Tests

- Low-density lipoprotein (LDL)
- Alkaline phosphatase (ALP)

PLANNING AND IMPLEMENTATION

- Assist with mobility
- Implement safety measures
- Treat pain as prescribed
- Monitor for vascular compromise to extremity (pain, pallor, pulse, paresthesia, or paralysis)
- Chemotherapy, radiation, surgery, palliative care, or a combination (depends on stage of cancer)
- Monitor for side effects of radiation and chemotherapy
- If amputation is necessary, anticipatory grieving counseling

SPECIAL CONCERNS

- See Special Procedures and Treatments for information on Cancer, Pain, and Palliative Care.

NURSING DIAGNOSIS

- Falls, Risk for
- Grieving, Anticipatory
- Pain, Acute
- Mobility, Impaired physical

Cancer, Ovarian

DEFINITION

- Ovarian cancer is the fifth most common cancer in women, and 85 percent of ovarian cancers are epithelial.
- Risk factors include increased age, early menstruation, late menopause, no children or first child after age of 30, prolonged use of clomiphene citrate, and family history of breast, ovarian, or colorectal cancer.

KEY ASSESSMENTS

- Asymptomatic (most patients)
- Abdominal pain and swelling
- Bloating
- Nausea and vomiting
- Change in bowel and bladder habits
- Leg and back pain

Diagnostics

- Ultrasound
- Computed tomography (CT)
- Colposcopy

Lab Tests

- Cancer antigen 125 (CA 125)
- Human chorionic gonadotropin (HCG)
- Acid-fast bacillus (AFB)
- BRAC1 or BRAC2

PLANNING AND IMPLEMENTATION

- Surgical removal of the ovaries and uterus. Chemotherapy and radiation may be indicated.
- Monitor for complications of surgery including hemorrhage, infection, and deep venous thrombosis (DVT) formation.
- Monitor intake and output (I & O).
- Promote adequate fluid and nutritional intake by mouth.
- Monitor for complications of radiation therapy and chemotherapy, if indicated.
- Monitor complete blood count (CBC) and electrolytes.

- Monitor vital signs.
- Promote early ambulation.
- Encourage deep breathing.
- Encourage discussing body image and sexuality changes.

SPECIAL CONCERNS

- See Special Procedures and Treatments for information on Cancer, Pain, and Palliative Care.

NURSING DIAGNOSIS

- Body image, Disturbed
- Sexual dysfunction
- Anxiety
- Knowledge, Deficient

Cancer, Prostate

DEFINITION

- Prostate cancer is a condition of abnormal cell growth of the prostate. It begins with epithelial abnormalities and continues until cellular changes are widespread. It is the second most commonly diagnosed cancer in men. Bone is the most common site of metastases.

KEY ASSESSMENTS

- Urinary incontinence

History and Examination

- Digital rectal exam reveals an enlarged, nodular hard prostate.

Diagnostics

- Rectal ultrasonography
- Postvoiding bladder scan
- Prostate biopsy (minimum of two performed)

Lab Tests

- Prostate-specific antigen ([PSA], biopsy usually performed for PSA greater than 4)

PLANNING AND IMPLEMENTATION

- Treatment is based on grading and staging.

Radiation Therapy

- Traditional external beam radiation
- Intensity modulated radiation therapy
- Brachytherapy (implantation of radioactive seeds)

Surgical Procedure

- Radical prostatectomy—removal of the entire prostate gland, seminal vesicles, and lymph nodes. It may be performed as a transabdominal, laparoscopic, transperitoneal, or extraperitoneal procedure.

SPECIAL CONCERNS

- See Special Procedures and Treatments for information on Cancer, Pain, and Palliative Care.
- Impotence and urinary incontinence is common after many treatments, and explaining this effect is paramount before initiating treatment.

Geriatric Considerations

- Eighty percent of men over the age of 80 have prostate cancer.

Teaching Considerations

- Recommend that men over the age of 50 have an annual screening digital rectal exam.

NURSING DIAGNOSIS

- Urinary elimination, Impaired
- Pain, Chronic
- Fear
- Sexual dysfunction

Cancer, Renal

DEFINITION

- Renal cancer is a malignancy in the kidney. Risk factors include cigarette smoking and obesity, and it is thought to have a genetic component.

KEY ASSESSMENTS

- Hematuria
- Flank or back pain
- Weight loss
- Testicular enlargement
- Fatigue
- Fever
- Anemia
- Abdominal swelling

Diagnostics

- Computed tomography (CT)
- Magnetic resonance imaging (MRI)
- Abdominal ultrasound

Lab Tests

- Complete blood count (CBC)
- Electrolytes
- Prothrombin time (PT), partial thromboplastin time (PTT), and international normalized ratio (INR)
- Blood urea nitrogen (BUN) and creatinine (Cr)
- Liver function tests

PLANNING AND IMPLEMENTATION

- Monitor renal labs
- Monitor intake and output (I & O)
- Daily weight
- Anticipate a nephrectomy (removal of the kidney) or chemotherapy
- Monitor for side effects of chemotherapy

SPECIAL CONCERNS

- See Special Procedures and Treatments for information on Cancer, Pain, and Palliative Care.

Cultural Considerations

- Renal cancer is more common in patients of Northern European ancestry.

Gender Considerations

- Men are twice as likely as women to develop renal cancer.

NURSING DIAGNOSIS

- Fear
- Knowledge, Deficient

Cancer, Stomach

DEFINITION

- Stomach cancer refers to the growth of an adenocarcinoma or lymphoma tumor in the stomach. *Helicobacter pylori* infection is a risk factor for developing stomach cancer. Stomach cancer is twice as common in men as it is in women.

KEY ASSESSMENTS

- Abdominal pain
- Anorexia
- Indigestion
- Fatigue
- Weight loss

Diagnostics

- Endoscopy with tissue biopsy
- Barium swallow

Lab Tests

- Hemoglobin and hematocrit

PLANNING AND IMPLEMENTATION

- Surgery, chemotherapy, or palliative care (depends on size and stage of cancer)
- Daily weight
- Monitor intake and output (I & O)
- Treat pain and nausea
- Offer frequent, small meals
- Calorie count
- Administer chemotherapy as indicated

Surgical Approaches

- Gastrectomy (removal of more than 80 percent of the stomach)
- Partial gastrectomy (removal of less than 80 percent of the stomach)

- Billroth I (removal of the lower stomach and anastomosis to the duodenum)
- Billroth II (removal of the lower stomach and anastomosis to the jejunum)

Postgastric Surgery

- Treat pain
- Monitor incision for signs of infection
- Monitor vital sounds
- Encourage deep breathing
- Administer oxygen
- Head of bed elevated 30 degrees
- Small, frequent meals
- No liquids with meals
- Maintain a patient IV
- Observe for dumping syndrome (nausea, vomiting, headache, flushing, abdominal cramping, hunger, diaphoresis, and borborygmi sounds [loud, hyperactive bowel sounds])
- Anticipate treating dumping syndrome with octreotide and acarbose
- Administer nutritional supplements
- Administer antacids, anticholinergics, and antibiotics as ordered

SPECIAL CONCERNS

- See Special Procedures and Treatments for information on Cancer, Pain, and Palliative Care.

Cultural Considerations

- Stomach cancer is more common in Japan, Korea, Eastern Europe, and Latin America.

NURSING DIAGNOSIS

- Pain, Acute
- Nutrition: less than body requirements, Imbalanced
- Knowledge, Deficient
- Fear
- Infection, Risk for

Cancer, Testicular

DEFINITION

- Testicular cancer is the most common form of cancer in men ages 15 to 35 years. There are two types—germinal and nongerminal.

Classifications

- Germinal tumors grow from the germinal cells of the testes and are the most common type of testicular cancer. Tumors may be seminomas or nonseminomas. Seminomas are the most common, are susceptible to treatment by radiation, and tend to stay localized. Nonseminomas are cancers of remaining embryonic tissue and are rapidly growing, aggressive tumors that metastasize.
- Nongerminal tumors originate in the epithelium and are extremely rare.

KEY ASSESSMENTS

- Painless lump or enlargement of a testicle

Diagnostics

- Scrotal ultrasonography
- Needle biopsy
- Computed tomography (CT) check for metastasis

Lab Tests

- Alpha-fetal protein (AFP)
- Beta human chorionic gonadotropin (HCG)
- L-lactate dehydrogenase (LDH)
- Tumor markers

PLANNING AND IMPLEMENTATION

- Treatment depends on cancer stage, lymph node involvement, and presence or absence of distant metastases and may include one or a combination of chemotherapy, radiation, and surgery (orchiectomy or surgical removal of the testes).

SPECIAL CONCERNS

- See Special Procedures and Treatments for information on Cancer, Pain, and Palliative Care.

- Males with untreated congenital cryptorchidism (undescended testis) have 10 to 40 times the risk of testicular cancer.
- Address infertility concerns before treatment begins.

Cultural Considerations

- Scandinavian and Swiss men have the highest incidence, while African and Asian men have the lowest incidence of testicular cancer.

Teaching Considerations

- Perform monthly testicular self-exams

NURSING DIAGNOSIS

- Sexual dysfunction
- Knowledge, Deficient
- Body image, Impaired
- Fear

Cancer, Thyroid

DEFINITION

- Thyroid cancer is a neoplasm of the thyroid gland. Predisposing factors include childhood exposure to radiation in the head or neck.

Classifications

- Papillary thyroid cancer tends to metastasize to regional lymph nodes in the neck.
- Follicular thyroid cancer metastasizes to the lungs or bone.

KEY ASSESSMENTS

- Firm nodule on thyroid gland
- Voice changes

Diagnostics

- Thyroid scan
- Fine needle biopsy

PLANNING AND IMPLEMENTATION

- Thyroid lobectomy or total thyroidectomy (depending on size)
- Thyroid suppression therapy with daily levothyroxine

- Radiation
- Monitor patient for signs of hypothyroidism

SPECIAL CONCERNS

- See Special Procedures and Treatments for information on Cancer, Pain, and Palliative Care.

NURSING DIAGNOSIS

- Anxiety
- Knowledge, Deficient

Cancer, Vaginal

DEFINITION

- Vaginal cancer is a malignancy of the vagina; 85–90 percent of vaginal cancers are squamous cell occurring in the upper area of the vagina, and approximately 10 percent are adenocarcinomas.
- Risk factors include Diethylstilbestrol (DES) exposure, human papillomavirus (HPV) infection, cervical cancer, smoking, and increased age.

KEY ASSESSMENTS

- Asymptomatic (some patients)
- Abnormal vaginal discharge
- Vaginal bleeding
- Vaginal mass
- Dyspareunia (painful intercourse)
- Dysuria
- Pelvic pain

Diagnostics

- Ultrasound
- Vaginal biopsy
- Ultrasound
- Computed tomography (CT)
- Colposcopy

C

Lab Tests

- Human chorionic gonadotropin (HCG)
- Cancer antigen 125 (CA 125)
- Alpha-fetoprotein (AFP)

PLANNING AND IMPLEMENTATION

- Surgical removal of the vagina, chemotherapy, and radiation
- Monitor for complications of surgery including hemorrhage, infection, and deep venous thrombosis (DVT) formation
- Monitor intake and output (I & O)
- Promote adequate fluid and nutritional intake by mouth
- Monitor for complications of radiation therapy and chemotherapy, if indicated
- Monitor complete blood count (CBC) and electrolytes
- Monitor vital signs
- Promote early ambulation
- Encourage deep breathing
- Encourage discussing body image and sexuality changes

SPECIAL CONCERNS

- See Special Procedures and Treatments for information on Cancer, Pain, and Palliative Care.
- Surgery alters the appearance of the vaginal opening and may result in scar tissue that causes painful intercourse and difficulties attaining orgasm.
- Discuss sexual concerns with the patient and significant other.

NURSING DIAGNOSIS

- Body image, Disturbed
- Sexual dysfunction
- Anxiety
- Knowledge, Deficient

Cancer, Vulvar

DEFINITION

- Vulvar cancer is a malignant neoplasm of the vulvar tissue, and when diagnosed early, the five-year survival rate is 90 percent.

Most vulvar cancers are squamous cell cancers and begin with precancerous changes to the epithelial layer called vulvar intraepithelial neoplasias (VIN).
- Risk factors for vulvar cancer include human papillomavirus (HPV) infection, human immunodeficiency virus (HIV) infection, smoking, and lichen sclerosis (a condition that makes the skin thin and atrophic).

KEY ASSESSMENTS

- Asymptomatic (most women)
- Persistent vulvar itching
- Vulvar skin color changes
- White watery bumps
- Vulvar sores that do not heal
- New or atypical vulvar mole

Diagnostics

- Ultrasound
- Biopsy
- Ultrasound
- Computed tomography (CT)
- Colposcopy

Lab Tests

- Human chorionic gonadotropin (HCG)
- Cancer antigen 125 (CA 125)
- Alpha-fetoprotein (AFP)

PLANNING AND IMPLEMENTATION

- Treatment is based on cancer extent and may include local laser excision, cryosurgery, hysterectomy, or pelvic exenteration (removal of the uterus, lymph nodes, bladder, vagina, and rectum) in combination with radiation and chemotherapy.
- Monitor for complications of surgery, including hemorrhage, infection, and DVT formation.
- Monitor intake and output (I & O).
- Promote adequate fluid and nutritional intake by mouth.
- Monitor for complications of radiation therapy and chemotherapy, if indicated.
- Monitor complete blood count (CBC) and electrolytes.
- Monitor vital signs.
- Promote early ambulation.

- Encourage deep breathing.
- Encourage discussing body image and sexuality changes.

SPECIAL CONCERNS

- See Special Procedures and Treatments for information on Cancer, Pain, and Palliative Care.
- Surgery alters the appearance of the vaginal opening and may result in scar tissue that causes painful intercourse and difficulties attaining orgasm.
- Discuss sexual concerns with the patient and significant other.

NURSING DIAGNOSIS

- Body image, Disturbed
- Sexual dysfunction
- Anxiety
- Knowledge, Deficient

Cardiomyopathy

DEFINITION

- Cardiomyopathy is a disease of the heart muscle that causes a decrease functioning of the heart.
- Decreased functioning results in:
  - Decreased cardiac output
  - Increased systemic vascular resistance
  - Decreased stroke volume
  - Activation of sympathetic nervous system
  - Activation of the rennin-angiotensin system
  - All eventually lead to heart failure

Classifications

- Dilated cardiomyopathy (DCM) results in a dilated heart chamber that decreases the ability of the heart to pump forcefully. DCM is associated with coronary artery disease (CAD), hypertension, valvular disease, family history, a history of Coxsackie B viral infection, autoimmune disease, toxins, and pregnancy.
- Hypertrophic cardiomyopathy (HCM) results in an increase to the size and thickness of the heart muscle, decreasing the volume of blood that can be pumped.

- HCM has a strong familial link, but in most cases, the cause is considered idiopathic.
- Myectomy, removal of scarred tissue, may be part of the medical treatment.
- Arrhythmogenic right ventricular cardiomyopathy (ARVC) results in a scarred and fatty tissue replacing normal heart muscle. The cause of ARVC is unknown but thought to have genetic links. The progressive loss of heart muscle affects the electrical functioning.
- Restrictive cardiomyopathy (RCM) results in a stiff muscle causing resistance and increased myocardial workload. The cause of RCM is unknown but may be a sequela of radiation therapy or metabolic disorders.

KEY ASSESSMENTS

- Crackles
- Decrease oxygen saturation
- Dyspnea
- Jugular vein distention
- Peripheral edema
- Cyanotic nail beds
- Circumoral pallor
- Confusion
- Abdominal distention, pain
- Auscultation of S_3
- Orthopnea
- Paroxysmal nocturnal dyspnea
- Tachycardia
- Weak distal pulses
- Fatigue
- Syncope
- Chest pain
- Hepatojugular reflux

PLANNING AND IMPLEMENTATION

- Electrocardiogram (ECG)
- Echocardiogram
- Stress test
- Brain natriuretic peptide ([BNP], useful to diagnose severity)
- C-reactive protein (CRP) and tumor necrotizing factor (TNF)
- Heart biopsy
- Electrophysiological studies
- Fluid restriction

- Implement safety measures
- Restrict sodium
- Head of bed elevated
- Oxygen administration
- Monitor pulmonary status
- Accurate intake and output (I & O)
- Daily weight
- Report to health care provider weight gain of 2 pounds in a day or 5 pounds in a week
- Medicine regimes—typically a combination of medications including diuretics, angiotensin-converting enzyme (ACE) inhibitors, vasodilators, beta blockers, digitalis, nitrates, antiarrhythmics, and aspirin
- Educate patients concerning restrictions and medications
- Pacemaker insertion, automatic internal defibrillation insertion, or heart transplantation

NURSING DIAGNOSIS

- Cardiac output, Decreased
- Activity intolerance
- Fluid volume, Risk for imbalanced
- Breathing pattern, Ineffective
- Tissue perfusion, Ineffective

Carpal Tunnel Syndrome

DEFINITION

- Carpal tunnel syndrome is an entrapment neuropathy caused by compression of the median nerve (usually from the carpal ligament) in the tunnel located in the wrist.

KEY ASSESSMENTS

- Pain exacerbated by flexion and dorsiflexion of the wrist
- Pain is usually worse at night
- Burning and tingling
- Sensory and motor loss of the palmar aspect of the first three fingers
- Positive Tinel's sign (pain elicited by tapping over the medial nerve at the wrist)
- Positive Phalen's sign (pain and numbness when the wrist is flexed for a minute)

History and Examination

- Patients with occupations including repetitive movements of the wrists for prolonged periods of time are at higher risk for carpal tunnel syndrome.

PLANNING AND IMPLEMENTATION

- Apply hand splints as ordered
- Administer nonsteroidal medications as prescribed
- Surgical release of the medial nerve

SPECIAL CONCERNS

- Patients may require modifications of occupational activities to relieve symptoms.

NURSING DIAGNOSIS

- Pain, Chronic
- Knowledge, Deficient

Cataracts

DEFINITION

- Cataracts result from the formation of protein clumps in the lens of the eye and are characterized by a yellowish haze and visual disturbances. Cataracts form as part of the normal aging process, after traumatic eye injury, and may be a congenital defect in children. The risk for cataract formation increases in patients with certain diseases, such as diabetes.

KEY ASSESSMENTS

- Decreased visual acuity
- Cloudy, yellowish, or brownish lens
- Blurry vision
- Reduced night vision
- Color distortion

Diagnostics

- A dilated eye exam

PLANNING AND IMPLEMENTATION

Preoperative

- Explain surgical procedure
- Teach the patient how to instill eye drops
- Anticipate administering eye drops and oral medications to reduce intraocular pressure

Postoperative

- Patch the surgical eye
- Prevent and treat nausea
- Instill eye drops as ordered

SPECIAL CONCERNS

Teaching Considerations

- Avoid activities that increase intraocular pressure, including bending over, vomiting, coughing, sneezing, and lifting heavy objects.
- Contact the health care provider if vision worsens or if there is sharp pain in the eye.

NURSING DIAGNOSIS

- Knowledge, Deficient
- Sensory perception, Disturbed

Cholecystitis

DEFINITION

- Cholelithiasis, or gallstones, forms in the gallbladder from cholesterol. Gallstones cause inflammation in the gallbladder and may cause cholangitis (inflammation of the bile duct) and cholestasis (impeding the flow of bile).

KEY ASSESSMENTS

- Clay-colored stools
- Dark urine
- Jaundice
- Midepigastric pain radiating to the right scapular region

- Anorexia
- Nausea and vomiting

Diagnostics

- Gallbladder ultrasound

PLANNING AND IMPLEMENTATION

- Treat pain
- Treat nausea
- Monitor intake and output (I & O)
- Monitor vital signs
- Monitor for signs of infection (fever or tachycardia)
- Anticipate laparoscopic cholecystectomy (removal of the gallbladder)

SPECIAL CONCERNS

Cultural Considerations

- Cholelithiasis is more common in people of Northern European descent.

Gender Considerations

- Cholelithiasis is more common in women than in men.

NURSING DIAGNOSIS

- Pain, Acute
- Infection, Risk for

Chronic Obstructive Pulmonary Disease (COPD)

DEFINITION

- COPD is a disease state characterized by progressive airflow limitation and an abnormal inflammatory response of the lungs that is not fully reversible. Smoking is the major cause of COPD.

Clinical Causes

- Chronic bronchiolitis is a disease of the lungs caused by an inflammatory process, which causes structural changes in the small airways.
- Chronic bronchitis is an inflammatory process accompanied by hypersecretion of mucus and a chronic cough.
- Asthma is a chronic inflammatory disorder with a hyperresponsiveness to stimuli and variable airflow obstruction.
- Alpha-1-antitrypsin deficiency is the genetic deficiency of a lung-protective protein that causes emphysema and COPD.
- Emphysema is a condition characterized by abnormal, permanent enlargement of the alveoli with destruction of the alveolar walls, and it may be considered panlobular emphysema when the destruction is on the entire lung (known as "blue bloaters") or centrilobular emphysema when the destruction is more in the distal alveoli (known as "pink puffers").

KEY ASSESSMENTS

- Dyspnea on exertion
- Accessory muscle usage for breathing
- Signs of right sided heart failure (Cor pulmonale)
- Increased A-P diameter (barrel chest)
- Clubbing of fingers
- Anxiety
- Fatigue
- Change in level of consciousness (LOC)
- Chronic cough with sputum production
- Chest hyperresonant to percussion
- Prolonged expiratory phase

History and Examination

- Frequent upper respiratory infections
- Cigarette smoking
- Exposure to environmental chemicals or irritants
- Weight loss

Diagnostics

- Pulmonary function tests
- Chest X-ray (CXR)
- Arterial blood gases ([ABGs], hypoxia and hypercapnia)
- Sputum cultures

PLANNING AND IMPLEMENTATION

- Encourage smoking cessation.
- Initiate low flow oxygen therapy; 2 L per nasal cannula. (Hypoxia is the stimulus for respiration in patients with COPD and too much O_2 will result in apnea.)
- Continuous pulse oximetry.
- Monitor LOC.
- Vaccinate against influenza and pneumococcus.
- Encourage adequate fluid and nutritional intake.
- Demonstrate and encourage purse lipped breathing.
- Provide frequent rest periods.
- Space activities.
- Promote self-care.
- Initiate safety measures.
- Prevent infections.
- Encourage pulmonary rehabilitation.
- Anticipate administering bronchodilators, corticosteroids, expectorants, mucolytics, and antibiotics if pulmonary infection is present.
- Lung transplantation is a treatment option in which one or both lungs may be transplanted. Infection and rejection are lifelong concerns after transplantation.
- Lung reduction surgery is a treatment in which 20–30 percent of the lung volume is excised, allowing the diaphragm to work more normally and assist in ventilation.

Discharge Planning

- If discharged on oxygen therapy, the patient must know how to use oxygen safely in and out of the home.
- Teach patients to never increase the flow of oxygen therapy beyond the prescribed rate.

SPECIAL CONCERNS

Genetic Considerations

- Alpha-1-antitrypsin deficiency affects approximately 1 in every 3,000 Caucasian Americans. Symptoms usually appear by the third decade of life. A blood test can determine if a person is a genetic carrier.

NURSING DIAGNOSIS

- Activity intolerance
- Breathing pattern, Ineffective

- Injury, Risk for
- Tissue perfusion, Ineffective

Cirrhosis

DEFINITION

- Cirrhosis is a progressive condition characterized by fibrotic tissue and remodeling of the liver.

Classifications

- Alcoholic cirrhosis (Laënnec's cirrhosis) is destruction of the liver from alcohol ingestion. The liver progresses from a fatty liver to cirrhosis. Fifty percent of alcoholics develop cirrhosis, and women are at a higher risk.
- Postnecrotic cirrhosis occurs as a result of hepatitis infection or drug induced liver damage.
- Biliary cirrhosis is caused by bile duct blockage that can be inherent or caused by surgery or trauma.
- Cardiac cirrhosis is caused by right-sided heart failure that increases portal pressure, increasing pressure in the liver.

KEY ASSESSMENTS

- Ascites (accumulation of fluid in the peritoneal cavity)
- Spontaneous bacterial peritonitis (increased fever, abdominal pain)
- Esophageal varices (distended veins in the esophagus caused by portal hypertension)
- Weight loss
- Nausea and vomiting
- Asterixis (hand flapping)
- Pruritus
- Petechiae
- Jaundice
- Dark urine
- Clay colored stools
- Peripheral edema
- Fetor hepaticus (fruity smelling breath)
- Palmar erythema (red palms)
- Shortness of breath (SOB)
- Portal systemic encephalopathy (PSE), (change in level of consciousness (LOC) ranging from mild confusion to coma)

Diagnostics

- Liver Biopsy

Lab Tests

- Aspartate transaminase (AST) and alanine aminotransferase (ALT)
- Ammonia levels
- Glucose
- Liver profile
- Prothrombin time (PT), partial thromboplastin time (PTT), and international normalized ratio (INR)
- Platelet count
- Complete blood count (CBC)
- Protein
- Blood urea nitrogen (BUN) and creatinine (Cr)
- Electrolytes

PLANNING AND IMPLEMENTATION

- Restrict fluids to 1,000–1,500 mL per day.
- Encourage no salt diet.
- Promote diuretic therapy.
- Promote antibiotic therapy.
- Encourage avoidance of alcohol.
- Carefully administer medications metabolized in the liver
- Implement safety measures.
- Measure abdominal girths.
- Monitor intake and output (I & O).
- Monitor vital signs frequently.
- Elevate head of bed.
- Monitor for cardiac arrhythmias.
- Monitor for bleeding.
- Monitor glucose levels.
- Treat coagulopathies.
- Monitor liver function tests, coagulation studies, and electrolytes.
- Encourage high protein diet until PSE occurs, then restrict protein.
- Administer lactulose and oral neomycin (to decrease ammonia levels).
- Paracentesis (removal of fluid from the peritoneum) may be indicated.
- LaVeen shunting (diverts fluid from the peritoneum into the superior vena cava) may be indicated.
- Transjugular intrahepatic portosystemic shunt (TIPS) may be indicated. The procedure, performed in the radiology

department, threads a catheter into the portal vein stenting to the hepatic vein to decrease portal hypertension.
- If a patient has known esophageal varices, do not insert nasogastric tubes and avoid any activity that would increase pressure in the esophagus (vomiting, straining for bowel movements).
- Endoscopic sclerotherapy (injecting sclerosing drugs into the esophageal varices) may be indicated.
- If esophageal varices rupture, it is a medical emergency. The health care provider will insert a gastric-esophageal balloon. Clearly label all lumina of the tube. If the patient develops respiratory difficulty, decompress the esophageal balloon.
- Liver transplantation may be indicated.

NURSING DIAGNOSIS

- Infection, Risk for
- Breathing pattern, Ineffective
- Injury, Risk for
- Confusion, Acute
- Nutrition: less than body requirements, Imbalanced
- Tissue perfusion, Ineffective
- Fluid volume, Risk for imbalanced

Compartment Syndrome

DEFINITION

- Compartment syndrome is the compression of nerves and blood vessels within enclosed tissue. The resulting pressure causes acute neurovascular compromise, and the affected structure will experience cellular death if it is not treated.

Clinical Causes

- Fracture
- Crush injuries
- Burns
- Casts

KEY ASSESSMENTS

- Pallor
- Decreased or absent pulse

- Paresthesia
- Pain
- Paralysis

PLANNING AND IMPLEMENTATION

- Notify the health care provider immediately
- Anticipate measures to relieve pressure (cut cast)
- With burns and crush injuries, a fasciotomy (surgical incisions made to release compartment restoring neurovascular function)
- Wound care
- Treat pain
- Frequent vital signs
- Frequent neurovascular checks
- Maintain adequate fluid balance
- Implement safety measures
- Monitor compartment pressure (normal is 0–10 mm Hg)

NURSING DIAGNOSIS

- Tissue perfusion, Ineffective
- Pain, Acute
- Mobility, Impaired physical

Conjunctivitis

DEFINITION

- Conjunctivitis, also known as pink eye, is inflammation of the conjunctiva caused by chemicals, allergens, or viral and bacterial infections. Conjunctivitis from a bacterial infection is easily transmitted.

KEY ASSESSMENTS

- Unilateral or bilateral red conjunctiva
- Purulent drainage from eye
- Pain

Diagnostics

- Diagnosis is made by physical exam
- Culture of eye drainage

PLANNING AND IMPLEMENTATION

- Instill antibiotic eye drops as ordered
- Use good hand-washing techniques
- Avoid touching the eye
- Refrain from using makeup
- Clean washcloths and towels after use

NURSING DIAGNOSIS

- Knowledge, Deficient

Coronary Artery Disease (CAD)

DEFINITION

- CAD is a blood vessel disease of the epicardial arteries responsible for supplying the myocardium with blood.
- The major contributor to CAD is atherosclerosis or hardening of the arteries. The cellular process of atheroma formation includes several progressive steps, beginning as fatty streaks of the arterial wall in adolescence that can progress to hard fatty plaques in adulthood.
- Nonmodifiable CAD risk factors include increased age, sex (male), and family history.
- Modifiable risk factors include hyperlipidemia, hypertension, cigarette smoking, obesity, and a sedentary lifestyle.
- These atherosclerotic plaques can rupture, leading to occlusions.
- Ischemia may occur when reduced blood supply through narrowed arteries does not meet myocardial oxygen demand.

Acute Coronary Syndromes (ACS)

- ACS is a life-threatening condition that can occur at any time in patients with CAD. ACS encompasses a continuum that ranges from unstable angina to an acute myocardial infarction.

Angina

- Angina is typically defined as chest pain that occurs when myocardial oxygen demand is unmet. Types of angina include:
  - Unstable angina—increased frequency, duration, or severity not relieved by rest or nitroglycerin
  - Stable angina—short, predictable episodes relieved by rest or nitroglycerin

- Prinzmetal's variant angina—usually occurs at rest; CAD may be undetectable
- Silent angina—no pain is present; common with diabetics
- Syndrome X—angina symptoms without radiographic evidence of CAD

Key assessments for angina

- P—precipitating event
- Q—quality
- R—radiation
- S—severity
- T—timing
- Angina typically is located substernal radiating to the epigastrium, neck, jaw, shoulders, arm, or back. Indigestion-like pain and pain between the shoulder blades may be cardiac in origin and should not be dismissed.

History and Examination

- Medical, surgical, family, or social history
- Review of systems
- Habits
- Current medications: prescribed, over-the-counter, and supplements
- Allergies
- Physical examination
- Vital signs

Diagnostics

- 12 lead electrocardiogram (ECG)
- Presence of ST segment depression (ischemia)
- Chest X-ray (CXR)
- Stress ECG
- Pharmacological stress tests
- Nuclear scans
- Coronary angiography

Lab Tests

- C-reactive protein (CRP)
- Homocysteine
- Cholesterol triglycerides
- Low-density lipoprotein (LDL)—"bad cholesterol"
- High-density lipoprotein (HDL)—"good cholesterol"

PLANNING AND IMPLEMENTATION

- Assist the patient in identifying and reducing modifiable risk factors.
- Explain purpose of and any preparation for laboratory and diagnostic tests.
- Teach the patient about nitroglycerin safety and use (see Table 6).
- Anticipate administering medications to treat CAD.
- Common medications include nitrates, beta blockers, calcium channel blockers, antiplatelet agents, angiotensin-converting enzyme (ACE) inhibitors, and lipid altering agents.
- Use stable angina mnemonic.
  - Aspirin and antianginal therapy
  - Beta blocker and blood pressure
  - Cigarette smoking and cholesterol
  - Diet and diabetes
  - Education and exercise

TABLE 6

Patient Education: Acute Angina and Sublingual Nitroglycerin

Acute Angina: Use of Nitroglycerin

- Stop activity; sit or lie down.
- Place one nitroglycerin tablet under the tongue and allow to dissolve. (Do not chew.)
- Tablet will cause a tingling sensation.
- Can cause feelings of heart pounding, flushing, and headache.
- Stay in resting position for 15–20 minutes and get up slowly after taking nitroglycerin to prevent fainting from postural hypotension.
- Relieves angina in approximately three seconds and lasts 20–45 minutes.
- If angina is not relieved in five minutes, the dose may be repeated two times at five-minute intervals for a total of three doses
- If angina is not relieved after three doses, seek immediate medical attention.
- For preventative use, take 5–10 minutes before activity that typically causes angina.
- Report angina that increases in frequency, last longer, limits previous level of activity, and occurs at rest.

Storage of Nitroglycerin

- Carry tablets at all times.
- Keep tablets tightly sealed in original dark bottle with metal cap.
- Protect from light and moisture.
- Store in a cool dry place.
- Be aware of expiration date.
- Replace six months after opening bottle.
- Plan ahead for refills.

SPECIAL CONCERNS

- See Special Procedures and Treatments for information on Coronary Angiogram, Coronary Angioplasty, and Coronary Artery Bypass Grafting (CABG).
- Use of phosphodiesterase inhibitors, such as Viagra and Cialis, may cause severe hypotension and cardiovascular collapse if taken within 24 hours of nitrate administration.
- See Special Procedures and Treatments for information on Coronary Angiography.

NURSING DIAGNOSIS

- Knowledge, Deficient
- Cardiac output, Decreased
- Pain, Acute
- Tissue perfusion, Ineffective

Crohn's Disease

DEFINITION

- Crohn's disease is a chronic inflammatory bowel disease (IBD) causing inflammation of the bowel. (The ileum is most commonly affected.) The etiology is unknown but is postulated to be autoimmune in nature. Initially, there is surface ulceration in patches of the bowel. Disease progression creates deep fissures through bowel layers, and inflammation narrows the bowel lumen.

KEY ASSESSMENTS

- Diarrhea
- Blood in the stool
- Abdominal pain
- Weight loss

Diagnostics

- Proctosigmoidoscopy (cobblestone appearance from fissures)
- Barium study—"string sign" revealing constriction of a small intestine segment

Lab Tests

- Complete blood count (CBC)

- IBD serology panel (antineutrophilic cytoplasmic antibodies [ANCA], immunoglobulin G [IgG], antisaccharomyces cerevisiae mannan antibodies [ASCA], immunoglobulin A [IgA], and alpha outer membrane protein C immunoglobin antibodies [OmpC IgA])

PLANNING AND IMPLEMENTATION

- Treatment depends on the severity of symptoms.
- Encourage smoking cessation.
- Monitor vital signs.
- Monitor intake and output (I & O).
- Monitor caloric intake.
- Encourage fluid and nutritional intake.
- Administer vitamins and nutritional supplements.
- Take daily weight.
- Administer antidiarrheal and antiperistaltic medications.
- Exacerbations may require administration of corticosteroids and immunosuppressant therapy (Imuran or methotrexate).
- Administer antibiotics if infection present.
- Monitor infections.
- Encourage stress reduction.
- Monitor for development of anal sphincter fissures (bleeding and pain with defecation).
- Monitor for the development of perirectal fistulas (abnormal tunneling surrounding the rectum).
- Monitor for the development of rectal abscesses (infections creating collections of pus in the rectal area).
- If therapies are unsuccessful in limiting symptoms, surgical resection of the diseased portion of the bowel may be necessary and may result in a permanent ostomy.

SPECIAL CONCERNS

- Refer to Cancer, Colorectal for a discussion concerning ostomies.

Gender Considerations

- Crohn's disease more commonly affects men.

NURSING DIAGNOSIS

- Pain, Chronic
- Diarrhea
- Nutrition: less than body requirements, Imbalanced
- Skin, Impaired integrity

- Infection, Risk for
- Fluid volume, Risk for deficient

Cushing's Disease

DEFINITION

- Cushing's disease is a state of hypercortisolism.

Clinical Causes

- Adrenocorticotropic hormone (ACTH) secreting adenomas
- Pituitary adenomas
- ACTH secreting neoplasm
- Iatrogenic effects of chronic glucocorticoid therapy

KEY ASSESSMENTS

- Hirsutism
- Thin skin than bruises easily
- Hypertension
- Arrhythmias (hypokalemia)
- Thin extremities
- Trunk obesity
- "Buffalo hump" (subclavicular fat pads)
- Amenorrhea, impotence

Diagnostics

- Dexamethasone ACTH suppression test
- Urine free cortisol test (high)
- ACTH and corticotropic releasing hormone (CRH) stimulation test
- Computed tomography (CT) or magnetic resonance imaging (MRI)

Lab Tests

- Serum ACTH high (Low ACTH may indicate an adrenal tumor.)
- Plasma cortisol level (high)
- Electrolytes

PLANNING AND IMPLEMENTATION

- Monitor vital signs

- Monitor for signs of infection
- Monitor electrolytes and treat imbalances
- Monitor intake and output (I & O)
- Monitor for signs of fluid overload
- Monitor glucose levels
- Implement safety measures
- Assist with activities of daily living
- Anticipate surgical removal of tumor, if present
- If caused by corticosteroids, monitor for effects and treat

NURSING DIAGNOSIS

- Fluid volume, Excess
- Infection, Risk for
- Knowledge, Deficient

Deep Vein Thrombosis (DVT)

DEFINITION

- DVT is the formation of a thrombus or clot in the venous system. If the thrombus dislodges, it may cause a pulmonary emboli (see Pulmonary Embolism). Risk factors for developing DVT are based on Virchow's triad: trauma to the vessel, venous stasis, and hypercoagulability.

Clinical Causes

- Immobility
- Bone fractures
- Pregnancy
- Hormone therapy
- Cancer
- Congestive heart failure
- Soft tissue damage
- Venous injury
- Obesity
- Surgery

KEY ASSESSMENTS

- May be asymptomatic
- Pain and tenderness below thrombus site

- Unilateral swelling
- Redness and warmth over site

Diagnostics

- Venous ultrasound

PLANNING AND IMPLEMENTATION

Prevention of DVTs

- Early ambulation
- Compression stocking
- Pneumatic compression devices to legs
- Aspirin, low molecular weight heparin, unfractioned heparin, or Coumadin
- Monitor anticoagulation status

Once DVT Is Diagnosed

- Do not massage or manipulate affected limb.
- Monitor for signs of a pulmonary emboli (hypoxemia or anxiety).
- Administer low molecular weight heparin, Coumadin, or unfractioned heparin as requested.
- Monitor partial thromboplastin time (PTT) levels (heparin).
- Monitor international normalized ration (INR) levels (Coumadin).
- Institute bleeding precautions.
- Institute safety measures.
- Have anticoagulant reverse agents (vitamin K for Coumadin and protamine sulfate for heparin) available.
- If patient cannot tolerate anticoagulation therapy, a vena cava filter may be inserted.

NURSING DIAGNOSIS

- Tissue perfusion, Ineffective
- Injury, Risk for
- Mobility, Impaired physical

Diabetes Insipidus

DEFINITION

- Diabetes insipidus results from insufficient antidiuretic hormone (ADH) occurring from posterior pituitary disturbances (central diabetes insipidus) or a lack of sensitivity to circulating ADH from the nephrons in the kidney (nephrogenic diabetes insipidus).

Clinical Causes

- Pituitary tumor
- Hypopituitarism
- Infections, thrombus or immunological disorders of the pituitary gland
- Medications
- Kidney disorder

KEY ASSESSMENTS

- Polydipsia
- Polyuria
- Level of consciousness (LOC)
- Hypovolemia (tachycardia, hypotension, dry mucous membranes, or weight loss)
- Visual disturbances

Diagnostics

- Specific gravity

Lab Tests

- Electrolytes

PLANNING AND IMPLEMENTATION

- Monitor LOC
- Monitor vital signs
- Implement safety precautions
- Treat hypovolemia with intravenous (IV) fluids
- Monitor intake and output (I & O)
- Daily weight
- Monitor vision
- Monitor electrolytes (hypokalemia, hypernatremia)
- Treat electrolyte imbalances
- Cardiac monitoring (if hypokalemic)
- Administer vasopressin as requested
- If tumor present, anticipate surgical removal

NURSING DIAGNOSIS

- Fluid volume, Deficient

- Knowledge, Deficient
- Injury, Risk for

Diabetes Mellitus

DEFINITION

- Diabetes mellitus (DM) refers to a group of chronic disorders of metabolism characterized by hyperglycemia, an elevated blood glucose level, and disturbances in metabolism of carbohydrates, fats, and proteins. Diabetes affects 16 million patients, and obesity is the number one modifiable risk factor.

Classifications

Type 1 diabetes: Juvenile onset diabetes

- Results from a defect or failure of the beta cells of the pancreas islet cells. The destruction is caused by genetic or environmental factors or autoimmunity. The loss of beta cells causes an absolute lack of insulin. Type 1 diabetes is more common in children but can develop at any time. It affects 1.4 million patients.

Type 2 diabetes: Adult onset diabetes

- Results from defective beta cell secretion, insulin resistance in the peripheral tissues, and an increase in production of glucose from the liver. Type 2 diabetes has a familiar tendency and is more common in older and obese patients. There has been a dramatic increase in type 2 diabetes in children, and it is linked with childhood obesity, diet, and inactivity. It affects 14.5 million patients.

Prediabetes

- Characterized by fasting blood glucose between 110 and 125 mg/dL. Lifestyle modifications are recommended to prevent or slow the development of type 2 diabetes.

Gestational diabetes

- Results from hyperglycemia during pregnancy. Glucose levels usually return to normal after delivery, but patients are at higher risk for developing type 2 diabetes.

Syndrome X: Insulin resistance syndrome

- A group of metabolic abnormalities that increases the risk for diabetes, cardiovascular disease, and stroke. It is characterized by increased waist/hip ratio, hypertension, increased triglycerides and glucose levels, and decreased high-density lipoprotein (HDL). Weight loss, exercise, and dietary changes can help prevent or delay the onset of type 2 diabetes in patients with syndrome X. It affects one in five adults.

KEY ASSESSMENTS

- Polydipsia (increased thirst)
- Polyuria (increased urine output)
- Polyphagia (increased hunger)
- Pain with urination (urinary tract infection)
- Weight loss
- Poor wound healing
- Numbness or tingling of the extremities (neuropathy)
- Kussmaul respirations (rapid, deep respirations)
- Signs of hypovolemia (weak pulse, hypotension, tachycardia, or dry mucous membranes)
- Fruity breath
- Irritability or confusion
- Slurred speech
- Fatigue

History and Examination

- Waist/hip ratio greater than 0.9 in men and 0.8 in women
- Obesity
- Family history of diabetes

Diagnostics

- Fasting glucose level greater than 126 mg/dL
- Random glucose level greater than 200 mg/dL with clinical signs of diabetes
- Two-hour oral glucose tolerance test greater than 200 mg/dL with a 75-g glucose load

Factors that increase blood glucose

- Stress (surgery, trauma, general anesthesia, or infection)
- Medications (tricyclic antidepressants or corticosteroids)
- Diet (excess refined sugar or excessive carbohydrate consumption)

Lab Tests

- Fasting blood glucose
- White blood count (WBC)
- Glycosylated hemoglobin (HgA1C)
- Cholesterol, triglycerides

- Low-density lipoprotein (LDL) and HDL
- C-reactive protein (CRP)
- Electrolytes

PLANNING AND IMPLEMENTATION

- Correct dehydration with administration of 0.9% normal saline (NS)
- Daily weight
- Monitor intake and output (I & O)
- Monitor glucose levels
- Monitor for and treat electrolyte imbalances
- Monitor for signs of infection (fever or elevated white blood count)
- Treat infection with appropriate antibiotic administration
- Provide American Diabetes Association (ADA) diet
- Encourage adequate exercise
- Monitor skin for breakdown and infection
- Wound care as ordered
- Monitor for neuropathy
- Institute safety measures
- Always perform Glucometer glucose testing prior to insulin or oral hypoglycemic administration to avoid hypoglycemia
- Hold insulin or oral hypoglycemic medications if patient is not to take anything by mouth (NPO) and prior to surgery
- Administer insulin as ordered (see Table 7)
- Administer oral hypoglycemic medications as ordered
- Monitor for signs of hypoglycemia (especially when antidiabetic medication is peaking), including tremors, tachycardia, diaphoresis, ataxia, seizures, confusion, lethargy, and coma
- Monitor for signs of hyperglycemia, including polydipsia, polyphagia, polyuria, fatigue, blurred vision, and confusion
- Monitor for Somogyi effect (hyperglycemia and headaches on waking from too much insulin promoting gluconeogenesis, hence hyperglycemia)
- Anticipate decreasing insulin doses if Somogyi effect occurs
- Monitor for dawn phenomenon (hyperglycemia from predawn release of cortisol and growth factors, common in adolescence)
- Anticipate increasing insulin dose for dawn phenomenon
- Promptly treat hypoglycemia in conscious patients with juice or a fast-acting carbohydrate
- Promptly treat hypoglycemia in the unconscious patient with IV dextrose administration

TABLE 7

Types of Insulin

Type	Onset	Peak	Duration
Humalog (Lispro)	Less than 15 minutes	30–90 minutes	4 hours
Regular	30–60 minutes	2–4 hours	5–7 hours
NPH	3–4 hours	6–12 hours	18–28 hours
Lente	1–3 hours	8–12 hours	18–28 hours
Ultra Lente	4–6 hours	18–24 hours	36 hours
70/30	15–30 minutes	2–3 hours and 8–12 hours	18–24 hours
Insulin glargine	1.1 hour	5 hours	24 hours

- Monitor for diabetic ketoacidosis and hyperosmolar hyperglycemic nonketonic syndrome (see Diabetic Ketoacidosis and Hyperosmolar Hyperglycemic Nonketonic Syndrome)
- Monitor for long-term complications of diabetes, including visual changes and development of cardiac disease

SPECIAL CONCERNS

Cultural Considerations

- African American, Hispanic (Americans), Native American, Asian (Americans), and Pacific Islanders are at higher risk for developing DM.

Geriatric Considerations

- Twenty percent of patients 65 and older have DM.

Teaching Considerations

Diet

- Carbohydrate caloric intake: 45–65 percent
- Protein caloric intake: 15–20 percent
- Encourage intake of fresh fruits, vegetables, and lean meats and fish
- Limit saturated fats and cholesterol intake
- Encourage using olive and canola oil
- Increase dietary fiber

- Moderate alcohol (only if glucose control is adequate)
- Encourage reading food labels
- Use the Food Pyramid Guide
- Adjust caloric intake to promote weight loss, if obese

Exercise

- Discuss exercise with the health care provider before starting
- Goal is 30 minutes a day of exercise
- Heart rate within target range (220 minus patient age, multiply by 60 for lower target limit and 80 percent for upper target limit)
- Stop exercising for shortness of breath, chest pain, dizziness, or palpitations
- If hypoglycemia occurs during exercise, stop and ingest one-half cup fruit juice or 8 oz. low fat milk

Glucose monitoring

- Perform throughout the day
- Log results
- Perform control testing to ensure the accuracy of reading
- Regulate diet and antidiabetic medications based on glucose monitoring as ordered by the health care provider

Insulin administration

- Keep a sharps container (needle-proof biohazard container) to avoid accidental needle sticks
- Identify and rotate administration sites
- Use pen insulin cartridges for visually impaired patients
- Store open at room temperature for up to four weeks
- Refrigerate insulin vials not in use

Insulin pumps

- Change insertion site every 48–72 hours
- Change batteries as instructed
- Count carbohydrates
- Program pump based on carbohydrates eaten at each meal

Foot care

- Inspect feet with a mirror daily to observer for injury or breakdown
- Trim toenails straight across
- Ensure shoes fit properly
- Wash and dry feet daily
- Encourage regular inspection of feet by a health care provider

Eye care

- Encourage annual eye exam
- If vision decreases, provide visual aids

Signs of hypoglycemia

- Tremors
- Tachycardia
- Diaphoresis
- Ataxia (gait disturbances)
- Seizures
- Confusion, lethargy, or coma
- Wear identification stating they are diabetic

Signs of hyperglycemia

- Polydipsia
- Polyphagia
- Polyuria
- Fatigue
- Blurred vision
- Confusion

Signs of infection

- Fever, hyperglycemia
- Skin infection or wounds with purulent draining
- Urinary tract infection or pain with urination

NURSING DIAGNOSIS

- Infection, Risk for
- Knowledge, Deficient
- Skin integrity, Risk for impaired
- Sensory perception, Disturbed
- Injury, Risk for
- Fluid volume, Risk for deficient
- Home maintenance, Impaired

Diabetic Ketoacidosis

DEFINITION

- Diabetic ketoacidosis (DKA) results in a quick, marked insulin deficiency and is typically associated with type 1 diabetes but may occur in type 2 diabetes. It is a life-threatening medical emergency associated with a mortality of 5 percent. Illness, infection, inadequate diabetes management, and undiagnosed type 1 diabetes contribute to DKA.

- In DKA, there is insufficient insulin to metabolize glucose, and the body breaks down protein for energy. Ketones are a by-product of protein breakdown and are acidic in nature. As the ketone levels increase in the blood, the pH is altered and metabolic acidosis develops.

KEY ASSESSMENTS

- Dehydration (hypotension, tachycardia)
- Nausea and vomiting
- Decrease in level of consciousness (LOC)
- Polydipsia
- Polyphagia
- Polyuria (leading to oliguria if dehydration is profound)
- Fruity breath
- Kussmaul's respirations (blow off CO_2 in acidotic state)
- Fever (infection may be precipitating cause)

Lab Tests

- Glucose
- Electrolytes (especially potassium)
- Urine for ketones
- Arterial blood gas ([ABGs], acidosis)
- Complete blood count (CBC)

PLANNING AND IMPLEMENTATION

- Insert two large-bore intravenous (IV) lines
- Prompt administration of 0.9% normal saline (NS)
- Frequent (every hour until stable) glucose monitoring
- Monitor LOC
- Implement safety precautions
- Frequent vital signs
- Monitor intake and output (I & O)
- Monitor electrolytes
- Monitor for signs of infection
- Leave patient flat if hypotension is profound
- Insert Foley catheter to closely monitor urine output
- Cardiac monitoring (hypokalemia causes ventricular arrhythmias)
- Anticipate administering short-acting insulin intravenously

- Anticipate administering potassium supplements (Insulin will decrease serum potassium levels.)
- Reinforce diabetic teaching

NURSING DIAGNOSIS

- Fluid volume, Deficient
- Infection, Risk for
- Knowledge, Deficient

Disseminated Intravascular Coagulation (DIC)

DEFINITION

- DIC is not a disease but a clinical syndrome related to an underlying condition. DIC is a disruption of the hematological system characterized by widespread intravascular bleeding and clotting. It can range from mild to life threatening.
- DIC is caused by abnormal clotting process in which a massive amounts of microclots form. The body responds by activating the fibrinolytic process, which attempts to break down the clots and contributes to bleeding. The cycle of clot formation impairs organ function and clumps clotting factors. Thus, when bleeding occurs, there are no clotting factors available for the site of bleeding.

Clinical Causes

- Aortic aneurysm
- Hemolytic uremic syndrome
- Burns
- Obstetric complications
- Bacterial and viral infections
- Sepsis
- Anything that causes prolonged bleeding or large blood volume loss

KEY ASSESSMENTS

- Decreased level of consciousness ([LOC], cerebral hemorrhage or anoxia)
- Oxygenation status
- Shock (tachycardia or decreased blood pressure)

- Cyanosis of extremities
- Hematuria
- Hematemesis
- Bloody stools
- Frank bleeding from incision, venipuncture, or any tube insertion site

Lab Tests

- Complete blood count (CBC)
- Platelet count
- Schistocytes (fragmented red blood cells [RBCs])
- Coagulation studies (prothrombin time [PT], partial thromboplastin time [PTT], international normalized ratio [INR], thrombin time, and fibrin degradation products)
- DIC panel

PLANNING AND IMPLEMENTATION

- Consents for blood and blood product administration
- Active type and cross-match for blood products
- Two patent large-bore intravenous (IV) lines
- Monitor and treat signs of shock
- Anticipate blood and blood product administration
- Administer oxygen
- Frequent vital signs including pulse oximetry
- Observe for organ dysfunction
- Observe neurological status
- Heparin—may be given to help prevent new clots from forming

SPECIAL CONCERNS

- While caring for a patient with DIC, it is essential for the nurse to use the proper personal protective equipment to avoid contact with blood.

NURSING DIAGNOSIS

- Fluid volume, Risk for deficient
- Tissue perfusion, Ineffective

Diverticulitis

DEFINITION

- Diverticulitis is the inflammation of diverticula, saclike out pouches of the mucosa of the bowel. Diverticulitis is closely associated with a diet low in fiber and high in refined foods, decreased activity levels, and constipation.

D

KEY ASSESSMENTS

- Constipation or diarrhea
- Lower abdominal pain and cramping
- Fatigue
- Low grade fever
- Bloody stools

Diagnostics

- Computed tomography (CT)
- Barium enema
- Abdominal X-rays

Lab Tests

- Complete blood count (CBC), increased white blood count

PLANNING AND IMPLEMENTATION

- Administer antibiotics.
- Monitor vital signs for signs hemorrhage or peritonitis.
- Monitor and treat pain.
- Administer nothing by mouth (NPO) or clear liquids during acute pain phase.
- Administer stool softeners and bulk-forming medications.
- Administer antispasmodics.
- Encourage high-fiber diet once inflammation is resolved.
- Encourage activity.
- Monitor for signs of peritonitis (infection of the peritoneal cavity), severe pain drawing knees to the chest, tachycardia, diaphoresis, or high fever.
- Monitor for signs of lower gastrointestinal (GI) bleed (melena).
- If the patient experiences hemorrhage: insert two large-bore intravenous (IV) lines, administer 5% albumin or 0.9% normal saline (NS) to maintain blood pressure, notify health care

provider, insert a nasogastric tube and apply low-intermittent suction, administer oxygen therapy, type and cross-match for blood transfusion, and anticipate administering H_2 antagonist intravenously and packed red blood cells.

- Surgical intervention may be required if peritonitis or hemorrhage occurs.

SPECIAL CONCERNS

Geriatric Considerations

- Diverticulitis affects 50 percent of patients over 80.

NURSING DIAGNOSIS

- Constipation
- Diarrhea
- Pain, Acute
- Knowledge, Deficient

Dysfunctional Uterine Bleeding

DEFINIION

- Dysfunctional uterine bleeding is abnormal uterine bleeding in the absence of pathology.

KEY ASSESSMENTS

- Menorrhagia (prolonged but regular menses)
- Metrorrhagia (bleeding between menstrual cycles)

History and Examination

- Menstrual cycle length
- Complete history and diagnostic workup to rule out Von Willebrand's, leukemia, and endometrial cancer

Diagnostics

- Endometrial biopsy
- Pelvic ultrasound
- Saline infused sonogram
- Dilatation and curettage (D & C)

Lab Tests

- Complete blood count (CBC)
- Von Willebrand's
- Testosterone
- Pregnancy testing
- Pap smear

PLANNING AND IMPLEMENTATION

- Antiprostaglandin therapy, cyclooxygenase inhibitors, or oral contraceptives may be indicated.
- Endometrial ablation (destruction of the uterine lining with heat) or hysterectomy (surgical removal of the uterus) may be indicated.

NURSING DIAGNOSIS

- Knowledge, Deficient

Ebola Virus

DEFINITION

- Ebola virus is a filovirus causing viral hemorrhagic fevers with a high mortality rate. Ebola virus outbreaks have been limited to Africa, and if seen outside of Africa, biological warfare must be considered.
- Spread is person to person.
- Average incubation period is 2–21 days.

KEY ASSESSMENTS

- Fever
- Headache
- Myalgias
- Sore throat
- Weakness
- Abdominal pain
- Diarrhea
- Vomiting
- Bleeding
- Hypotension
- Hemorrhagic shock

History and Examination

- Recent travel to Africa

Lab Tests

- Enzyme-linked immunosorbent assay (ELISA)
- IgM ELISA
- Specimens—must be sent to a biolevel-4 lab for analysis; the Centers for Disease Control (CDC) will advise on packaging and transporting the specimen
- International normalized ratio (INR), prothrombin time (PT), and partial thromboplastin time (PTT)

PLANNING AND IMPLEMENTATION

- Isolate patient
- Standard, droplet, and airborne precautions
- Treatment is supportive
- Initiate intravenous (IV) access
- Maintain adequate fluid balance with IV fluids
- Monitor intake and output (I & O)
- Monitor vital signs
- Monitor oxygenation status
- Monitor for signs of overt and internal bleeding
- Monitor white blood count (WBC), PT, PTT, and INR
- Replace blood as requested
- Monitor and treat diarrhea
- Monitor and treat electrolyte imbalances
- If respiratory status deteriorates, anticipate intubation and ventilation

NURSING DIAGNOSIS

- Diarrhea
- Fluid volume, Deficient
- Breathing pattern, Ineffective

Endometriosis

DEFINITION

- Endometriosis is a condition in which segments of the endometrium implant outside of the uterus in the pelvis or abdomen. The cause and the mechanism of implantation are unknown. Between 5 and 15 percent of women are affected during their reproductive years. It is common among family members, and 30–40 percent of affected women will become infertile from the condition.

E

KEY ASSESSMENTS

- Excessive bleeding during menstruation
- Dysmenorrhea (pain during menses)
- Dyspareunia (painful intercourse)
- Abdominal cramping
- Diarrhea or constipation
- Inflammation

Diagnostics

- Diagnosis is difficult because there are no specific tests (other than surgery) to diagnose the condition.

PLANNING AND IMPLEMENTATION

- Laparoscopic surgery is indicated to remove the implants.

SPECIAL CONCERNS

- Infertility is a major concern in patients with endometriosis. Address fears honestly and openly.

NURSING DIAGNOSIS

- Pain, Acute
- Family processes, Interrupted
- Fear

Epididymitis

DEFINITION

- Epididymitis is inflammation of the epididymis and vas deferens, usually from a bacterial infection and commonly from contracting a sexually transmitted disease (chlamydia or gonorrhea).

KEY ASSESSMENTS

- Fever
- Erythema and edema of the groin, testicle, and scrotum
- Pain of the groin, testicle, and scrotum
- Dysuria
- Urethral discharge

History and Examination

- Recent unprotected sex

Diagnostics

- Doppler ultrasonography (rule out testicular torsion)

Lab Tests

- Complete blood count (CBC)
- Urine and urethral discharge cultures

PLANNING AND IMPLEMENTATION

- Identify causative organism and initiate appropriate pharmacological interventions
- Antipyretics for fever
- Treat pain
- Elevate scrotum
- Monitor intake and output (I & O)
- Monitor vital signs

NURSING DIAGNOSIS

- Pain, Acute
- Hyperthermia
- Infection
- Knowledge, Deficient

Fat Embolism

DEFINITION

- Fat embolism is the release of fat globules into the blood stream, which then travel to the lungs or brain causing ischemia. It may occur 24–72 hours after fractures or surgical manipulation of the long bones, pelvis, or ribs. The severity ranges from mild to death.

KEY ASSESSMENTS

- Hypoxemia
- Mental status changes
- Petechiae to the upper body
- Accessory muscle use
- Dyspnea
- Anxiety
- Fever
- Retinal hemorrhages

Diagnostics

- Chest X-ray (CXR)
- Computed tomography (CT) of brain

Lab Tests

- Arterial blood gases ([ABGs], metabolic acidosis)
- Complete blood count (CBC)

PLANNING AND IMPLEMENTATION

- High Fowler's position
- Supplemental oxygen to maintain O_2 saturation above 90 percent
- Anticipate intubation and mechanical ventilation
- Insert two large-bore peripheral intravenous (IV) lines
- Fluid resuscitation with 0.9% normal saline (NS) for hypotension
- Frequent vital signs
- Monitor neurological status and report any changes
- Implement safety measures

NURSING DIAGNOSIS

- Tissue perfusion, Ineffective
- Anxiety
- Fluid volume, Risk for deficient

Fatty Liver

DEFINITION

- Fatty liver (hepatic steatosis) occurs when lipids account for more than 5 percent of the weight of the liver.

Clinical Causes

- Obesity
- Pregnancy
- Poorly controlled diabetes
- Malnutrition
- Corticosteroid use
- Prolonged treatment with total parental nutrition
- Side effect of bariatric surgery
- Exposure to chemicals toxic to the liver
- Chronic alcohol ingestion

KEY ASSESSMENTS

- Hepatomegaly (enlarged liver)
- Right upper quadrant pain
- Fatigue
- Jaundice nausea and vomiting

Diagnostics

- Liver biopsy
- Computed tomography (CT) of abdomen

Lab Tests

- Lipid profile
- Alanine aminotransferase (ALT) and aspartate transaminase (AST)

PLANNING AND IMPLEMENTATION

- Low-fat diet
- Weight loss if obese
- Avoid alcohol
- Monitor for signs of worsening liver function (ascites, confusion)

NURSING DIAGNOSIS

- Fatigue
- Nutrition, Readiness for enhanced

Fibroadenomas

DEFINITION

- Fibroadenomas are benign, fibrous growths, or tumors, of the glandular epithelium in the breast tissue, occurring in women between the ages of 15 and 30.

KEY ASSESSMENTS

- Solid, rubbery, painless movable tumor

Diagnostics

- Mammogram
- Needle biopsy

PLANNING AND IMPLEMENTATION

- Anticipate surgical removal with a local anesthetic

NURSING DIAGNOSIS

- Knowledge, Deficient
- Anxiety

Fibrocystic Breast

DEFINITION

- Fibrocystic breast is a condition in which there are round, fluid-filled movable cysts in the breast tissue. The etiology is unknown but appears to be hormonally related, and there is no treatment.

KEY ASSESSMENTS

- Round, fluid-filled movable cysts bilaterally in the breasts
- Mastalgia (breast pain), worse premenstrual

Diagnostics

- Self-breast exam
- Mammogram
- Needle biopsy

PLANNING AND IMPLEMENTATION

- Encourage patients to perform self-breast exams regularly and obtain routine mammogram.
- Contact the health care provider for breast changes.

NURSING DIAGNOSIS

- Pain, Chronic
- Knowledge, Deficient

Fibromyalgia

DEFINITION

- Fibromyalgia is a clinical syndrome that involves diffuse musculoskeletal pain, stiffness, and tenderness that is accompanied by fatigue and insomnia. The etiology is unclear and appears to be multifactorial, and currently, the role of infectious agents is being investigated. Fibromyalgia differs from other musculoskeletal disorders because it lacks inflammatory and structural pathology.

KEY ASSESSMENTS

- Fatigue
- Insomnia
- Widespread musculoskeletal pain, stiffness, and tenderness

Diagnostics

- Diagnosis is based on history of widespread pain and pain in 11 of 18 tender point sites on palpation.

Lab Tests

- No test confirms fibromyalgia. Testing may be used to rule out other diagnoses.

PLANNING AND IMPLEMENTATION

- Administer analgesics, antidepressants, and muscle relaxants as ordered
- Promote exercise

- Encourage nutritious diet
- Limit alcohol and caffeine
- Employ stress-reducing techniques
- Establish regular sleep schedule

NURSING DIAGNOSIS

- Pain, Chronic
- Sleep pattern, Disturbed
- Coping, Ineffective

Flail Chest

DEFINITION

- Flail chest is rib cage instability resulting from multiple broken ribs. The instability causes hypoxia and inadequate ventilation. It is usually caused by severe trauma.

KEY ASSESSMENTS

- Paradoxical movement over affected area (chest wall goes in with inspiration and out with expiration)
- Dyspnea
- Hypotension
- Chest pain
- Tachycardia and tachypnea
- Decreased pulse oximetry

Diagnostics

- Chest X-ray (CXR) confirms diagnosis
- Arterial blood gases (ABGs)
- Complete blood count (CBC)

PLANNING AND IMPLEMENTATION

- High Fowler's position if the patient is not hypotensive
- Administer oxygen
- Anticipate intubation and mechanical ventilation
- Insert two large-bore intravenous (IV) lines
- Treat pain and anxiety
- Patient may have surgical stabilization of the fractures

NURSING DIAGNOSIS

- Breathing pattern, Ineffective
- Tissue perfusion, Ineffective

Fracture

DEFINITION

- A fracture is any disruption in the continuity of a bone.

Classifications

- Stress—a fracture that occurs as a result of repetitive use and is common in track and field sports.
- Pathological—a fracture that occurs to a bone weakened by an underlying disease process.
- Transverse—the fracture line is horizontal or straight across the bone.
- Oblique—the fracture line is at a 45-degree angle.
- Spiral—a fracture that partially encircles the bone.
- Comminuted—a fracture with crushed or splintered bone.
- Segmental—a fracture involving two or more pieces of bone segment.
- Compression—a fracture caused by the compression of one bone with another.
- Complete—the fracture completely breaks the bone in two pieces.
- Incomplete—the fracture extends through part of the bone.
- Open—the fracture penetrates the skin.
- Closed—the skin remains intact over the fracture site.

KEY ASSESSMENTS

- Pulse, color, temperature, distal to fracture
- Deformity
- Numbness
- Pain
- Hypotension, tachycardia (shock)
- Hemorrhage
- Airway

Diagnostics

- X-ray

Lab Tests

- Complete blood count (CBC)

PLANNING AND IMPLEMENTATION

- Cover open wounds.
- Splint fracture.
- Insert two large-bore peripheral intravenous (IV) lines.
- Check vital signs frequently.
- Treat pain.
- Elevate extremity.
- Monitor neurovascular status (pain, pallor, pulse, paresthesia, or paralysis).
- If neurovascular status is compromised, notify health care provider immediately.
- Administer wound care as indicated.
- Pin site care for external fixation.
- Monitor for fat emboli (shortness of breath, decreased pulse oximetry, or chest pain).
- Monitor for malunion (fracture healing in an abnormal position).
- Monitor for deep vein thrombosis (thrombus in venous system causing swelling and pain to affected limb).
- Monitor for delayed union (healing does not advance).
- Monitor for nonunion (healing ceases and the fracture union unlikely).
- Monitor for compartment syndrome (increased pressure causing vascular and nerve compression).
- Monitor site for infection.
- Depending on the type of fracture, treatment may consist of:
  - Open reduction—the surgical reduction of a fracture through an incision.
  - Closed reduction—realigning the bone using a cast or traction.
  - Internal fixation—using pins, rods, screws, or nails to support the bone directly.
  - External fixation—the use of pins or wires through the bone connecting to a rigid external frame.
- Traction principles—allow weight to hang freely, keep the line of pull continuous, keep ropes free of knots, and maintain the patient's body in good alignment.

Teaching Considerations

- Teach cast care.
- Keep plaster casts dry.

- Synthetic casts can be dried with a hairdryer on low setting.
- Elevate the limb above the level of the heart when possible.
- Do not put anything down the cast.
- Call the health care provider if cast becomes tight or for numbness or extreme pain.

NURSING DIAGNOSIS

- Pain, Acute
- Mobility, Impaired physical
- Tissue perfusion, Ineffective
- Infection, Risk for

Fracture, Hip

DEFINITION

- Hip fracture is a fracture within the femoral head, neck, intertrochanteric, subtrochanteric, or acetabular area. It is a common injury in the elderly, and osteoporosis and a subsequent fall are usually the cause. Women have four times more hip fractures than men do.

KEY ASSESSMENTS

Initial

- Affected leg shortened and externally rotated
- Hypotension, tachycardia, or tachypnea (hypovolemic shock)
- Neurovascular checks to extremity (pain, pallor, pulse, paralysis, or paresthesia)
- Pain level

Postoperative

- Neurovascular checks to extremity (pain, pallor, pulse, paralysis, or paresthesia)
- Pain level
- Vital signs
- Oxygenation status
- Wound drainage (color or amount)
- Level of consciousness (LOC)

Diagnostics

- X-ray
- Magnetic resonance imaging (MRI)

Lab Tests

- Complete blood count (CBC)
- Type and cross-match for packed red blood cells
- Blood urea nitrogen (BUN) and creatinine (Cr)
- Glucose
- Electrolytes

PLANNING AND IMPLEMENTATION

Initial

- Frequent vital signs
- Insert two large-bore peripheral intravenous (IV) lines
- Initiate fluid resuscitation with 0.9% normal saline (NS)
- Administer blood products as requested
- Blood and surgical consents
- Treat pain
- Maintain alignment of extremity
- Anticipate treatment consisting of hemiarthroplasty (replace femoral head with an implant) or internal fixation of hip fracture with rods, screws, or pins

Postoperative

- Frequent vital signs
- Monitor oxygenation status
- Wound care as ordered
- Observe for signs of infection (common sites are wound, urinary tract, and pulmonary)
- Monitor breath sounds and pulse oximetry
- Encourage deep breathing and coughing
- Treat pain
- Monitor bowel sounds
- Implement safety measures
- Prevent abduction
- Use adduction pillow while turning
- Administer prophylactic antibiotics
- Prevent patient from bending hips at a greater than 90-degree angle
- Encourage early, safe mobility with physical therapy
- Encourage quadriceps exercises

SPECIAL CONCERNS

- See Special Procedures and Treatments for information on Joint Replacement.

Geriatric Considerations

- One in three people over the age of 64 fall each year and are at highest risk for hip fracture.
- Elderly patients with comorbid factors are at higher risk for postoperative complications.

NURSING DIAGNOSIS

- Pain, Acute
- Fluid volume, Risk for deficient
- Infection, Risk for
- Falls, Risk for
- Mobility, Impaired physical

Fracture, Nasal

DEFINITION

- A nasal fracture is the most commonly broken bone in the body and should be suspected with any blunt trauma to the face.

KEY ASSESSMENTS

- Bleeding from the nose
- Pain
- Black eyes
- Deformity, instability, crepitus, or point tenderness of the nose during palpation
- X-ray will confirm diagnosis and rule out other facial fractures

PLANNING AND IMPLEMENTATION

- Control bleeding and swelling with ice packs
- Administer analgesics for pain
- Rinse oral cavity
- Surgical correction may be necessary
- Surgical postoperative care includes:

- Check nasal packing or "moustache dressing" for signs of bleeding
- Observe for frequent swallowing that may indicate bleeding
- Monitor vital signs for indications of hemorrhage
- Treat pain
- Frequent oral care because of mouth breathing

NURSING DIAGNOSIS

- Pain, Acute
- Body image, Disturbed

G

Gastritis

DEFINITION

- Gastritis is the inflammation of the stomach lining and may be acute or chronic. If untreated, gastritis can lead to ulcer formation. If hemorrhage occurs, it is an emergent medical condition.

Classifications

- Nonatrophic associated with *Helicobacter pylori* infection
- Atrophic associated with *H. pylori* infection and environmental factors
- Special forms associated with chemicals (i.e., nonsteroidal anti-inflammatory drugs [NSAIDS] or acid reflux), radiation, and autoimmune (i.e., Vitamin B_{12} deficiency) causes

KEY ASSESSMENTS

- Epigastric pain
- Weight loss
- Poor appetite
- Bloating
- Nausea and vomiting
- Signs of ulcer hemorrhage: melena (blood in the feces), hematemesis (vomiting blood), and hemorrhagic shock (low blood pressure [BP] or tachycardia)
- Signs of ulcer perforation: melena (blood in the feces), hematemesis (vomiting blood), hemorrhagic shock (low BP, tachycardia), and a rigid, intensely painful abdomen

Diagnostics

- Endoscopy with testing for *H. pylori*
- Barium swallow
- Hemoglobin and hematocrit

PLANNING AND IMPLEMENTATION

- Treat nausea and vomiting.
- Encourage smoking cessation.
- Discontinue NSAIDs.
- Administer antacids, H_2 receptor antagonists, and proton pump inhibitors.
- If *H. pylori* present, anticipate administering antibiotics (bismuth subsalicylate, metronidazole, and tetracycline).
- Take daily weight.
- Monitor stools for melena.
- Monitor for hematemesis.
- Monitor vital signs for signs of shock.
- Monitor intake and output (I & O).
- Monitor caloric intake.
- Offer small, frequent meals.
- If the patient experiences hemorrhage: insert two large-bore intravenous (IV) lines, administer 5% albumin or 0.9% normal saline (NS) to maintain BP, notify health care provider, insert a nasogastric tube and apply low-intermittent suction, administer oxygen therapy, type and cross-match for blood transfusion, and anticipate administering H_2 antagonist IV and packed red blood cells.

NURSING DIAGNOSIS

- Pain, Acute
- Nutrition: less than body requirements, Imbalanced
- Knowledge, Deficient
- Fluid volume, Risk for deficient

Gastroesophageal Reflux Disease (GERD)

DEFINITION

- GERD refers to the backing up of gastric contents into the esophagus causing pyrosis (heartburn); 15–20 percent of adults experience GERD.

KEY ASSESSMENTS

- Pyrosis (heartburn or low sternal or epigastric pain), especially after a large meal or with bending forward
- Esophagitis
- Pharyngitis
- Hoarseness
- Brash water (excess saliva stimulated by acid reflux)

Diagnostics

- Endoscopy with esophageal biopsy (checking for Barrett's esophagus, cellular changes in the esophageal tissue [metaplasia], which increases the chance of developing esophageal cancer)
- Barium swallow

PLANNING AND IMPLEMENTATION

- Provide small meals.
- Encourage sitting in upright position while eating and for one hour after meals.
- Encourage weight loss if obese.
- Avoid hot and cold beverages.
- Avoid alcohol, caffeine, and tobacco.
- Avoid eating before bedtime.
- Administer antacids, H_2 blockers, and proton pump inhibitors as ordered.
- Surgery to tighten the lower esophageal sphincter may be necessary.

NURSING DIAGNOSIS

- Pain, Acute
- Knowledge, Deficient

Glaucoma

DEFINITION

- Glaucoma is a group of diseases that causes an increase in intraocular pressure, resulting in optic nerve damage and subsequent vision loss. Glaucoma is irreversible, and there is no cure.

Classifications

- Open angle glaucoma occurs as channels that drain fluid within the eye are blocked increasing the intraocular pressure. The pressure builds slowly, causing a gradual loss of vision.
- Closed angle glaucoma occurs when channels, which drain fluid within the eye, are blocked, increasing the intraocular pressure. The pressure rises quickly, causing an acute loss of vision.

KEY ASSESSMENTS

- Eye pain
- Blurred vision
- Headache
- Decrease in visual acuity

Diagnostics

- Visual acuity and field testing
- Tonometry (measures intraocular pressure)

PLANNING AND IMPLEMENTATION

- Provide a safe environment.
- Do not move patient items or furniture.
- Instill timolol eye drops as ordered.
- Anticipate administering systemic medications to decrease intraocular pressure, including sympathomimetic, parasympathomimetic, beta-adrenergic antagonist, carbonic anhydrase inhibitor, and prostaglandin analogue medications.
- Anticipate possible trabeculectomy (creation of a fistula to allow the aqueous humor to drain).

SPECIAL CONCERNS

Cultural Considerations

- Open angle glaucoma more commonly affects people of African or European descent.

- Closed angle glaucoma more commonly affects people of Asian descent.

NURSING DIAGNOSIS

- Falls, Risk for
- Sensory perception, Disturbed
- Knowledge, deficient

Glomerulonephritis

DEFINITION

- Glomerulonephritis is the inflammation of the glomerular capillaries and may lead to renal failure. It is caused by a variety of conditions.

Clinical Causes

- Bacterial infections (postgroup A beta hemolytic streptococcus or bacterial endocarditis)
- Viral infections (human immunodeficiency virus [HIV] or hepatitis B or C)
- Immune disorders (lupus or vasculitis)
- Diabetes
- Hypertension

KEY ASSESSMENTS

- Nephrotic syndrome (hematuria, edema, and hypertension)
- Flank pain
- Malaise, weakness
- Nausea and vomiting
- Low urine output

Diagnostics

- Throat culture (rule out strept infection)
- Urinalysis
- Urine culture and sensitivity
- Blood cultures

Lab Tests

- Blood urea nitrogen (BUN) and creatinine (Cr)
- Complete blood count (CBC)

PLANNING AND IMPLEMENTATION

- Monitor intake and output (I & O)
- Daily weight
- Monitor edema
- Monitor vital signs (especially blood pressure)
- Encourage low-sodium diet
- Fluid restriction (1 Liter/day)
- Administer antibiotics as ordered
- Administer diuretics
- Monitor electrolytes

SPECIAL CONCERNS

- See Special Procedures and Treatments for information on Dialysis.

NURSING DIAGNOSIS

- Fluid volume, Excess
- Infection
- Knowledge, Deficient

Goodpasture's Syndrome

DEFINITION

- Goodpasture's syndrome is a glomerular basement membrane disease that causes vascular membrane destruction of the capillary beds of the lungs and the kidneys. The etiology is unknown. There is no cure, and the mortality rate is approximately 50 percent.

KEY ASSESSMENTS

- Shortness of breath
- Hemoptysis
- Hematuria
- Peripheral edema
- Hypertension
- Report of decreased urine output

Diagnostics

- Chest X-ray (CXR)

Lab Tests

- Positive antiglomerular basement membrane (GBM) antibodies
- Urinalysis
- Complete blood count(CBC)
- Blood urea nitrogen (BUN) and creatinine (Cr)

PLANNING AND IMPLEMENTATION

- High Fowler's position
- Monitor respiratory status
- Monitor hemoptysis
- Administer oxygen therapy
- Monitor CBC
- Anticipate administering packed blood cells
- Monitor renal labs
- Monitor blood pressure
- Monitor intake and output (I & O)
- Daily weight
- Monitor peripheral edema
- Low-sodium diet
- Administer corticosteroid and antihypertensive medications
- Plasmapheresis may be indicated

NURSING DIAGNOSIS

- Airway clearance, Ineffective
- Fluid volume, Risk for imbalance
- Tissue perfusion, Ineffective

Gout

DEFINITION

- Gout is a metabolic disorder with a hereditary tendency causing hyperuricemia (excessive uric acid) producing nodules or tophi consisting of uric acid. The tophus may be found in the joints and cause an acute foreign body reaction.
- Hyperuricemia may cause the production of kidney stones and predispose the patient to renal failure.

KEY ASSESSMENTS

- Pain
- Swelling
- Decreased range of motion to affected joint
- Affected joints commonly include ears, hands, or feet

History and Examination

- Family history of gout
- Previous gout episodes
- History of high-purine diet

Lab Tests

- Uric acid level (increased)
- Urine albumin and uric acid (increased)
- X-ray (identify tophi)
- Complete blood count (CBC)
- Blood urea nitrogen (BUN) and creatinine (Cr)
- Urinalysis

PLANNING AND IMPLEMENTATION

- Bedrest (first 24 hours)
- Heat
- Ice
- Elevation of extremity
- Low-purine diet
- Administer nonsteroidal anti-inflammatory drugs (NSAIDs) as ordered
- Administer corticosteroids during acute phase
- Monitor for side effects of steroid therapy
- Administer colchicines and allopurinol as prescribed
- Monitor intake and output (I & O)

SPECIAL CONCERNS

Teaching Considerations

- Avoid foods high in purine, including alcohol, organ meats, anchovies, sardines, herring, mussels, codfish, scallops, trout, haddock, bacon, turkey, veal, and venison.

NURSING DIAGNOSIS

- Pain, Acute

- Knowledge, Deficient
- Mobility, Impaired physical

Graft-versus-Host Disease (GVHD)

DEFINITION

- GVHD results when transfused blood or transplanted tissue is incompatible with the patient and the body attempts to reject the substance. GVHD may be considered acute or chronic. Acute rejection occurs within 7 to 30 days and chronic rejection occurs 100 days or greater after a transplant. Allograft or homograft transplantation (tissue from a donor with a similar type of cell compatibility) decreases the chance of GVHD.

KEY ASSESSMENTS

- Rash
- Edematous extremities
- Pruritus
- Jaundice
- Dermatitis
- Enteritis (diarrhea)
- Signs of infection (elevated temperature or productive cough)

Diagnostics

- Liver enzymes
- Serum electrolytes
- Blood cultures
- Skin biopsy (confirms diagnosis)

PLANNING AND IMPLEMENTATION

- Meticulous skin care
- Cool baths for pruritus
- Encourage adequate fluid intake
- Document skin assessments
- Monitor signs of infection
- Aseptic technique
- Avoid the use of indwelling catheters
- Monitor white blood count (WBC) count, electrolyte, and liver function tests

- Antidiarrheal medications
- Monitor intake and output (I & O)
- Daily weight
- Monitor stool consistency
- Anticipate administering corticosteroids and immunosuppressive medications (the patient is at a higher risk for infection during this time)
- Neutropenic precautions
- Good hand washing
- Apheresis (withdrawing blood and removing a component and retransfusing) or plasmapheresis (removing plasma and replacing with albumin or saline) may be performed

SPECIAL CONCERNS

Teaching Considerations

- Thoroughly wash all fruits and vegetables
- Avoid raw animal meat and fish
- Do not change litter boxes
- Avoid people who are ill
- Use good hand washing
- Recognize signs of infection

NURSING DIAGNOSIS

- Infection, Risk for
- Skin integrity, Impaired
- Diarrhea
- Fluid volume, Risk for deficient

Guillain-Barré Syndrome

DEFINITION

- Guillain-Barré syndrome is an acute idiopathic polyneuropathy that often follows an infective illness. It is believed that the illness triggers a demyelinization of the nerves. The neuropathy begins distally and ascends to the hands and face. Paralysis may affect the respiratory muscles, and ventilator support may be required. The severity of weakness varies widely, and most patients fully recover.

KEY ASSESSMENTS

- Recent illness
- Respiratory status with continuous pulse oximetry
- Frequent vital signs
- Dyspnea
- Cyanosis
- Autonomic dysfunction
    - Tachycardia
    - Hypotension or hypertension
    - Facial flushing
    - Sweating
- Distal extremity weakness moving toward arms and face
- Absent or weak deep tendon reflexes
- Dysphagia
- Paralysis of vocal cords
- Pain and paresthesia

Diagnostics

- Cerebrospinal fluid tap (high protein)
- Rule out other causes for symptoms (spinal cord tumor or botulism)

PLANNING AND IMPLEMENTATION

- Monitor and support airway
- Keep emergency intubation equipment near
- Frequent vital signs (autonomic dysfunction)
- Monitor for cranial nerve deficits
- Monitor ability to speak and swallow
- Treat pain
- Monitor bowel and bladder function
- Meticulous skin care
- Turn every two hours
- Head of bed elevated at least 30 degrees
- Teach patient about disease process
- Treat anxiety
- Prevent all complications of immobility
- Monitor intake and output (I & O) to prevent fluid volume deficit (FVD)
- Monitor fluid and nutritional intake
- Prevent infections (urinary or pulmonary)
- Provide a means of communication

- Frequent range of motion and physical therapy
- Monitor for deep venous thrombosis (DVT) formation
- Compression boots and antiembolic stockings.
- Anticipate plasmapheresis or intravenous immune globulin

NURSING DIAGNOSIS

- Gas exchange, Impaired
- Ventilation, Impaired spontaneous
- Mobility, Impaired physical

Gynecomastia

DEFINITION

- Gynecomastia is the enlargement of male breast tissue. It may be transitory (with puberty), related to a shift in estrogen/androgen ratio due to illness or medication, or the result of increased fatty tissue. It occurs in 40–60 percent of men and may cause embarrassment.

KEY ASSESSMENTS

- Enlarged breasts

PLANNING AND IMPLEMENTATION

- Assess for pain or unilateral breast enlargement (Men can have breast cancer.)
- Assess for cause
- If obesity is the cause, promote weight loss and increased physical exercise

NURSING DIAGNOSIS

- Body image, Disturbed

Headache

DEFINITION

- A headache is any reported type of pain in the head. Headaches are the most common form of chronic pain.

Classifications

- Tension-type headaches are caused by irritation of the pain-sensitive structures of the brain and may be episodic or chronic and are the most common type of headache.
- Migraine headaches are caused by vasodilatation of dural blood vessels and are episodic with severe pain.
- Cluster headaches are believed to be a variant of migraines headaches. The headaches have a rapid onset with intense pain that occurs at least once a day for 4 to 12 weeks.

KEY ASSESSMENTS

- Photophobia
- Phonophobia
- Nausea and vomiting
- Assess pain using quality, radiation, severity, and timing (QRST)
- Triggers (food, nicotine, alcohol, emotional stress, fatigue, or drugs)
- Aggravating and alleviating factors

Diagnostics

- Computed tomography (CT), electromyography (EMG), electroencephalogram (EEG), or magnetic resonance imaging (MRI) may be performed to rule out underlying pathology.

PLANNING AND IMPLEMENTATION

- Identify and avoid triggers
- Administer medications as ordered
- Monitor for side effects of medication administration
- Monitor pain levels
- Supportive care during episodes of severe pain

SPECIAL CONCERNS

- Alternative therapy, such as yoga, biofeedback, acupuncture, acupressure, and hypnosis, are commonly used as nonpharmacological treatment of headaches.

Gender Considerations

- Migraine headaches are more common in women than in men.

NURSING DIAGNOSIS

- Pain, Acute
- Knowledge, Deficient
- Home maintenance, Impaired

Heart Failure

DEFINITION

- Heart failure (HF), also known as congestive heart failure (CHF), is a condition in which the heart cannot pump enough blood throughout the body.
- When HF occurs the body attempts to compensate by:
  - Increasing heart rate
  - Increasing the size and strength of the ventricular muscle
  - Increasing the capacity of the ventricle
  - Activating the sympathetic nervous system
  - Activating the rennin-angiotensin system

Clinical Causes

- Normal aging
- Chronic lung disease
- Pulmonary hypertension
- Congenital heart disease
- Valvular disease
- Coronary artery disease (CAD)
- High blood pressure
- Excessive alcohol consumption
- Myocardial infarction (MI)
- Liver failure
- Kidney failure
- Hypothyroidism
- Heart muscle infection
- Abnormal blood vessel connections

Classifications

(See Figure 1)

- Diastolic heart failure occurs because of the heart's inability to relax, causing a decrease in ventricular filling.

- Systolic heart failure occurs when there is an inability of the ventricles to contract and pump blood adequately.
- Right-sided heart failure occurs when the right ventricle loses its ability to pump efficiently, backing up into the systemic circulation. This causes congestion that affects the liver, the gastrointestinal (GI) tract, and the periphery (peripheral edema). Patients display systemic symptoms (peripheral edema, abdominal distention, jugular vein distension [JVD]).
- Left-sided heart failure occurs when the left ventricle loses its ability to effectively pump oxygenated blood into the system, causing pulmonary congestion and decreased oxygenation.

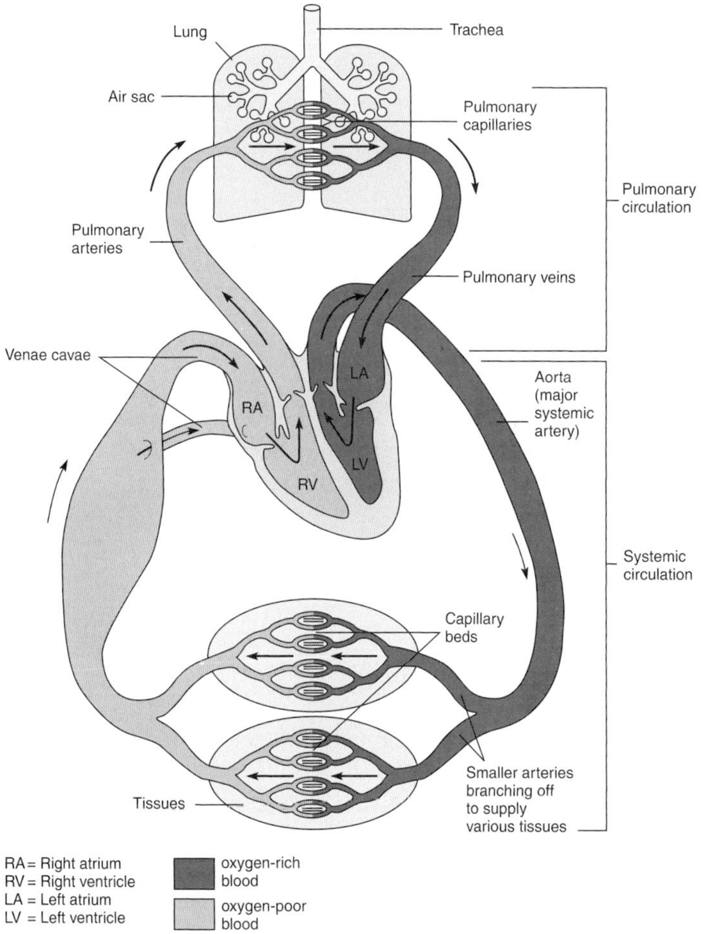

Figure 1 Schematic drawing of blood flow through the heart, showing pulmonary and systemic circulation.

Patients display pulmonary symptoms (shortness of breath [SOB], crackles).

KEY ASSESSMENTS

- Crackles
- Decrease oxygen saturation
- Dyspnea
- JVD
- Peripheral edema
- Cyanotic nail beds
- Circumoral pallor
- Confusion
- Abdominal distention, pain
- Auscultation of S_3
- Orthopnea
- Paroxysmal nocturnal dyspnea
- Tachycardia
- Weak distal pulses
- Hepatojugular reflux

PLANNING AND IMPLEMENTATION

- Electrocardiogram (ECG)
- Echocardiogram
- Stress test
- Brain natriuretic peptide ([BNP], useful to diagnose severity)
- C-reactive protein (CRP) and tumor necrosis factor (TNF)
- Fluid restriction
- Implement safety measures
- Restrict sodium
- Head of bed elevated
- Oxygen administration
- Monitor pulmonary status
- Monitor intake and output (I & O)
- Take daily weight
- Educate patients concerning restrictions and medications
- Medicine regimes: combination of medications including diuretics, angiotensin-converting enzyme (ACE) inhibitors, vasodilators, beta blockers, digitalis, nitrates, and aspirin

NURSING DIAGNOSIS

- Cardiac output, Decreased

- Fluid volume, Excess
- Breathing pattern, Ineffective
- Tissue perfusion, Ineffective

Heat Stroke

DEFINITION

- Heat stroke is the loss of thermoregulation, causing hyperthermia and dehydration. It can lead to death if not promptly treated.

KEY ASSESSMENTS

- Hot, dry skin
- Acute painful muscle spasms
- Hyperthermia
- Tachypnea
- Initial hypertension followed by hypotension
- Tachycardia
- Confusion or coma

Lab Tests

- Electrolytes
- Glucose
- Blood urea nitrogen (BUN) and creatinine (Cr)
- Osmolality

PLANNING AND IMPLEMENTATION

- Insert two large-bore intravenous (IV) lines
- Initiate fluid resuscitation
- Frequent vital signs
- Anticipate administering low-dose corticosteroids
- Monitor neurological status
- Implement safety precautions
- Monitor for evidence of organ damage (renal, oliguria, and increased serum creatinine)
- Monitor and treat electrolyte imbalances

NURSING DIAGNOSIS

- Hyperthermia
- Fluid volume, Deficient

Hemochromatosis

DEFINITION

- Hemochromatosis is a genetic disorder causing excessive iron extraction from food. The excessive iron eventually causes cardiac and liver failure.

KEY ASSESSMENTS

- Bronze skin color
- Abdominal pain
- Joint pain
- Ascites
- Clay colored stools
- Dark urine
- Cardiac arrhythmias
- Shortness of breath

Lab Tests

- Positive HFE (hemochromatosis gene)
- Liver biopsy
- Aspartate aminotransferase (AST) and alanine aminotransferase (ALT)
- Transferrin and ferritin

PLANNING AND IMPLEMENTATION

- Monitor intake and output (I & O)
- Treat pain
- Monitor cardiac rhythm
- Anticipate phlebotomy
- Avoid foods high in iron
- Avoid food high in vitamin C (increases iron absorption)
- Avoid alcohol

NURSING DIAGNOSIS

- Pain, Chronic
- Knowledge, Deficient

Hemophilia

DEFINITION

- Hemophilia is a group of hereditary diseases that results in a deficiency of clotting factors. Depletion of factors VIII, IX, and X collectively make up approximately 95 percent of the bleeding disorders. The lack of clotting factor puts patients with hemophilia at higher risk for bleeding.

Classifications

- Hemophilia A is a factor VIII deficiency known as classic hemophilia and may be considered severe, moderate, or mild.
- Hemophilia B is a factor IX deficiency also known as Christmas disease.
- Hemophilia C is a factor XI deficiency.
- Von Willebrand's disease is a decrease in the quantity of von Willebrand's factor, a substance that helps platelets stick at the site of injury or bleeding. It may be classified as mild or severe.

KEY ASSESSMENTS

- Joint or muscle pain
- Bruising
- Hemarthrosis (bleeding into joints); weight-bearing joint most commonly affected
- Hemorrhage (may be fatal after trauma or surgery)
- Signs of hemorrhagic shock (tachycardia or hypotension)
- Oxygenation status

History and Examination

- Obtaining a family history may aid in the diagnosis of hemophilia and prevent hemorrhage.

Lab Tests

- Serum platelet levels
- Factor assay tests
- Coagulation serum tests (prothrombin time [PT], partial thromboplastin time [PTT], and bleeding time)
- Chorionic villus sampling (may detect genetic abnormality in utero)

PLANNING AND IMPLEMENTATION

(See Table 8)

- Frequent vital signs (signs of shock-hypotension and tachycardia)
- Blood consents
- Active type and cross-match for blood products
- Anticipate blood and factor replacement
- Avoid administering medications that interfere with platelet aggregation
- Observe for hemorrhage, especially at surgical site
- Avoid invasive procedures that may cause bleeding
- Monitor clotting factors
- Monitor patient for hypersensitivity reactions to factor replacement (chest tightness, urticaria, or hypotension)

SPECIAL CONCERNS

Cultural Considerations

- Hemophilia C primarily affects Ashkenazi Jews and may affect both men and women.

Genetic Considerations

- Hemophilia A affects 1 in 10,000 males and is a cross-linked recessive disorder transmitted from mother to son.
- Hemophilia B affects 1 in 40,000 males and is a cross-linked recessive disorder transmitted from mother to son.
- Von Willebrand's disease is a hereditary disease that affects approximately 1 percent of the population (men and women).

TABLE 8

Pharmacology Management of the Types of Hemophilia

Type of Hemophilia	Medication
Hemophilia A	Heat-treated factor VIII concentrate or cryoprecipitate
Mild Hemophilia A	Desmopressin acetate (DDAVP, Stimate)
Hemophilia B	Factor IX (IV); fresh-frozen plasma when necessary
Hemophilia C (Factor XI deficiency)	Fresh-frozen plasma
von Willebrand's disease	Cryoprecipitate and DDAVP

NURSING DIAGNOSIS

- Fluid volume, Risk for deficient
- Knowledge, Deficient
- Pain, Acute

Hepatitis

DEFINITION

- Hepatitis is inflammation of the liver that commonly occurs from a viral infection and may be acute or chronic. Acute viral hepatitis occurs initially after infection, and chronic hepatitis occurs when symptoms continue beyond six months.

Classifications

Hepatitis A (HAV)

- HAV is spread via fecal-oral route.
- Infection may occur from eating food or drinking water contaminated with the virus; eating raw shellfish may lead to infection (if the shellfish was caught in contaminated water).
- HAV vaccine is available.
- Hand washing after toileting reduces spread.
- Symptoms appear 15–50 days after exposure.
- Symptoms are usually mild and flu-like.
- Immune globulin (IG) given within two weeks of exposure effectively treats the virus.

Hepatitis B (HBV)

- HBV is spread through blood and body fluids via skin and mucous membranes.
- Infection may occur through unprotected sex, mother to baby, needle sharing, and accidental needle sticks.
- HBV vaccine is available.
- Symptoms appear 48–180 days after exposure.
- HBV is 100 times more infectious than human immunodeficiency virus (HIV).
- Fifteen percent of HBV infections progress to a chronic state.
- Hepatitis IG given within two weeks of exposure effectively treats the virus.

Hepatitis C (HCV)

- HCV is spread through blood and body fluids via skin and mucous membranes.
- Infection may occur through unprotected sex, mother to baby, needle sharing, and accidental needle sticks.
- No vaccine is available.
- Symptoms appear 14–180 days after exposure.
- Eighty-five percent of HCV infections progress to a chronic state.
- Seventy percent of chronically infection patients develop liver disease.
- HCV patients account for 50 percent of all liver transplants.
- No postexposure prophylaxis has been proven effective.

Hepatitis D (HDV)

- HDV is spread through blood and body fluids via skin and mucous membranes.
- Infection may occur through unprotected sex, mother to baby, needle sharing, and accidental needle sticks.
- Coinfection with HBV is common.
- Symptoms appear 14–56 days after exposure; some patients are asymptomatic.
- Most with HDV progress to a chronic state.
- HBV IG given within two weeks of exposure effectively treats the virus.

Hepatitis E (HEV)

- HEV is spread via fecal-oral route.
- Infection may occur from eating food or drinking water contaminated with the virus; eating raw shellfish (if caught in contaminated water) may lead to infection.
- Most often associated with water-born epidemics in Asia, Africa, and Central and South America.
- Hand washing after toileting can reduce spread.
- Symptoms appear 15–64 days after exposure.
- Symptoms are usually mild and flu-like.
- IG given within two weeks of exposure effectively treats the virus.

Alcoholic hepatitis

- Alcoholic hepatitis is inflammation of the liver by alcohol consumption.

Toxic hepatitis

- Toxic hepatitis is inflammation of the liver from a toxic substance or a prescribed medication, including carbon tetrachloride, amanita mushrooms, acetaminophen, halothane, methyldopa, phenytoin, and monoamine oxidase (MAO) inhibitors.

Autoimmune hepatitis

- Autoimmune hepatitis is inflammation of the liver from autoimmune diseases, such as Graves' disease, ulcerative colitis, and autoimmune anemia.

KEY ASSESSMENTS

- Acute infection
- Anorexia
- Nausea and vomiting
- Jaundice
- Fatigue
- Fever
- Arthralgias
- Light colored stools
- Dark color urine

History and Examination

- Drug use
- Sexual behaviors
- Living conditions
- Foreign travel
- Recent body piercing or tattoos
- Occupational hazards
- Alcohol consumption
- Recent shellfish consumption

Diagnostics

- Liver biopsy may be performed to confirm diagnosis.

Lab Tests

- Anti-HAV, -HBV, -HCV, -HDV, and -HEV antibodies
- Aspartate aminotransferase (AST) and alanine aminotransferase (ALT)
- Bilirubin
- Prothrombin time (PT), partial thromboplastin time (PTT), and international normalizing ratio (INR)

PLANNING AND IMPLEMENTATION

- Monitor intake and output (I & O).

- Daily weight
- Small frequent meals
- Enforce hand washing after toileting
- Use standard precautions
- Clean blood spills with bleach solution
- Provide rest periods
- Do not administer acetaminophen
- Administer postexposure IG
- Administer vitamins and dietary supplements
- Avoid alcohol
- Monitor liver function tests
- Monitor color of stool and urine
- Tepid baths (if pruritus is present)
- Monitor for signs of worsening liver function (ascites, confusion, coagulopathies, malnutrition, or increased susceptibility to infection)
- Careful administration of medications that are metabolized in the liver
- If chronic infection occurs, administer interferon-alpha, ribavirin, lamivudine, and adefovir dipivoxil as ordered

SPECIAL CONCERNS

Teaching Considerations

- Avoid sharing personal items like razors
- Use safe sex practices
- Wash hands after toileting
- Avoid alcohol
- Avoid acetaminophen
- When traveling, drink bottled water
- Avoid raw shellfish

NURSING DIAGNOSIS

- Activity intolerance
- Fatigue
- Nutrition: less than body requirements, Imbalanced
- Infection, Risk for
- Knowledge, Deficient

Hiatal Hernia

DEFINITION

- A hiatal hernia is the protrusion of the stomach above the diaphragm. It occurs more commonly in the elderly and in patients experiencing increased intra-abdominal pressure (i.e., obesity, pregnancy, and ascites).

Classifications

- Sliding hiatal hernia—the upper stomach slides upward through the gastroesophageal junction.
- Paraesophageal hiatal hernia—the stomach herniates through the esophageal hiatus.

KEY ASSESSMENTS

- Pyrosis (heartburn or low sternal or epigastric pain), especially after a large meal or with bending forward
- Esophagitis
- Pharyngitis
- Hoarseness
- Brash water (excess saliva stimulated by acid reflux)

Diagnostics

- Endoscopy
- Barium swallow

PLANNING AND IMPLEMENTATION

- Provide small meals
- Upright position while eating and for one hour after meals
- Encourage weight loss if obese
- Avoid hot and cold beverages
- Avoid alcohol, caffeine, and tobacco
- Avoid eating before bedtime
- Administer antacids, H_2 blockers, and proton pump inhibitors as ordered
- Surgery to tighten the lower esophageal sphincter

NURSING DIAGNOSIS

- Pain, Acute
- Knowledge, Deficient

Human Immunodeficiency Virus (HIV)

DEFINITION

- HIV is a retrovirus infection that replicates rapidly, destroys CD4 T cells (helper cells), and renders the body at risk for opportunistic infections. The virus spreads though unsafe sexual contact, parental (blood), and perinatal exposure. Initial infection causes illness, usually mistaken for the flu. Many patients with HIV infection maintain good health with the use of antiviral medications, but others develop acquired immunodeficiency syndrome (AIDS).
- AIDS is present when a patient with HIV infection has a CD4 level below 200 cells/μL and the presence of an opportunistic infection or cancer, wasting syndrome, or the development of AIDS dementia complex.
- Opportunistic infections are caused by organisms that are part of the normal environment and occur when the immune system is not working properly.

KEY ASSESSMENTS

Neurological

- AIDS dementia complex (mental changes associated with HIV infection; etiology is not well understood)
- Headaches
- Fatigue
- Seizures
- Gait disturbance
- Memory loss
- Visual loss or blindness

Integumentary

- Kaposi's sarcoma (blue or red patches on the skin)
- White patches on tongue (candida infection)
- AIDS wasting syndrome (loss of more than 10 percent of body weight)
- Peripheral neuropathy
- Skin rash
- Chills and fever
- Night sweats

Respiratory

- SOB
- Productive cough

Cardiovascular

- Tachycardia

Gastrointestinal/Genitourinary

- Nausea
- Vomiting
- Abdominal pain
- Diarrhea

Immunological

- Opportunistic infections
- Lymphadenopathy (swollen lymph glands)

Lab Tests

- Enzyme-linked immunosorbent assay (ELISA)
- Western blot
- CD4 cell count
- HIV-ribonucleic acid (RNA) concentration (viral load testing, useful to mark progression of the infection)
- Deoxyribonucleic acid-polymerase chain reaction (DNA-PCR) amplification
- Complete blood count ([CBC], anemia)
- White blood count ([WBC], leucopenia)

PLANNING AND IMPLEMENTATION

- Monitor neurological status
- Monitor intake and output (I & O)
- Monitor WBC
- Aseptic technique
- Avoid indwelling catheters
- Elevate head of bed
- Offer small frequent meals
- Implement complementary therapy (massage or music)
- Standard precautions
- If neutropenic, implement neutropenic precautions
- Monitor respiratory status
- Emotional support
- Assist with activities of daily living
- Meticulous skin and oral care

- Encourage fluids and nutritional intake
- Daily weight
- Frequent rest periods
- Treat diarrhea
- Implement safety measures
- Monitor for signs of depression
- Monitor for opportunistic infections including:
  - Mycobacterium avium complex (MAC), salmonellosis, syphilis, tuberculosis, aspergillosis, candidiasis, histoplasmosis, primary central nervous system (CNS) lymphoma, non-Hodgkin's lymphoma, Kaposi's sarcoma, pneumocystic carinii pneumonia (PCP), cytomegalovirus, herpes simplex, herpes zoster, human papilloma virus (HPV), or oral hairy leukoplakia
- Administer highly active antiviral therapy (HAART), including nucleoside reverse transcriptase inhibitor (NRTI), nonnucleoside reverse transcriptase inhibitors (NNRTI), protease inhibitors (PI), and fusion inhibitor medications
- Monitor and treat side the effects of HAART, including hypertension, diabetes, osteopenia, hyperlipidemia, nausea, vomiting, diarrhea, fatigue, headache, peripheral neuropathy, abdominal pain, and liver dysfunction
- Administer antibiotic medications if bacterial infection is present

SPECIAL CONCERNS

- See Special Procedures and Treatments for information on Pain and Palliative Care.

Cultural Considerations

- AIDS is sixth leading cause of death in African American males ages 25–44.

Teaching Considerations

- Medication compliance is necessary but difficult because of the unpleasant side effects the medications cause.
- Contact the health care provider if signs of infection arise.
- Practice safe sex.
- Thoroughly wash all fruits and vegetables.
- Avoid raw animal meat and fish.
- Do not change litter boxes.
- Do not share toothbrushes or razors.
- Clean blood spills with bleach.
- Avoid people who are ill.
- Avoid crowded places, especially during flu season.

NURSING DIAGNOSIS

- Pain, Acute
- Diarrhea
- Activity intolerance
- Fluid volume, Risk for deficient
- Fatigue
- Infection, Risk for
- Knowledge, Deficient
- Oral mucous membrane, Impaired

Huntington's Disease

DEFINITION

- Huntington's disease, also called Huntington's chorea, is a rare, hereditary disease affecting the central nervous system (CNS) in which cells in the basal ganglia and extrapyramidal motor system are destroyed. There is also a decrease in the neurotransmitters gamma-aminobutyric acid (GABA) and acetylcholine (Ach), resulting in chronic, progressive chorea (involuntary, rapid, purposeless movements) and dementia. The disease has a late onset, usually between the ages of 30 and 50 and progresses until the patient is totally dependent. Death is usually from pneumonia or sepsis.

KEY ASSESSMENTS

- Family history of Huntington's disease
- Intellectual decline from forgetfulness to dementia
- Facial grimacing
- Jerky movements
- Gait disturbances

Diagnostics

- Genetic testing

PLANNING AND IMPLEMENTATION

- Monitor mental status
- Implement safety measures
- Monitor fluid and nutritional intake
- Monitor ability to swallow

- Monitor bowel and bladder function
- Inspect and document skin assessment
- Meticulous skin care
- Frequent oral care
- Anticipate administering muscle relaxant, antipsychotic, and antidepressant medications

SPECIAL CONCERNS

- Huntington's disease is caused by autosomal dominant gene transmission. Children have a 50 percent chance of inheriting the gene. Genetic testing is available for the Huntington's gene. Testing is a difficult choice because if it is positive, the patient must cope with knowing that he or she will develop the disease.

Teaching Considerations

- Teaching should address the physical, emotional, and social aspects of the disease.
- In the early stages of the disease, encourage the patient to address long-term issues, such as advanced directives, estate planning, and care options.

NURSING DIAGNOSIS

- Injury, Risk for
- Confusion, Chronic
- Mobility, Impaired physical

Hydrocele

DEFINITION

- Hydrocele is a fluid-filled sack located on the spermatic cord within the scrotum and may be associated with an inguinal hernia, adjacent infection, scrotal trauma, or a systemic infection.

KEY ASSESSMENTS

- Painless swelling or bulging in the scrotum
- Pain (scrotal trauma)
- History of trauma or infection

Diagnostics

- Scrotal ultrasonography

PLANNING AND IMPLEMENTATION

- No treatment may be indicated.
- Surgical repair is indicated if it becomes uncomfortably large or blood flow is disrupted (spermatocelectomy [removal of the spermatic cord]).
- Treat infection, if present, with appropriate antibiotics.
- If pain is present, treat and monitor.

NURSING DIAGNOSIS

- Knowledge, Deficient
- Body image, Disturbed

Hypercalcemia

DEFINITION

- Hypercalcemia is an excess of calcium with a serum calcium level greater than 10.5 mEq/L. Hypercalcemia may result from excess calcium intake or the inability to excrete calcium. Excess calcium suppresses cellular excitability, resulting in muscle weakness.

Clinical Causes

- Immobility (calcium released from the bone)
- Hyperparathyroidism
- Malignancy
- Excessive ingestion of calcium

KEY ASSESSMENTS

- Respiratory status for apnea and weakness
- Cardiac status for dysrhythmias and pulse strength
- Neurological status for confusion
- Muscle strength
- Bowels sounds (decreased)

PLANNING AND IMPLEMENTATION

- Monitor respiratory status.
- Limit activity if weakness is present.
- Monitor cardiac status and pulse strength.
- Monitor serum calcium levels.
- Anticipate administration of diuretics and fluids.
- With significant hypercalcemia, IV sodium phosphate may be administered to quickly bind calcium.

NURSING DIAGNOSIS

- Falls, Risk for
- Cardiac output, Decreased

Hyperkalemia

DEFINITION

- Hyperkalemia is a potassium level greater than 4.5 mEq/L, resulting from an excessive ingestion of potassium or when excretion of potassium is impaired. Hyperkalemia may cause death and should be treated promptly.

Clinical Causes

- Overmedication with potassium supplements
- Ingestion of excessive dietary potassium
- Kidney impairment
- Metabolic acidosis (shifts potassium from intracellular to extracellular)

KEY ASSESSMENTS

- Assess cardiac status
- Electrocardiogram (ECG) may show tall, tented T waves
- Monitor for abnormal muscle function ranging from twitching to paralysis
- Abdominal cramping and diarrhea

PLANNING AND IMPLEMENTATION

- Remove all sources of potassium (intravenous [IV] and medications)

- Monitor potassium levels
- Monitor cardiac status
- Place on cardiac monitor with potassium greater than 5 mEq/L
- Monitor gait
- Monitor respiratory status
- Anticipate administering medications to lower potassium:
  - Kayexalate (by mouth [PO] or rectally [PR]) exchanges sodium and potassium in the gastrointestinal (GI) tract.
  - IV calcium interrupts the action of potassium.
  - IV regular insulin and glucose pushes the potassium in the cell.
  - Sodium bicarbonate IV pushes the potassium in the cell.

NURSING DIAGNOSIS

- Cardiac output, Decreased
- Injury, Risk for

Hypermagnesemia

DEFINITION

- Hypermagnesemia is an excess of the magnesium ion with a serum magnesium level greater than 2.6 mEq/L. Elevated magnesium levels may be due to an excessive ingestion of magnesium or failure to excrete magnesium. High levels of magnesium are associated with muscle weakness and suppression of electrical impulses.

Clinical Causes

- Excess ingestion of magnesium
- Renal failure

KEY ASSESSMENTS

- Respiratory status for apnea and weakness
- Arrhythmias
- Decreased pulse strength
- Confusion and lethargy
- Muscle weakness
- Bowels sounds (decreased)
- Parentheses
- Hyporeflexia

PLANNING AND IMPLEMENTATION

- Monitor respiratory status
- Limit activity if weakness is present
- Monitor cardiac status and pulse strength
- Monitor neurological status
- Monitor gastrointestinal (GI) status
- Monitor magnesium levels

SPECIAL CONCERNS

- Patients with renal failure have a decreased ability to excrete magnesium and should avoid medications that contain magnesium, such as milk of magnesia and magnesium-based antacids, to avoid hypermagnesemia.

NURSING DIAGNOSIS

- Cardiac output, Decreased
- Injury, Risk for

Hypernatremia

DEFINITION

- Hypernatremia is an excess of sodium ions with a serum sodium level greater than 145 mEq/L. Hypernatremia is rarely caused by an excess of sodium; it is more commonly a sign of insufficient water in the body, resulting in a high sodium level due to concentration.

Clinical Causes

- Elderly patients unable to ingest water independently or communicate their need for water
- Excessive diuretic use
- Diabetes insipidus
- High sodium intake
- Excess administration of hypertonic solutions
- Excessive insensible loss
- Salt water drowning
- Severe gastrointestinal (GI) loss

KEY ASSESSMENTS

- Change in level of consciousness (LOC), ranging from restlessness to seizures
- Increased muscle tone
- Hyperreflexia
- Flushed dry skin, poor skin turgor
- Dry mucous membranes
- Weight loss
- Output greater than input

PLANNING AND IMPLEMENTATION

- Monitor LOC
- Seizure precautions
- Monitor intake and output (I & O)
- Daily weight
- Frequent oral care
- Replacement of isotonic fluids
- Increase in oral intake of free water
- Monitor for postural hypotension
- Anticipate administering desmopressin in patients with diabetes insipidus

NURSING DIAGNOSIS

- Fluid volume, Risk for imbalanced
- Injury, Risk for

Hyperosmolar Hyperglycemic Nonketonic Syndrome (HHNS)

DEFINITION

- HHNS results in a decrease of circulating insulin with profound hyperglycemia that may develop over days to weeks. It is a life-threatening medical emergency associated with profound fluid volume deficiency that occurs in the elderly with type 2 diabetes and is often preceded by infection or recent surgery.
- The insulin deficiency is less profound than in diabetes ketoacidosis, and protein is not broken down for energy, resulting in the absence of ketones and acidosis.
- Symptoms may be mistaken for a stroke in the elderly patient.

KEY ASSESSMENTS

- Dehydration (hypotension or tachycardia)
- Nausea and vomiting
- Decrease in level of consciousness (LOC)
- Polydipsia
- Polyphagia
- Polyuria (leading to oliguria if dehydration is profound)
- Seizures
- Aphasia
- Coma
- Fever (infection)

Lab Tests

- Glucose
- Electrolytes (especially potassium)
- Serum osmolality
- Complete blood count (CBC)

PLANNING AND IMPLEMENTATION

- Insert two large-bore intravenous (IV) lines
- Prompt administration of 0.9% normal saline (NS)
- Frequent (every hour until stable) glucose monitoring
- Monitor electrolytes
- Monitor breath sounds
- Monitor pulse oximetry readings
- Monitor intake and output (I & O)
- Monitor LOC
- Implement safety precautions
- Frequent vital signs
- Monitor for signs of infection
- Leave patient flat if hypotension is profound
- Insert Foley catheter to closely monitor urine output
- Cardiac monitoring (hypokalemia causes ventricular arrhythmias)
- Anticipate administering short-acting insulin intravenously
- Anticipate administering potassium supplements (insulin will decrease serum potassium levels)
- Reinforce diabetic teaching

NURSING DIAGNOSIS

- Fluid volume, Deficient
- Infection, Risk for
- Knowledge, Deficient

Hyperparathyroidism

DEFINITION

- Hyperparathyroidism is a clinical state of oversecretion of parathyroid hormone by the parathyroid gland.

Clinical Causes

- Enlarged parathyroid gland
- Adenoma of the parathyroid
- Parathyroid cancer

KEY ASSESSMENTS

- Lethargy
- Fatigue
- Paresthesia
- Dyspepsia
- Nausea
- Constipation
- Polyuria
- Coma
- Muscle weakness
- Osteoporosis (over time)

Diagnostics

- Computed tomography (CT)

Lab Tests

- Calcium (high)
- Parathyroid hormone (PTH) levels
- Phosphorus (low)

PLANNING AND IMPLEMENTATION

- Monitor level of consciousness (LOC)
- Administer 0.9% normal saline (NS) intravenously
- Monitor electrolytes and treat imbalances
- Monitor intake and output (I & O)
- Administer vitamin A and D supplements
- Avoid calcium containing medications
- Anticipate parathyroidectomy for adenoma

NURSING DIAGNOSIS

- Injury, Risk for
- Constipation
- Confusion

Hyperphosphatemia

DEFINITION

- Hyperphosphatemia is a phosphorus level of greater than 4.5 mEq/L. Hyperphosphatemia may result from the excess intake of phosphorus or the inability to excrete phosphorus. Effects of high phosphorus are due to the associated hypocalcaemia resulting from the reciprocal relationship of the two ions.

Clinical Causes

- Excessive phosphorus intake
- Renal failure

KEY ASSESSMENTS

- Paresthesias
- Twitching
  - Trousseau's sign—inflate blood pressure cuff on the arm and hand will spasm
  - Chvostek's sign—tapping on the facial nerve and spasm of facial muscle on tapped side
- Hyperactive reflexes
- ST segment lengthened and prolonged PR interval on electrocardiogram (ECG)
- Tetany of respiratory muscles (causing respiratory arrest)
- Increased GI motility, cramping, and diarrhea

PLANNING AND IMPLEMENTATION

- Monitor level of consciousness (LOC)
- Monitor respiratory status
- Monitor cardiac status
- Monitor gastrointestinal (GI) status
- Monitor calcium levels
- Anticipate calcium replacements

- Monitor gait and musculoskeletal status
- Anticipate administering phosphate binders
- In the renal patient, dialysis may be required

NURSING DIAGNOSIS

- Cardiac output, Decreased
- Ventilation, Impaired spontaneous

Hyperprolactinemia

DEFINITION

- Hyperprolactinemia is a prolactin secreting pituitary tumor.

Clinical Causes

- Pituitary adenoma
- Primary hypothyroidism
- Injury or surgery to the pituitary stalk
- Estrogen therapy
- Pregnancy
- Multiple sclerosis
- Medications (dopamine antagonist, haloperidol, risperidone, metoclopramide, and opioids)

KEY ASSESSMENTS

- Amenorrhea or galactorrhea (women)
- Erectile dysfunction or gynecomastia (men)
- Infertility
- Headaches
- Visual field defect

Diagnostics

- Computed tomography (CT)
- Magnetic resonance imaging (MRI)

Lab Tests

- Basal prolactin level
- Thyroid panel
- Blood urea nitrogen(BUN) and creatinine (Cr)
- Aspartate aminotransferase (AST) and alanine aminotransferase (ALT)

PLANNING AND IMPLEMENTATION

- Anticipate administering dopaminergic medications (bromocriptine or cabergoline).
- Monitor neurological status.
- Monitor prolactin levels.
- If tumor is large or does not respond to medication, a transsphenoidal hypophysectomy (surgical removal of the tumor through the nose to reach the pituitary gland) may be warranted.

SPECIAL CONCERNS

- Discuss sexual function and infertility issues with the patient.

NURSING DIAGNOSIS

- Sexual dysfunction
- Knowledge, Deficient
- Body image, Disturbed

Hypertension

DEFINITION

- Hypertension is a sustained elevation of systemic blood pressure. Hypertension places the patient at risk for organ damage to eyes, brain, heart, kidneys, and great vessels.

Classifications

- Primary, or essential, with unknown etiology and risk factors that are:
  - Modifiable—obesity, substance abuse, stress, diet, and sedentary lifestyle
  - Nonmodifiable—family history, increasing age, gender, and ethnicity (African Americans are at higher risk)
- Secondary, or related to another disease
  - Diseases may include renal artery narrowing, chronic kidney disease, endocrine disease (hyperaldosteronism or pheochromocytoma), neurological (head trauma or brain tumor), sleep apnea, pregnancy-induced hypertension, and certain medication therapy.

Classifications of Blood Pressure in Adults

	Systolic pressure mm Hg	Diastolic pressure mm Hg
Normal	less than 120	less than 80
Prehypertension	120–139	80–90
Stage 1 hypertension	140–159	90–99
Stage 2 hypertension	greater than 160	greater than 100

KEY ASSESSMENTS

- Family history
- Presence of primary risk factors or secondary diseases or conditions
- Neurological status
- Vital signs with blood pressure in both arms
- Respiratory status

PLANNING AND IMPLEMENTATION

- Monitor blood pressure frequently
- Monitor intake and output (I & O)
- Institute safety precautions
- Administer antihypertensive therapy

SPECIAL CONCERNS

Teaching Considerations

- Teach patients about modifiable risk factors including weight reduction, smoking cessation, stress reduction, and dietary changes.
- Recommend and educate patients about the dietary approaches of stopping hypertension (DASH)—diet that is rich in grains, fruits, vegetables, and low-fat dairy products.
- Recommend and educate patients about moderate alcohol consumption and caffeine and sodium restriction.
- Encourage moderate exercise and stress reduction.
- Educate patients about antihypertensive medicines and side effects.
- Teach patients to get up slowly to avoid postural hypotension.
- Educate patients on complications associated with untreated hypertension.

NURSING DIAGNOSIS

- Knowledge, Deficient
- Therapeutic regimen management, Ineffective

Hyperthyroidism

DEFINITION

- Hyperthyroidism is the continuous secretion of thyroid hormones resulting in elevated triiodothyronine (T_3) and thyroxine (T_4) hormone and low thyroid-stimulating hormone (TSH) levels. Thyrotoxic crisis is a life-threatening complication of hyperthyroidism.

Classifications

- Thyrotoxicosis—the acceleration of metabolism elevating thyroid hormone levels with toxic manifestations
- Graves' disease—a diffuse toxic goiter that is the most common cause of thyrotoxicosis
- Hashimoto's thyroiditis—an autoimmune-mediated destruction of the thyroid gland with subsequent release of stored hormones
- Subclinical hyperthyroidism—defined as a low TSH and normal T_3 and T_4 levels

KEY ASSESSMENTS

- Enlarged thyroid
- Palpitations
- Fatigue
- Heat intolerance
- Weight loss
- Exophthalmos
- Tachycardia

Diagnostics

- Thyroid scan
- Computed tomography (CT)

Lab Tests

- T_3 and T_4
- TSH
- Thyroid antibodies (Graves' and Hashimoto's)

- Radioactive iodine uptake
- Complete blood count (CBC)
- Liver function tests

PLANNING AND IMPLEMENTATION

- Space activities.
- Provide frequent rest periods.
- Monitor oxygenation status.
- Monitor for cardiac arrhythmias.
- Take daily weight.
- Ensure adequate fluid and nutritional intake.
- Reinforce relaxation techniques.
- Anticipate administer beta blockers.
- Provide eye care (artificial tears, shielding at night).
- Administer antithyroid medications (propylthiouracil [PTU], methimazole, and potassium iodide [SSKI]).
- Monitor for side effects of medications.
- Radioiodine therapy is indicated for patients who do not respond to medications (I 131). Sodium iodide (I 131) is an orally ingested substance that irradiates the thyroid gland.
- Monitor for hypothyroidism after radioiodine therapy.
- Thyroidectomy may be indicated.
- Postthyroidectomy, monitor for airway edema, hemorrhage, and hypocalcemia.
- Monitor for thyrotoxic crisis or thyroid storm (brought on by infection, stress, or pregnancy).
    - Extreme fever
    - Restlessness, agitation, or coma
    - Atrial fibrillation, heart failure, or angina
    - Hypertension quickly deteriorating to hypotension
    - Diaphoresis
- Anticipate treatment for thyroid storm.
    - Transfer to intensive care unit
    - Oxygen therapy
    - Insert two large-bore peripheral intravenous (IV) lines
    - Administer IV fluid
    - Cooling blanket and acetaminophen for fever
    - Administer antibiotics
    - Frequent vital signs including temperature
    - Cardiac monitoring
    - May require plasmapheresis or dialysis to remove circulating antibodies

Discharge Planning

- Patients receiving radioactive iodine therapy need discharge instructions, including:
  - Sleep alone
  - No close contact with children
  - Practice personal hygiene
  - Launder linens, towels, and clothes daily
  - Avoid preparing food with bare hands

SPECIAL CONCERNS

Gender Considerations

- Hashimoto's thyroiditis is six times more common in women than in men.

Teaching Considerations

- Use radioactive iodine therapy safety.
- Keep outer door closed.
- Flush twice after using bathroom.
- Only disposable items are allowed in the patient's room.
- Bathe and wash hands frequently.
- Children and pregnant women visitors are restricted.
- Nurses and health care providers must wear gloves, gown, and mask when in the room.
- Monitor radiation levels, and discharge only when levels are acceptable as deemed by the radiation officer.

NURSING DIAGNOSIS

- Nutrition: less than body requirements, Imbalanced
- Anxiety
- Fatigue
- Knowledge, Deficient

Hypocalcemia

DEFINITION

- Hypocalcemia is a deficit of calcium with a serum calcium level of less than 4.5 mEq/L. Hypocalcemia may result from inadequate calcium intake or excessive calcium ingestion. Calcium suppresses electrical activity in the cell when low electrical activity occurs spontaneously.

Clinical Causes

- Crohn's disease
- Inadequate calcium intake
- Renal disease
- Diarrhea
- Excessive wound drainage
- Alkalosis
- Pancreatitis
- Increased phosphorus levels (calcium and phosphorus have a reciprocal relationship)
- Removal of the parathyroid gland

KEY ASSESSMENTS

- Paresthesias
- Twitching
  - Trousseau's sign—inflate blood pressure cuff on the arm and hand will spasm
  - Chvostek's sign—tapping on the facial nerve and spasm of facial muscle on tapped side
- Hyperactive reflexes
- ST segment lengthened and prolonged PR interval on electrocardiogram (ECG)
- Tetany of respiratory muscles (causing respiratory arrest)
- Increased GI motility, cramping, or diarrhea

PLANNING AND IMPLEMENTATION

- Monitor level of consciousness (LOC)
- Monitor respiratory status
- Monitor cardiac status
- Monitor gastrointestinal (GI) status
- Monitor calcium levels
- Anticipate calcium replacements
- Monitor gait and musculoskeletal status

NURSING DIAGNOSIS

- Injury, Risk for
- Ventilation, Impaired spontaneous

Hypokalemia

DEFINITION

- Hypokalemia is a potassium level lower than 3.5 mEq/L. Hypokalemia results from an excessive loss of potassium from the body or from a prolonged decrease in the ingestion of potassium. Never push intravenous (IV) potassium with this condition.

Clinical Causes

- Diuretics
- Heart failure (due to excess aldosterone release)
- Diarrhea
- Vomiting
- Nasogastric suctioning
- Drainage from large wounds
- Diets without foods rich in potassium
- Metabolic acidosis (potassium and bicarbonate ions are excreted and hydrogen ions shift into the cells forcing potassium out)

KEY ASSESSMENTS

- Poor muscle contraction
- Hyporeflexia
- Fatigue
- Decreased GI motility
- Nausea
- Vomiting
- Paresthesias
- Confusion
- Lethargy
- Cardiac arrhythmias (including premature ventricular contractions and ventricular tachycardia)
- Flattened T waves on the ECG
- Increased sensitivity to digitalis and risk of toxicity

PLANNING AND IMPLEMENTATION

- Monitor serum potassium levels.
- Frequent auscultation of the apical pulse.
- Place patient on the cardiac monitor if potassium level is less than 3 mEq/L.

- Limit patient activities until level is within normal.
- Assess gait.
- Closely monitor respiratory status.
- Anticipate potassium replacement.
- Oral potassium replacements may cause GI upset.
- IV potassium must be given with extreme caution per IV pump.
- Potassium is irritating, and the IV site should be watched closely for infiltration.
- If metabolic alkalosis is present, anticipate treating it as well.

NURSING DIAGNOSIS

- Cardiac output, Decreased
- Injury, Risk for

Hypomagnesemia

DEFINITION

- Hypomagnesemia is a deficit of magnesium ions with serum magnesium levels of less than 2.1 mEq/L. Magnesium levels may be deficient due to insufficient intake or poor absorption. Hypomagnesemia is associated with increased cellular excitability and often occurs simultaneously with hypokalemia and hypocalcemia.

Clinical Causes

- Alcoholism
- Inadequate magnesium intake
- Diuretic use
- Diabetes

KEY ASSESSMENTS

- Hyperreflexia
- Twitching
- Cardiac arrhythmias
- Seizures
- Confusion or lethargy
- Respiratory (arrest may occur)
- Nausea and vomiting
- Diarrhea

PLANNING AND IMPLEMENTATION

- Monitor cardiac status
- Limited activities
- Monitor neurological status
- Anticipate replacing magnesium
- Monitor muscle strength
- Monitor respiratory status
- Monitor serum magnesium levels
- Monitor calcium and potassium levels

NURSING DIAGNOSIS

- Cardiac output, Decreased
- Injury, Risk for

Hyponatremia

DEFINITION

- Hyponatremia is a deficiency of sodium ions with a serum sodium level of less than 135 mEq/L. This deficiency may be from a loss of sodium ions or from excess body water that dilutes the sodium in the bloodstream. Excess antidiuretic hormone (ADH) causes water retention with dilution of serum sodium.

Clinical Causes That Increase ADH Secretions

- Elective surgery
- Pain and nausea
- Head injuries or tumors (syndrome of inappropriate antidiuretic hormone [SIADH])
- Lung conditions, such as cancer or tuberculosis
- Patients receiving hypotonic solutions
- Diuretic use, especially thiazide diuretics
- Excessive free water ingestion
- Renal disorders
- Loss of gastrointestinal (GI) secretions (vomiting, diarrhea, bulimia, or tap water enemas)
- Burns
- Congestive heart failure (CHF)

KEY ASSESSMENTS

- Change in level of consciousness (LOC), ranging from headaches to seizures
- Muscle weakness
- Signs of fluid volume overload (edema, distended neck veins, or crackles)
- Nausea, vomiting, diarrhea, or abdominal cramps
- Serum sodium levels
- Decreased urine output

PLANNING AND IMPLEMENTATION

- Monitor LOC
- Monitor for weakness or unsteady gait
- Monitor vital signs for signs of fluid volume overload or deficiency
- Monitor intake and output (I & O)
- Daily weight
- Restrict fluids if excess water exists
- Seizure precautions
- Monitor sodium levels
- Judicious replacement of sodium
- Diuretic administration
- Restrict all free water (fluids that are hypotonic)
- Administer medications to counteract ADH
- Teach patient about cause of hyponatremia

NURSING DIAGNOSIS

- Injury, Risk for
- Fluid volume, Risk for imbalanced

Hypoparathyroidism

DEFINITION

- Hypoparathyroidism is the clinical state in which there is a failure to secrete parathyroid hormone (PTH) or to respond to PTH.

Clinical Causes

- Idiopathic
- Infections

- Accidental surgical removal of the parathyroid glands with thyroid surgery

KEY ASSESSMENTS

- Laryngospasm
- Tetany
- Trousseau's sign (carpopedal spasms)
- Chvostek's sign (facial twitching)
- Muscle cramping
- Lethargy
- Numbness of lips and hands
- Prolonged QT intervals on electrocardiogram (ECG)

Lab Tests

- Calcium (low)
- Phosphorus (high)

PLANNING AND IMPLEMENTATION

- Monitor for Chvostek's and Trousseau's sign
- Keep emergency tracheotomy equipment
- Monitor respiratory status
- Monitor deep tendon reflexes
- Initiate intravenous (IV) line
- Administer calcium gluconate intravenously
- Monitor muscle strength and for the presence of tetany
- Administer calcium and vitamin D supplements
- Restrict foods high in calcium
- Monitor calcium and phosphorus levels

NURSING DIAGNOSIS

- Injury, Risk for
- Knowledge, Deficient

Hypophosphatemia

DEFINITION

- Hypophosphatemia is a deficiency of phosphorus ions with a serum phosphorus level less than 2.5 mEq/L. Hypophosphatemia may be caused by a decreased ingestion of phosphate or by increased renal excretion. Phosphorus is important in neuromuscular and cellular energy.

Clinical Causes

- Diet poor in phosphorus
- Chronic alcoholism
- Excessive intake of magnesium or calcium antacids

KEY ASSESSMENTS

- Muscle weakness
- Respiratory failure
- Irritability and confusion
- Hyporeflexia
- Poor muscle tone
- Decreased bowel sounds
- Cardiac monitoring for arrhythmias

PLANNING AND IMPLEMENTATION

- Cardiac monitoring
- Limit activities due to weakness
- Monitor neurological status
- Monitor respiratory status
- Monitor gastrointestinal (GI) status
- Anticipate administering phosphorus
- Monitor phosphorus levels

NURSING DIAGNOSIS

- Cardiac output, Decreased
- Injury, Risk for

Hypopituitarism

DEFINITION

- Hypopituitarism is the inability to synthesize and secrete hormones from the pituitary gland.

Clinical Causes

- Invasive—space lying lesion
- Infarction—ischemic damage to the pituitary

- Infiltrative disease—sarcoidosis or hemochromatosis
- Injury—traumatic head injury
- Iatrogenic—surgical and radiation
- Infections
- Idiopathic
- Immunological—autoimmune process

KEY ASSESSMENTS

- Fatigue
- Weakness
- Sensitivity to cold
- Infertility
- Hypotension
- Visual disturbances
- Short stature

Diagnostics

- Computed tomography (CT)
- Magnetic resonance imaging (MRI)

Lab Tests

- Growth hormone
- Thyroid-stimulating hormone (TSH)
- Prolactin
- Luteinizing hormone
- Follicle-stimulating hormone
- Antidiuretic hormone

PLANNING AND IMPLEMENTATION

- If tumor present, anticipate surgical removal
- Anticipate administering supplemental hormones (thyroid, sex, and growth)
- Monitor blood pressure
- Discuss infertility concerns

NURSING DIAGNOSIS

- Knowledge, Deficient
- Sexual pattern, Ineffective

Hypothyroidism

DEFINITION

- Hypothyroidism is the clinical state in which there is deficient production of thyroid hormone by the thyroid gland. The disease may range from mild symptoms to myxedema coma, a medical emergency.

Clinical Causes

- Hashimoto's thyroiditis
- Thyroidectomy
- Radioiodine therapy
- Medications (lithium or antithyroid medications)
- Pituitary disturbances

KEY ASSESSMENTS

- Fatigue
- Weight gain
- Dry skin
- Cold intolerance
- Bradycardia
- Constipation
- Paresthesia
- Muscle weakness
- Confusion

Lab Tests

- Low thyroxine (T_4)
- Elevated thyroid-stimulating hormone (TSH)
- Normal triiodothyronine (T_3)

PLANNING AND IMPLEMENTATION

- Provide frequent rest periods
- Monitor vital signs
- Monitor for symptomatic bradycardia (dizziness or confusion)
- Provide warm environment
- Encourage fluid intake
- Monitor and treat constipation
- Monitor effects of mediations (increased sensitivity to sedatives and narcotics)

- Monitor for paresthesias
- Daily weight
- Administer medications (Levothyroxine [T_4] is the drug of choice; liothyronine [T_3] may be administered as well.)
- Monitor for side effects of therapy
- Monitor for myxedema coma—decreased level of consciousness (LOC), hypothermia, hypotension, bradycardia, or hypoventilation
- Anticipate treatment for myxedema coma: admit to the intensive care unit, administer oxygen therapy, initiate IV therapy, begin fluid resuscitation, cardiac monitoring, frequent vital signs, thyroid replacement IV, maintain adequate body temperature, and monitor LOC

SPECIAL CONCERNS

Gender Considerations

- Women are more commonly affected with hypothyroidism.

Geriatric Considerations

- Elderly patients are more commonly affected with hypothyroidism.

NURSING DIAGNOSIS

- Constipation
- Activity intolerance
- Fatigue

Inflammatory Process

DEFINITION

- The inflammatory process is a protective mechanism the body mounts in response to an injury. The injury may be from bacteria, trauma, chemicals, heat, cold, surgery, and many other agents.
- Leukocytes, the general name for all white blood cells, make up a defense system that responds to any invasion by an organism. Neutrophils are rapidly released when an invasion first occurs, and once they are depleted, the body will put out immature cells known as bands.

- A rise in bands and neutrophils is often called *a shift to the left* and is a lab marker of an acute infection.
- The leukocytes carry out phagocytosis, a process in which foreign substances are ingested and destroyed.
- Chronic inflammation is greater than two weeks in duration and is often caused by a persistent irritant, such as a foreign body or bacteria like mycobacterium tuberculous. The body will try to wall off the area with fibrous tissue and form a granuloma.
- Many diseases produce an inflammatory response, including infectious diseases like bacteria, viruses, and fungi.
- Many diseases are caused by an inflammatory response, such as arthritis, obesity, and asthma.

Antibiotic Resistant Organisms

- Antibiotic resistant organisms are no longer destroyed by usual antibiotic therapy. This is a special concern with patients with human immunodeficiency virus (HIV) because of antibiotic resistant strains of mycobacterium tuberculosis. In acute care settings three specific antibiotic resistant organisms are of concern.
  - Methicillin-resistant staphylococcus aureus (MRSA)
  - Vancomycin-resistant enterococcus (VRE)
  - Vancomycin-resistant staphylococcus aureus (VRSA)
- To prevent the emergence of new antibiotic resistant organisms, health care professionals need to be vigilant in using infection control measures and proper antibiotic therapy treatment.

Transmission Routes for Infection

- Direct contact transmission—there is body surface–to–body surface contact.
- Indirect contact transmission—there is an inanimate object involved in the transfer, such as handling contaminated instruments.
- Droplet transmission—infectious particles are propelled through the air short distances and deposited on the host.
- Airborne transmission—the infectious particle is trapped on dust and carried on air currents. (They can travel much farther than droplets.) Special air filtration equipment is required.
- Common vehicle transmission—the infectious material is the organism that is carried in food, water, or other commonly shared materials.
- Vector borne transmission—the infectious material is carried by a living organism, such as a rat or mosquito.

KEY ASSESSMENTS

- Monitor temperature for elevation, respirations for increase, blood pressure for decrease, and heart rate for increase, because all may be signs of infection.
- Any fever more than 101° F (38.3° C) should be reported to the health care provider.
- Cultures should be obtained before antipyretics or antibiotics are given with a new fever.
- The most common sites for infection include respiratory, urinary tract blood (sepsis), and wounds.
- Neurological—check orientation status. A decrease in level of consciousness (LOC) may be related to infection.
- Respiratory—auscultate breath sound for advantageous sounds, the rate, and quality and observe for the presence of sputum. Check pulse oximetry readings.
- Cardiovascular—auscultate heart sounds for rate, rhythm, and quality. Tachycardia may be present with infection.
- Gastrointestinal (GI)—check abdomen for distention, pain, or presence of bowel sounds.
- Genitourinary (GU)—check color, odor, and amount of urine; question pain with urination.
- Skin—check for intactness, redness, swelling, pain, drainage, and turgor and assess mucous membranes for dry lips and mouth.
- Monitor laboratory reports for leukocyte count and any culture reports.
- Monitor creatinine levels with nephrotoxic antibiotics.
- Monitor chest X-rays (CXRs) for pneumonia.

PLANNING AND IMPLEMENTATION

(See Tables 9–11)

Preventing Infections

- Use good hand-washing and frequent use of alcohol-based hand cleaner
- Follow Centers for Disease Control (CDC) guidelines for infection control
- Assume every patient is at risk for infection
- Discontinue unnecessary invasive lines when possible; rotate intravenous (IV) sites per CDC guidelines

Managing Infections

- Treat with medication appropriate for the infection (i.e., antibiotics with bacterial infection or antivirals for viral infections)

- Treat any pain associated with the infection
- Treat fevers with antipyretics
- Keep the room cool and provide tepid baths
- Closely monitor intake and output (I & O) for fluid volume deficit
- Encourage fluids by mouth when appropriate
- Encourage adequate diet intake

NURSING DIAGNOSIS

- Infection, Risk for
- Body temperature, Risk for imbalanced
- Pain
- Skin integrity, Risk for impaired
- Tissue perfusion, Ineffective

Irritable Bowel Syndrome (IBS)

DEFINITION

- IBS is a motility disorder with an unknown cause. Stress, smoking, alcohol consumption, and a diet high in fat exacerbate IBS symptoms.

KEY ASSESSMENTS

- Abdominal pain
- Diarrhea
- Constipation
- Bloating
- Flatulence

Diagnostics

- Health history and diagnostic tests ruling out other gastrointestinal (GI) disorders

PLANNING AND IMPLEMENTATION

- Administer bulk-forming laxatives and antispasmodics as ordered
- Encourage fluid and food intake by mouth
- Monitor intake and output (I & O)
- Take daily weight
- Monitor stools

TABLE 9

Concept Map: Inflammatory Process

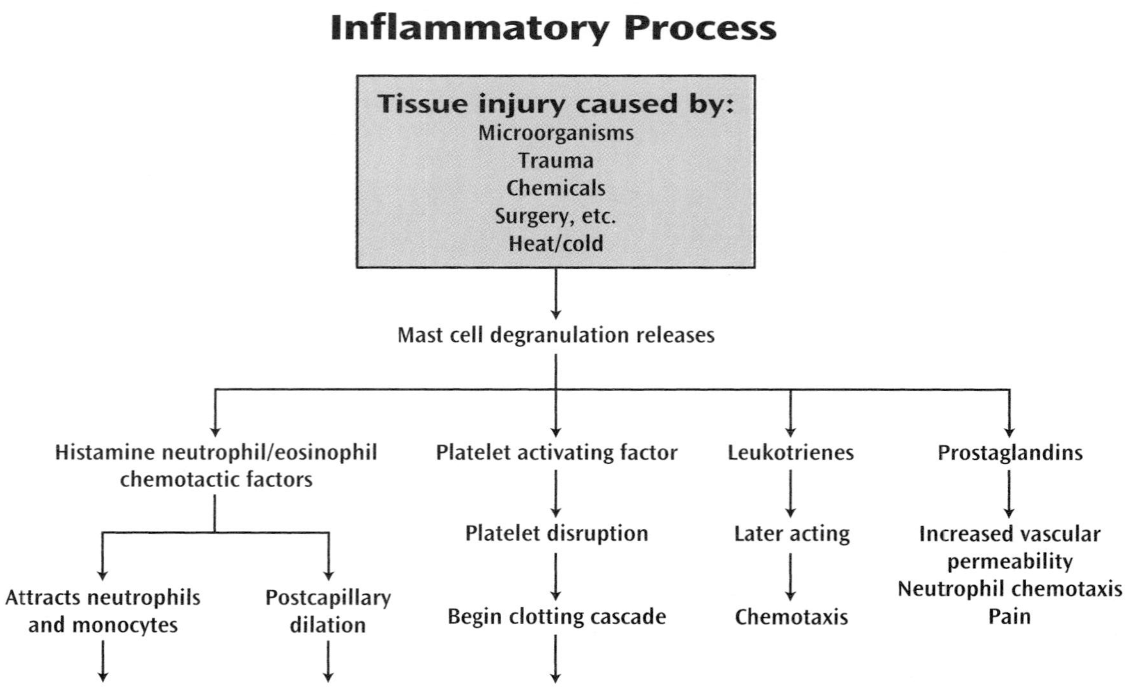
Inflammatory Process
Tissue injury caused by:
Microorganisms
Trauma
Chemicals
Surgery, etc.
Heat/cold
Mast cell degranulation releases
Histamine neutrophil/eosinophil chemotactic factors
Attracts neutrophils and monocytes
Postcapillary dilation
Platelet activating factor
Platelet disruption
Begin clotting cascade
Leukotrienes
Later acting
Chemotaxis
Prostaglandins
Increased vascular permeability
Neutrophil chemotaxis
Pain

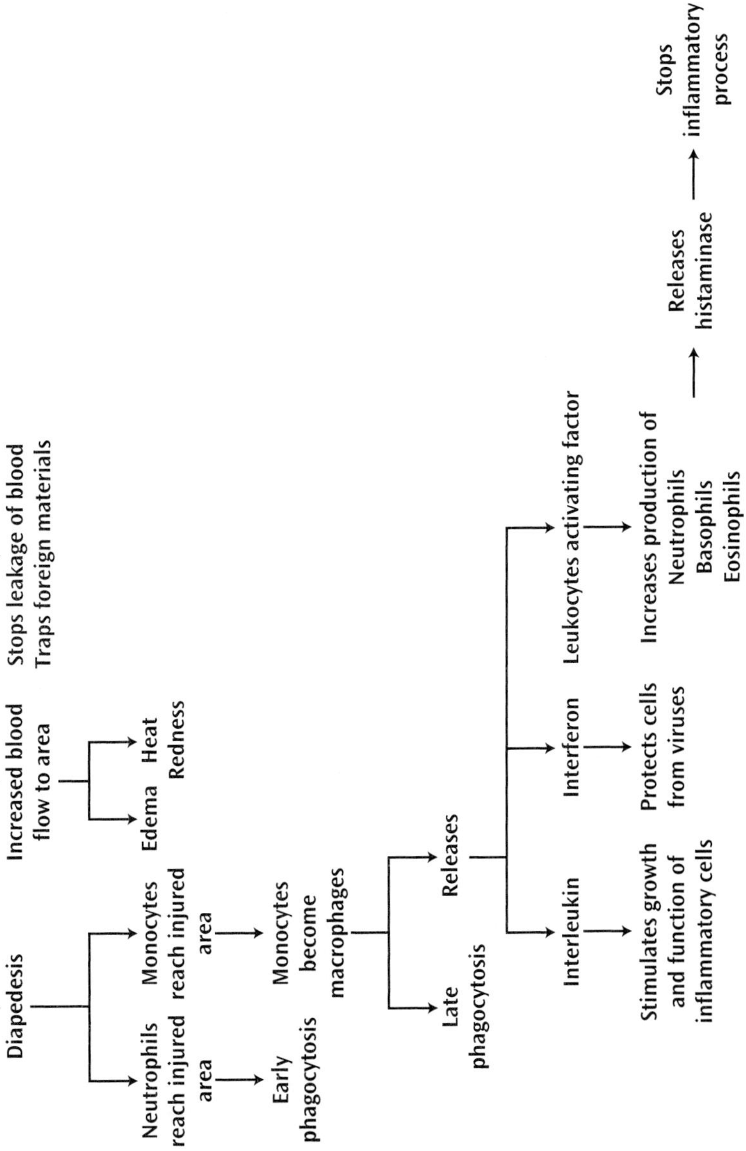
Diapedesis
Neutrophils reach injured area
Monocytes reach injured area
Early phagocytosis
Monocytes become macrophages
Late phagocytosis
Releases
Interleukin
Interferon
Leukocytes activating factor
Stimulates growth and function of inflammatory cells
Protects cells from viruses
Increases production of Neutrophils Basophils Eosinophils
Releases histaminase
Stops inflammatory process
Increased blood flow to area
Edema
Heat
Redness
Stops leakage of blood
Traps foreign materials

TABLE 10

Guidelines for Infection Control: Standard Precautions for All Patients in a Health Care Setting

Situation	Action
When touching any body fluid, secretion, or contaminated item	Nonsterile gloves Wash hands after removing gloves
Possibility of splashes or sprays from body fluids	Masks, eye protection, or face shields
Exposure to blood, body fluids, secretions, excretions	Gown: Remove before leaving patient room Wash hands after gown removal
Patient care equipment exposed to body fluids and secretions	Clean before use with another patient
Linens	Transport in closed containers Laundry facilities adequate to destroy pathogens

TABLE 11

Center for Disease Control (CDC) Guidelines

Situation	Action
Airborne transmission	Place patient in room in which air is filtered before entering general circulation. Keep door shut. Use respiratory mask with high-efficiency particulate air (HEPA) filter. Patient transport must be limited. Patient must wear mask during transport.
Droplet transmission	Place patient in private room if possible, or keep patient at least three feet from another patient. Room door can remain open. Staff must wear mask if working within three feet of patient. Limit patient transport. Patient must wear mask during transport.
Contact transmission	Place patient in private room if possible. Wear gown and gloves when contacting patient. Change gloves and wash hands during dressing changes: after removing old dressing and before applying new dressing. Use of equipment should be dedicated to one patient. Equipment must be cleaned before use with another patient.

SPECIAL CONCERNS

- Women are affected three times more often than men.

Teaching Considerations

- Avoid alcohol
- Promote smoking cessation
- Use stress-reducing techniques
- Identify food and stress triggers that exacerbate symptoms
- Avoid gas-forming foods
- Encourage a low-fat diet
- Encourage adequate water intake

NURSING DIAGNOSIS

- Constipation
- Diarrhea
- Pain, Acute
- Therapeutic regimen management, Ineffective

Labyrinthitis

DEFINITION

- Labyrinthitis is inflammation of the labyrinth section of the inner ear; causes include bacterial or viral infection and head trauma.

KEY ASSESSMENTS

- Vertigo
- Hearing loss
- Nystagmus
- Nausea and vomiting
- Recent head trauma
- Recent upper respiratory infection or ear infection
- Otoscopic examination—reveals inflammation of the labyrinth

PLANNING AND IMPLEMENTATION

- Decrease stimuli
- Administer antibiotics and anticholinergic medications
- Monitor hearing
- Assist with activities of daily living

- Provide small, frequent meals
- Implement safety measures

NURSING DIAGNOSIS

- Falls, Risk for
- Sensory perception, Disturbed

Laryngitis

DEFINITION

- Laryngitis is inflammation of the larynx from infection, voice misuse, environmental pollutants, or exposure to noxious agents. It may be acute and self-limiting or chronic.

KEY ASSESSMENTS

- Hoarseness or dysphonia (complete loss of voice)
- Sore throat
- Fatigue
- Fever

PLANNING AND IMPLEMENTATION

- Encourage resting the voice
- Encourage smoking cessation
- Encourage avoidance of environmental irritants
- Promote rest
- Encourage increased intake of cool liquids
- Administer appropriate antibiotics if the cause is bacterial

NURSING DIAGNOSIS

- Fatigue
- Pain, Acute

Latex Allergy

DEFINITION

- Latex allergy is an allergic reaction to proteins found in latex rubber. Risk for developing allergic symptoms increases with repeated latex exposure. Symptoms range from mild to anaphylaxis (a severe reaction that may result in death).

KEY ASSESSMENTS

Mild

- Skin redness, rash, hives, and pruritus
- Rhinitis, sneezing, or sore throat

Anaphylaxis

- Dyspnea
- Wheezing
- Airway angioedema
- Tachycardia
- Hypotension
- Chest pain
- Cardiac arrest

PLANNING AND IMPLEMENTATION

Mild Symptoms

- Remove latex product
- Anticipate administering antihistamines and topical steroids

Anaphylaxis

- Administer high-flow oxygen
- Keep intubation equipment at bedside
- Initiate two large-bore peripheral intravenous (IV) lines
- Maintain blood pressure with isotonic IV fluids
- Administer epinephrine, histamine (H_1, H_2) antagonist, and steroids IV as ordered
- Anticipate administering inhaled beta agonists
- Stop offending agent if possible
- Place patient in recumbent position
- Monitor cardiac status
- Monitor pulse oximetry continuously
- Monitor vital signs every two to three minutes until resolved

SPECIAL CONCERNS

- Use latex-free products in the hospital to prevent the possibility of developing a latex allergy
- Avoid latex condom use

NURSING DIAGNOSIS

- Airway clearance, Ineffective
- Skin integrity, Risk for impaired
- Knowledge, Deficient

Leukemia

DEFINITION

- Leukemia is a malignancy of bone marrow cells that occurs when stem cells lose the ability to differentiate into white blood cells (WBCs), red blood cells (RBCs), and platelets. Instead, an abnormal white blood count prevails and normal cell line development declines. No single factor has been identified as the cause of leukemia. The type of onset and the predominant cell involved classifies leukemia.

Classifications

- Acute myeloid leukemia is characterized by an abrupt onset and rapid progression, and the incidence rises sharply at age 60 years.
- Acute lymphocytic leukemia is characterized by an acute onset and rapid progression, most commonly affects children younger than 15 years, and has an 85 percent cure rate.
- Chronic myeloid leukemia has a gradual onset and relatively long survival period with increased incidence at ages 45 to 50 years.
- Chronic lymphocytic leukemia usually affects people older than age 65 years, may be symptomless, and may be discovered during routine blood work.

KEY ASSESSMENTS

- Anemia with fatigue
- Dyspnea
- Frequent infections and flu-like symptoms
- Enlarged lymph nodes

- Bleeding, bruising, and petechiae
- Bone and joint pain

Lab Tests

- Complete blood count (CBC), red blood count, and platelet count
- Bone marrow biopsy is necessary for definitive diagnosis to determine cell type

PLANNING AND IMPLEMENTATION

- Implement infection control and prevention
- Treat nausea
- Space activities to prevent further fatigue
- Monitor for stomatitis
- Monitor nutritional intake
- Monitor for dehydration from poor oral intake
- Use aseptic technique on all invasive lines
- Monitor for signs of bleeding
- Place patient in private room if possible
- Monitor white and red blood counts and platelet count
- Monitor dyspnea and administer oxygen if needed
- Administer blood and blood products
- Treat leukemia—radiation therapy, chemotherapy, stem cell transplant, or bone marrow transplant depending on the type of leukemia

SPECIAL CONCERNS

- See Special Procedures and Treatments for information on Cancer, Pain, and Palliative Care.

Teaching Considerations

- Teach patients about the effects of leukemia and its treatments
- Encourage emotional support
- Stress infection prevention
- Tell patients that chemotherapy may cause hair loss and skin changes
- Inform patients that frequent rest periods are necessary to combat fatigue
- Address possible sterility and reproductive issues resulting from chemotherapy
- Instruct patients about frequent oral care to prevent stomatitis

NURSING DIAGNOSIS

- Nausea
- Nutrition, less than body requirements, Imbalanced
- Fatigue
- Infection, Risk for

Liver Trauma

DEFINITION

- Liver trauma occurs as the result of a blunt or penetrating injury to the liver.

KEY ASSESSMENTS

- Right upper quadrant pain
- Hypovolemic shock (tachycardia, hypotension, or tachypnea)
- Abdominal distention or rigidity

Diagnostics

- Computed tomography (CT) of the abdomen

Lab Tests

- Liver function tests
- Complete blood count (CBC)
- Prothrombin time (PT), partial thromboplastin time (PTT), and international normalized ratio (INR)
- Type and cross-match for blood products

PLANNING AND IMPLEMENTATION

- Insert two large-bore peripheral intravenous (IV) lines
- Obtain blood consents
- Fluid volume replacement
- Administer blood products
- Monitor CBC
- Frequent vital signs
- Oxygen therapy
- Monitor pulse oximetry
- Treat pain
- Stop bleeding with exploratory laparotomy if indicated

NURSING DIAGNOSIS

- Fluid volume, Deficient
- Pain, Acute
- Tissue perfusion, Ineffective
- Infection, Risk for

Lyme Disease

DEFINITION

- Lyme disease is caused by the spirochete *Borrelia burgdorferi* and is transmitted to humans by the bite of a deer tick. The tick is the size of a pinhead, and the bite often goes unnoticed. The tick attaches to the host and remains in place 36–48 hours to transmit the spirochete. Symptoms develop in 7–14 days.

KEY ASSESSMENTS

First Stage

- Low-grade fever
- Fatigue
- Muscle and bone aches
- Chills
- Malaise
- Erythema migrans (a circular rash that continues to grow resembling a bulls-eye)

Second Stage

- Numbness and pain in the arms and legs
- Unilateral facial paralysis
- Meningitis
- Cardiac arrhythmias

Third Stage

- Arthritis
- Chronic pain
- Restless sleep
- Memory loss
- Keratitis (inflammation of the cornea)
- Papilledema (edema of the optic disk)
- Conjunctival erythema

Lab Tests

- Enzyme-linked immunosorbent assay (ELISA), positive two to six weeks after transmission
- Western blot

PLANNING AND IMPLEMENTATION

- Promote rest
- Monitor cardiac status
- Administer antipyretics for fever and nonsteroidal anti-inflammatory drugs (NSAIDS) for arthralgias
- Administer doxycycline (drug of choice)

SPECIAL CONCERNS

Teaching Considerations

- Wear long-sleeve tops and long pants if tick exposure is likely
- Use insect repellents that contain N,N-diethyl-meta-toluamide (DEET)
- Check for the presence of ticks after exposure
- Observe for erythema migrans

NURSING DIAGNOSIS

- Infection, Risk for
- Knowledge, Deficient
- Skin integrity, Risk for impaired

Lymphomas

DEFINITION

- Lymphomas are malignancies in the lymph tissue. Increased levels of lymphocytes, histocytes, and their precursors define lymphomas. The lymphomas are the sixth leading cause of death, and the incidence has increased in the past 35 years.

Classifications

- Hodgkin's disease is a lymphatic cancer that develops in lymph nodes. Affected lymph nodes contain Reed-Sternberg cells. Hodgkin's disease is labeled in stages I through IV. The earlier it is diagnosed the better the prognosis.

- Non-Hodgkin's lymphoma is characterized by a malignant mutation of the lymphoid system and may be considered aggressive or indolent. It may involve extranodal areas including soft tissue and bones.

KEY ASSESSMENTS

- Lymph node enlargement, painless or painful
- Fever, weight loss
- Night sweats
- Generalized malaise

Diagnostics

- Computed tomography (CT)
- Chest X-ray (CXR)
- Positron emission tomography (PET) of the body
- Lymph node biopsy
- Bone marrow biopsy

Lab Tests

- Complete blood count (CBC)
- Sedimentation rate
- Beta$_2$-microglobulin

PLANNING AND IMPLEMENTATION

- Anticipate treatment to include radiation, chemotherapy, or both
- Provide meticulous skin care
- Monitor for infection
- Use aseptic technique for all invasive lines
- Treat nausea
- Promote adequate nutritional intake
- Discuss reproductive concerns
- Monitor glucose levels
- Monitor CBC
- Promote rest periods to combat fatigue
- Monitor respiratory system and teach to report dyspnea
- Anticipate administering blood products, granulocyte colony-stimulating factor, and Epogen products

SPECIAL CONCERNS

- See Special Procedures and Treatments for information on Cancer, Pain, and Palliative Care.

NURSING DIAGNOSIS

- Fatigue
- Infection, Risk for nausea
- Nutrition: less than body requirements, Imbalanced

Macular Degeneration

DEFINITION

- Macular degeneration is a painless, gradual breakdown of the macula from metabolic wastes that accumulate in the retina. Family history is a significant risk factor. Progression is slow and results in mild to moderate visual loss.

KEY ASSESSMENTS

- Blurred vision
- Blind spot in the middle of the visual field

Diagnostics

- Ophthalmological examination of macular degeneration
- Eye angiography

PLANNING AND IMPLEMENTATION

- Use visual aids
- Monitor visual acuity
- Laser treatment (may slow progression)

SPECIAL CONCERNS

Gender Considerations

- Women are at greater risk than men to develop macular degeneration.

NURSING DIAGNOSIS

- Sensory perception, Disturbed
- Knowledge, Deficient

Malnutrition

DEFINITION

- Malnutrition is an altered nutritional state in which there is a deficiency of one or more nutrients.

Clinical Causes

- Malnutrition arises from various conditions that either increase nutritional needs, decrease the ability to ingest nutrients, or decrease the ability to absorb nutrients.
- Some conditions that may cause malnutrition include cancer, chemotherapy, depression, pain, infection, burns, Crohn's disease, pancreatitis, liver disease, acquired immunodeficiency syndrome (AIDS), gastrectomy, anorexia nervosa, and myasthenia gravis.

KEY ASSESSMENTS

- Marasmus (long-term undernutrition of calories and protein), severe muscle wasting, weakness, and a decrease in functioning
- Kwashiorkor weakness (short-term protein depletion), lethargy, and peripheral edema
- Weight loss
- Inadequate oral intake of protein, carbohydrates, fats, vitamins, and minerals
- Dry skin
- Delayed wound healing
- Hair loss
- Decrease in level of consciousness (LOC), impairing ability to ingest by mouth (PO)
- Difficulty swallowing or chewing

Lab Tests

- Albumin
- Transferrin
- Prealbumin (more sensitive for short-term changes in nutritional status)
- Hemoglobin and hematocrit (anemia)

PLANNING AND IMPLEMENTATION

- Take daily weight
- Monitor intake & output (I & O)

- Monitor caloric intake
- Monitor labs
- Provide frequent oral hygiene
- Monitor ability to swallow
- Treat nausea and vomiting
- Monitor LOC
- Provide meticulous skin care and document assessments
- Monitor for diarrhea and treat if present
- Provide oral supplements including high-calorie foods and beverages, adding vitamin and mineral supplements
- Offer small, frequent meals that are easy to chew and swallow
- Provide enteral or parental nutrition if patient unable to ingest oral supplements

SPECIAL CONCERNS

- Obese patients can experience malnutrition when intake is less than the body requirements.

Cultural Considerations

- Most hospital diets do not offer culturally appropriate foods. Encourage family members to bring food from home for the patient.

Geriatric Considerations

- Poor dentition is a cause of malnutrition in the geriatric population.

NURSING DIAGNOSIS

- Knowledge, Deficient
- Nutrition: less than body requirements, Imbalanced
- Infection, Risk for
- Swallowing, Impaired

Mammary Duct Ectasia

DEFINITION

- Mammary duct ectasia is a noncancerous breast condition in which the milk ducts beneath the nipple become dilated. It occurs most often during or after menopause.

Clinical Causes

- Smoking, hormonal changes, vitamin A deficiency, or inverted nipples

KEY ASSESSMENTS

- Breast and nipple tenderness
- White or green nipple discharge
- Redness or lump noted near nipple

Diagnostics

- Mammogram
- Needle biopsy

PLANNING AND IMPLEMENTATION

- Administer oral antibiotics.
- Apply warm compresses over affected area.
- If conservative treatment is not effective, surgical excision of the affected ducts may be indicated.

NURSING DIAGNOSIS

- Pain, Acute
- Infection, Risk for
- Knowledge, Deficient

Mastoiditis

DEFINITION

- Mastoiditis is an infection of the mastoid sinus, which occurs two to three weeks after otitis media, a middle ear infection.

KEY ASSESSMENTS

- Ear pain
- Headache
- Redness behind the ear
- Fever
- Ear drainage
- History of recent ear infection
- Hearing loss

Diagnostics

- Skull X-ray or computed tomography (CT)

PLANNING AND IMPLEMENTATION

- Treat pain.
- Monitor for hearing loss.
- Monitor for facial paralysis.
- Anticipate administering long-term antibiotics.
- Rarely, a mastoidectomy (removal of infected bone tissue) is performed.

NURSING DIAGNOSIS

- Pain, Acute
- Knowledge, Deficient

Menière's Disease

DEFINITION

- Menière's disease is a disorder thought to be caused by a range of inflammatory, traumatic, autoimmune, or idiopathic events that lead to the eventual dysfunction for the vestibulocochlear nerve (cranial nerve eight [CN 8]). It is characterized by episodic vertigo, hearing loss, tinnitus, and nystagmus.

Clinical Causes

- Syphilis and head trauma are known causes of Menière's disease.
- Higher incidence of Menière's disease is present in patients with herpes simplex virus and hypothyroidism.

KEY ASSESSMENTS

- Vertigo
- Reports of ear fullness
- Hearing loss
- Tinnitus
- Nystagmus

Diagnostics

- Hearing tests
- Caloric test

- Magnetic resonance imaging (MRI), to rule out tumors
- Electrocochleography, assesses electrical activity of the inner ear

PLANNING AND IMPLEMENTATION

- Implement safety measures.
- Assess and monitor gait.
- Speak slowly and clearly.
- Monitor and treat nausea.
- Encourage a low-sodium diet.
- Anticipate administering diuretics, antihistamines, antiemetics, or corticosteroids.
- Surgical interventions removing the vestibular portion of CN 8 may be necessary.

Discharge Planning

- Consider home safety and driving concerns before discharge.

SPECIAL CONCERNS

- Actively listen to patients concerns because the disease can be disabling.

Geriatric Considerations

- Menière's disease occurs more commonly in patients older than 60 years.

NURSING DIAGNOSIS

- Sensory perception, Disturbed
- Injury, Risk for
- Home maintenance, Impaired

Metabolic Acidosis

DEFINITION

- Metabolic acidosis is a metabolic state in which there is an addition of acid to the body or a loss of base. Regardless of the cause, there is an accumulation of acid, which is a central nervous system (CNS) depressant. Guidelines to determine metabolic acidosis are pH less than 7.35, HCO_3 less than 24, and CO_2 less than 22.

Clinical Causes

- Renal failure
- Diabetes
- Diabetes ketoacidosis
- Inadequate oxygenation of tissues
- Severe diarrhea
- Anaerobic metabolism
- Salicylate or methanol overdose

KEY ASSESSMENTS

- Kussmaul respirations (deep, rapid respirations)
- Respiratory and oxygenation status
- Diarrhea
- Abdominal pain
- Nausea and vomiting
- Warm, flushed skin
- Bradycardia or arrhythmias
- Decreased peripheral pulses

PLANNING AND IMPLEMENTATION

- Institute safety measures
- Treat underlying cause
- Administer oxygen
- Monitor arterial blood gases (ABGs)
- Encourage fluids
- Administer insulin to diabetics if necessary
- Treat diarrhea if present
- Monitor cardiac status and report arrhythmias
- Order sodium bicarbonate

NURSING DIAGNOSIS

- Cardiac output, Decreased
- Breathing pattern, Ineffective

Metabolic Alkalosis

DEFINITION

- Metabolic alkalosis is a metabolic state in which there is a loss of acid or an accumulation of base. Regardless of cause, there is an acid deficit. Alkalosis results in central nervous system (CNS) irritability. Guidelines to determine metabolic alkalosis are pH greater than 7.45, HCO_3 greater than 28, and normal CO_2 reading of 35–45.

Clinical Causes

- Vomiting
- Aspiration of gastrointestinal (GI) contents
- Overuse of antacid medications

KEY ASSESSMENTS

- Confusion, irritability
- Hyperreflexia
- Observe for respiratory distress
- Vomiting

PLANNING AND IMPLEMENTATION

- Institute safety measures
- Control vomiting
- Monitor intake and output (I & O)
- Monitor neurological status
- Monitor respiratory status
- Monitor arterial blood gases (ABGs)

SPECIAL CONCERNS

- Avoid using baking soda as an antacid medication because this can put a patient at risk for metabolic alkalosis.

NURSING DIAGNOSIS

- Injury, Risk for
- Confusion, Acute

Mitral Regurgitation

DEFINITION

- Mitral regurgitation is a disorder in which the blood pumped from the left ventricle backs up into the left atrium during systole. Increased left atrium workload can lead to hypertrophy over time.

Mitral regurgitation stems from dysfunction of the mitral valve leaflets, the chordae tendinea, the annulus, or the papillary muscle.

- Streptococcal infection (rheumatic fever) is the most common cause of acquired mitral regurgitation.

KEY ASSESSMENTS

- May be asymptomatic
- Systolic murmur
- Fatigue
- Shortness of breath (SOB)
- Dizziness or syncope
- Palpitations
- Chest pain
- Anxiety

PLANNING AND IMPLEMENTATION

- Perform echocardiogram.
- Teach patients to avoid caffeine, alcohol, and smoking.
- Monitor vital signs.
- Monitor cardiac status.
- Administer prophylactic antibiotics before dental procedures.
- Encourage weight loss if patients are obese.
- Promote exercise.
- Educate patients and family about treatments.
- Surgical valve replacement may be necessary.
- If a mechanical valve is inserted, lifelong anticoagulation therapy may be necessary.

SPECIAL CONCERNS

- See Special Procedures and Treatments for information on Valve Repair and Valve Replacement.

NURSING DIAGNOSIS

- Knowledge, Deficient
- Anxiety

Mitral Stenosis

DEFINITION

- Mitral stenosis is a narrowing or constriction of the mitral valve opening. Increased resistance of the mitral valve causes increased pressure of the left atrium causing hypertrophy over time. Mitral stenosis is most commonly caused by rheumatic heart disease and can cause pulmonary hypertension if untreated.

KEY ASSESSMENTS

- May be asymptomatic
- Diastolic murmur
- Fatigue
- Shortness of breath (SOB)
- Peripheral edema
- Mitral facies (a dusky appearance with cyanosed cheeks)
- Cough with hemoptysis
- Chest pain
- Dysphagia

PLANNING AND IMPLEMENTATION

- Perform echocardiogram.
- Monitor vital signs.
- Monitor cardiac status.
- Educate patients and family about treatments.
- Surgical valve replacement may be necessary.
- If a mechanical valve is inserted, lifelong anticoagulation therapy may be necessary.
- Valvuloplasty is a procedure where a balloon-tipped catheter is inserted via a peripheral artery into the heart, and the balloon is inflated in the mitral valve. The inflation increases the diameter of the mitral valve.

SPECIAL CONCERNS

- See Special Procedures and Treatments for information on Valve Repair and Valve Replacement.

Gender Considerations

- Two thirds of all patients with mitral stenosis are female.

NURSING DIAGNOSIS

- Fatigue
- Breathing pattern, Ineffective

Mitral Valve Prolapse (MVP)

DEFINITION

- MVP is usually an asymptomatic condition in which the mitral valve leaflets stretch into the atria during systole. Long-term stretching keeps the leaflet unable to close during systole, allowing blood from the left ventricle to back up into the left atrium.

KEY ASSESSMENTS

- Patients may be asymptomatic
- Murmur, midsystolic click
- Fatigue
- Shortness of breath (SOB)
- Dizziness or syncope
- Palpitations
- Chest pain
- Anxiety

PLANNING AND IMPLEMENTATION

- Perform echocardiogram.
- Teach patients to avoid caffeine, alcohol, and smoking.
- Treat pain.
- Monitor vital signs.
- Monitor cardiac status.
- Prophylactic antibiotics are required before going through dental procedures.
- If patients are obese, encourage weight loss.
- Promote exercise.
- Educate patients and family about treatments.
- Medications such as beta blockers, calcium channel blockers, or antiarrhythmics may be ordered.
- Surgical valve replacement may be necessary.
- If a mechanical valve is inserted, lifelong anticoagulation therapy may be necessary.

SPECIAL CONCERNS

- See Special Procedures and Treatments for information on Valve Repair and Valve Replacement.

Gender Considerations

- Females are three times more likely to have MVP than males. The typical age of onset for MVP is between 10 and 16 years of age.

NURSING DIAGNOSIS

- Knowledge, Deficient
- Activity intolerance

Multiple Sclerosis (MS)

DEFINITION

- MS is an inflammatory disease of the white matter of the central nervous system (CNS). The inflammation destroys the myelin sheath, which alters impulse transmission. The cause of MS is unknown, and onset is usually between the ages of 20 and 40 years. MS is characterized by remissions and exacerbations, and disease progression varies from patient to patient.

Classifications

Clinical course of MS has four classifications or categories.

- Relapsing-remitting is characterized by recurrent episodes with either partial or complete recovery during remissions.
- Secondary progressive is characterized by gradual deterioration with or without remissions.
- Progressing-relapsing is characterized by gradual deterioration without remissions.
- Primary progressive is characterized by gradual deterioration with exacerbations.

KEY ASSESSMENTS

- Assessments vary among patients and are worse during exacerbations and usually better during remissions. Symptoms may include:
  - Numbness, paresthesia, or pain
  - Paresis or paralysis

- Diplopia
- Incontinence
- Loss of balance and coordination
- Nystagmus
- Speech disturbances
- Fatigue

Diagnostics

- There is no single diagnostic test that confirms or rules out MS. Lesions called plaques found on magnetic resonance imaging (MRI) help confirm the diagnosis in conjunction with physical symptoms.
- Lumbar puncture reveals oligoclonal bands on 85–90 percent of people with MS but may be present in other inflammatory diseases.

PLANNING AND IMPLEMENTATION

- Care is centered on the patient's symptoms.
- Implement safety precautions.
- Assist with activities of daily living.
- Monitor the ability to swallow.
- Use appropriate assistive devices to aid in mobility.
- Encourage range-of-motion exercises.
- Implement stress-reducing techniques.
- Anticipate administering medications including immunomodulators, immunosuppressants, corticosteroids, muscle relaxants, antiepileptics, antidepressants, and stimulant.
- An implantable baclofen pump may be inserted for severe spasticity.

Discharge Planning

- MS is a debilitating disease that may cause changes in employment status, socioeconomic status, personal relationships, and ability to parent effectively. All of these changes are stressful, and stress can cause exacerbations of the disease. Explore stress-reduction techniques that can be implemented in the home setting before discharge.

SPECIAL CONCERNS

Cultural Considerations

- MS occurs twice as frequently in Caucasians than in non-Caucasians.

Gender Considerations

- MS occurs seven times more frequently in Caucasian women than in Caucasian men.

NURSING DIAGNOSIS

- Fatigue
- Activity intolerance
- Health maintenance, Impaired
- Knowledge, Deficient

Myasthenia Gravis (MG)

DEFINITION

- MG is a chronic, progressive neuromuscular disease and is theorized to be caused by an autoimmune process. There is destruction and blockage of acetylcholine receptor sites and structural changes that diminish acetylcholine at the postsynaptic muscle junction. The loss of acetylcholine results in decreased muscle strength and profound fatigue. A thymoma (thymus gland tumor) is present in 10 percent of MG patients.

Classifications

- Ocular—weakness affects the eye and eyelid muscles only
- Bulbar—weakness affects muscles involved in breathing, swallowing, and speech
- Generalized—weakness affects the proximal muscles of the limbs and neck and has ocular and bulbar manifestations

KEY ASSESSMENTS

- Ptosis (eyelid drooping)
- Diplopia (double vision)
- Fatigue
- Muscle weakness
- Loss of facial expression
- Slurred speech
- Difficulty swallowing or eating
- Respiratory difficulty

Diagnostics

- Serum assay for circulating acetylcholine receptor antibodies.
- Electromyography (EMG).
- Computed tomography (CT).
- Tensilon test—the patient is given Tensilon intravenously. In patients with MG there is a rapid improvement of symptoms within 15 to 30 seconds. The nurse closely monitors the patient's heart rate (for bradycardia) and respiratory status (for respiratory arrest) during the testing. Atropine and airway equipment should be at the bedside during testing.

PLANNING AND IMPLEMENTATION

- Monitor airway and respiratory status.
- Monitor the ability to swallow.
- Monitor fluid and nutritional intake.
- Promote frequent oral care.
- Monitor gag reflex.
- Use nonverbal techniques and communication boards.
- Monitor for pulmonary infections (productive cough or fever).
- Provide frequent rest periods.
- Assist with activities of daily living.
- Keep emergency airway equipment on the unit in case of respiratory distress.
- Implement safety measures.
- Anticipate administering anticholinesterase and immunosuppressive medications.
- Observe for side effects of medications.
- Thymectomy may be performed if thymoma is present.
- Plasmapheresis may be performed.
- Monitor for signs of myasthenic crisis and cholinergic crisis (see Table 12).

SPECIAL CONCERNS

- The issue of ventilation and long-term ventilatory support should be addressed with the patient early in the disease. If the patient does not wish to receive mechanical ventilation, obtain advanced directives and do not intubate orders.

Gender Considerations

- More women than men (3:2) are diagnosed with MG.

TABLE 12

Clinical Comparisons of Myasthenic Crisis and Cholinergic Crisis

Myasthenic Crisis	Cholinergic Crisis
Respiratory distress	Increased muscle weakness
Apnea	Abdominal discomfort ■ Nausea or vomiting ■ Diarrhea ■ Abdominal cramps
Increased muscle weakness	Dysphagia
Dysarthria	Dysarthria
Anxiety	Apprehension; restlessness Respiratory distress

Teaching Considerations

- Teaching should address the physical, emotional, and social aspects of the disease.
- In the early stages of the disease encourage the patient to address long-term issues, such as estate planning and care options.
- Reinforce medication, nutrition, and safety teaching.
- Teach patients and families signs of myasthenic and cholinergic crisis.

NURSING DIAGNOSIS

- Fatigue
- Breathing pattern, Ineffective
- Ventilation, Impaired spontaneous
- Activity intolerance

Myocarditis

DEFINITION

- Myocarditis is an inflammation of the myocardium, the middle layer of the heart. Myocarditis may result from infectious agents (virus, bacteria, or fungus), parasitic agents (parasites, protozoa, or spirochetes), or toxic agents (poison, allergens, or immunosuppressants).

- Myocarditis may cause dilation of the heart, thrombi on the heart wall, and degeneration of the muscle fibers.

KEY ASSESSMENTS

- Fatigue
- Dyspnea
- Palpitations
- Chest discomfort
- Murmurs

PLANNING AND IMPLEMENTATION

- Treat underlying cause
- Monitor for signs of heart failure
- Monitor vital signs
- Monitor tissue perfusion
- Teach patient and family about treatments

NURSING DIAGNOSIS

- Fatigue
- Breathing pattern, Ineffective
- Knowledge, Deficient

Nephrosclerosis

DEFINITION

- Nephrosclerosis is sclerosing (scarring) of the small arteries in the kidney. This occurs with age and as atherosclerosis progresses.

KEY ASSESSMENTS

- Hypertension
- Renal failure (decreased urine output and increased creatinine [Cr])

Diagnostics

- Test urine for 24 hours for Cr clearance
- Intravenous pyelogram (IVP)
- Computed tomography (CT) of the kidney

Lab Tests

- Blood urea nitrogen (BUN), Cr, and glomerular filtration rate (GFR)

PLANNING AND IMPLEMENTATION

- Monitor blood pressure
- Administer antihypertensive agents
- Monitor urine output
- Monitor renal function labs and test
- May lead to renal failure requiring dialysis

SPECIAL CONCERNS

- See Special Procedures and Treatments for information on Dialysis.

NURSING DIAGNOSIS

- Urinary elimination, Impaired
- Fluid volume, Risk for imbalanced

Nephrotic Syndrome

DEFINITION

- Nephrotic syndrome refers to a group of symptoms including proteinuria, hypoalbuminemia, edema, hypercholesterolemia, and normal renal function caused by another illness.

Classifications

- Primary nephrotic syndrome is caused by collagen vascular disease, lupus, rheumatoid arthritis, sickle cell disease, diabetes mellitus, amyloidosis malignancies, medications, and heroin use.
- Secondary nephrotic syndrome occurs after infections including group A beta-hemolytic streptococci, syphilis, malaria, tuberculosis, human immunodeficiency virus (HIV), hepatitis B, and infectious mononucleosis.

KEY ASSESSMENTS

- Edema
- Anasarca (generalized edema throughout the body)

- Foamy urine
- Anorexia
- Irritability
- Fatigue
- Abdominal discomfort

Lab Tests

- Proteinuria
- Low serum albumin levels
- Hyperlipidemia
- Chest X-ray (CXR) may show pleural effusion

PLANNING AND IMPLEMENTATION

- Monitor intake and output (I & O)
- Take daily weight
- Encourage sodium restricted diet
- Monitor edema
- Monitor respiratory status
- Provide frequent rest periods
- Monitor serum and urine protein levels
- Administer steroid therapy
- Monitor for side effects of steroid therapy (sad, sugar, or sick)
- Surveil for infection
- Administer antibiotics if infection is present
- Administer diuretics

Discharge Planning

- Monitor edema
- Measure urine protein in the first void of the day and record
- Maintain a low-sodium diet
- State symptoms of infection and when to contact the health care provider
- Adhere to medication regimen

NURSING DIAGNOSIS

- Knowledge, Deficient
- Infection, Risk for
- Therapeutic regimen management, Ineffective
- Fluid volume, Risk for imbalanced

Obesity

DEFINITION

- Obesity is a body mass index (BMI) greater than 30. The cause of obesity is multifactorial, including excessive caloric consumption and inadequate exercise.
- Bariatrics is the field of medicine that offers treatment and support to obese patients. Obesity is a major public health concern. Approximately 66 percent of adults are obese, and the rate of childhood obesity has tripled over the last 30 years.

KEY ASSESSMENTS

- BMI greater than 30
- Waist circumference greater than 40 inches in men and 35 inches in women

Lab Tests

- Low-density lipoproteins (LDL), high-density lipoproteins (HDL), and cholesterol
- C-reactive protein (CRP)
- Glucose

PLANNING AND IMPLEMENTATION

- Use medical equipment that is safe for the bariatric patient (the weight load limit for medical equipment, such as wheelchairs and beds, is usually 250 pounds [113 kg])
- Take daily weight
- Elevate head of bed 30 degrees
- Implement safety measures
- Monitor glucose
- Monitor intake and output (I & O)
- Offer low-calorie foods
- Encourage physical activity
- Thoroughly assess skin
- Wash and dry under skin folds

SPECIAL CONCERNS

- See Special Procedures and Treatments for information on Bariatric Surgery.

Teaching Considerations

- Reduce body weight 10 percent within six months
- Reduce caloric intake
- Increase physical activity
- Modify behaviors to improve eating habits
- Read labels on food items
- Eat only a standard portion size
- Eat slowly
- Avoid high-calorie snacks
- Increase intake of vegetables and salads
- Do not skip meals (eat three balanced meals)

NURSING DIAGNOSIS

- Nutrition: more than body requirements, Imbalanced
- Lifestyle, Sedentary
- Knowledge, Deficient

Obstruction, Intestinal

DEFINITION

- An intestinal obstruction is the partial or complete obstruction of any portion of the bowel from a structural or functional impairment.

Clinical Causes

- Causes include abdominal surgery, presence of adhesions, pelvic malignancies, complete bedrest, opiate use, and abdominal infections.

Classifications

- Ileus, or paralytic ileus, refers to an intestinal obstruction due to a decrease or absence of intestinal peristalsis.
- Acute colonic pseudo obstruction (ACPO), or Ogilvie's syndrome, is an obstruction due to massive dilation of the colon.
- Malignant bowel obstruction is an obstruction caused by a tumor compressing the bowel.
- Simple obstruction refers to an obstruction in one site.
- Closed-loop obstruction is characterized by two sites of obstruction.
- Strangulated obstruction is an obstruction in which there is vascular compromise and lack of blood flow to the affected bowel.

KEY ASSESSMENTS

- Abdominal distention
- High-pitched, tinkling bowel sounds (early)
- Absence of bowel sounds (late)
- Abdominal pain and cramping
- Nausea
- Vomiting (may have stool in vomitus)
- No bowel movements (complete obstruction)
- Watery diarrhea (stool leaking around partial obstruction)
- Electrolyte imbalance
- Fluid volume deficit (hypotension or tachycardia)

Diagnostics

- Abdominal X-rays
- Abdominal ultrasound
- Computed tomography (CT) of abdomen

Lab Tests

- Electrolytes
- Arterial blood gases ([ABGs], metabolic acidosis with strangulated obstruction)
- Complete blood count ([CBC], increased white blood cells)

PLANNING AND IMPLEMENTATION

- Insert peripheral intravenous (IV) line.
- Administer isotonic fluids.
- Correct electrolyte imbalance.
- Monitor cardiac status.
- Frequently monitor vital signs.
- Initiate nothing by mouth (NPO).
- Insert nasogastric tube and apply low intermittent suction (LIS).
- Monitor intake and output (I & O).
- Monitor and document bowel movements.
- Frequently assess bowel sounds.
- Administer appropriate medications including prokinetic agents (metoclopramide), anticholinesterases, anticholinergics, antiemetics, analgesics, and antibiotics.
- If conservative treatment fails for strangulated obstruction, endoscopic or surgical intervention may be required.

NURSING DIAGNOSIS

- Pain, Acute
- Infection, Risk for
- Pain, Acute
- Fluid volume, Risk for deficient

Obstruction, Laryngeal

DEFINITION

- Laryngeal obstruction is a medical emergency causing airway obstruction. Swelling of the mucous membranes may cause obstruction from infection, a severe allergic reaction, or aspiration of a foreign body. Regardless of cause, if not promptly treated, death occurs.

KEY ASSESSMENTS

- Stridor
- Wheezing
- Dyspnea
- Cyanosis
- Patient's hands around throat signifying airway obstruction
- Loss of consciousness

PLANNING AND IMPLEMENTATION

- If obstruction is suspected, perform abdominal thrusts or the Heimlich maneuver.
- If swelling is suspected, anticipate administering epinephrine and steroids intravenously.
- If attempts to maintain airway are not quickly successful, contact health care provider to perform an emergency tracheostomy.
- Provide a calm environment because the patient will be anxious.
- Monitor vital signs frequently including continuous pulse oximetry.
- Administer oxygen.
- If patient becomes pulseless, initiate cardiopulmonary resuscitation (CPR).

SPECIAL CONCERNS

- See Special Procedures and Treatments for information on Intubation and Mechanical Ventilation.

NURSING DIAGNOSIS

- Ventilation, Impaired spontaneous
- Tissue perfusion, Ineffective
- Anxiety, Death

Orchitis

DEFINITION

- Orchitis is an acute inflammation of the testes usually caused by a viral, spirochetal, parasitic, or bacterial infection. Mumps is the most common viral cause, and 30 percent of orchitis is a result of a sexually transmitted disease.

KEY ASSESSMENTS

- Fever
- Erythema and edema of the groin, testicle, and scrotum
- Pain of the groin, testicle, and scrotum
- Dysuria
- Urethral discharge

History and Examination

- Recent mumps infection or unprotected sexual contact

Diagnostics

- Doppler ultrasonography (rule out testicular torsion)

Lab Tests

- Complete blood count (CBC)
- Urine and urethral discharge cultures

PLANNING AND IMPLEMENTATION

- Identify causative organism and initiate appropriate pharmacological interventions
- Administer antipyretics for fever
- Treat pain
- Elevate scrotum
- Monitor intake and output (I & O)
- Monitor vital signs

SPECIAL CONCERNS

- Thirty percent of men with orchitis from the mumps develop testicular atrophy and subsequent sterility.
- Explain infertility concerns with patients with mumps.

NURSING DIAGNOSIS

- Pain, Acute
- Hyperthermia
- Infection
- Knowledge, Deficient

Osteoarthritis (OA)

DEFINITION

- OA or degenerative joint disease (DJD) is a noninflammatory DJD characterized by degeneration of the articular cartilage, hypertrophy of the bone at margins, and changes in the synovial membrane. The incidence of OA increases with age, weight, and joint injury.

Classifications

- Primary OA refers to the development without any known reason.
- Secondary OA refers to the development of OA with a known cause, such as history of joint trauma or mechanical stressors (obesity or athletics).

KEY ASSESSMENTS

- Pain (aching)
- Stiffness
- Increased pain with use
- Mild joint swelling
- Warmth over joint
- Heberden's nodes (hard nodules of the tubercles of the fingers)
- Bouchard's nodes (bony enlargement of the proximal interphalangeal joints)
- Obesity

History and Examination

- History of trauma or mechanical stressor

Diagnostics

- X-ray of affected joint
- Magnetic resonance imaging (MRI)

Lab Tests

- Synovial fluid analysis

PLANNING AND IMPLEMENTATION

- Promote weight control if obese.
- Encourage exercise.
- Apply heat or cold compresses.
- Administer acetaminophen and nonsteroidal medications as ordered.
- Monitor for side effects of medications.
- Joint replacement may be indicated.

SPECIAL CONCERNS

- See Special Procedures and Treatments for information on Joint Replacement.

NURSING DIAGNOSIS

- Pain, Chronic
- Mobility, Impaired physical
- Knowledge, Deficient
- Activity intolerance

Osteomalacia

DEFINITION

- Osteomalacia is a metabolic disease that causes poor mineralization of the bone cells. It is caused by vitamin D deficiency.

Clinical Causes

- Inadequate vitamin D intake
- Strict macrobiotic diet
- Lack of exposure to sunlight
- Malabsorption
- Renal tubule disease
- Anticonvulsant therapy
- Liver disease

KEY ASSESSMENTS

- Pain in the hips, back, ribs, or feet
- Pain with ambulation
- Waddling gait

Diagnostics

- Dual energy X-ray absorptiometry (DEXA) scan

Lab Tests

- Calcium
- Phosphate
- Alkaline phosphatase (ALP)
- Parathyroid hormone
- Vitamin D
- Blood urea nitrogen (BUN) and creatinine (Cr)

PLANNING AND IMPLEMENTATION

- Treat underlying cause
- Administer vitamin D supplements, ergocalciferol, and calcium citrate as prescribed
- Provide diet high in vitamin D, including milk fortified with vitamin D
- Institute safety precautions
- Assist with ambulation

NURSING DIAGNOSIS

- Activity intolerance
- Pain, Chronic
- Nutrition: less than body requirements, Imbalanced
- Knowledge, Deficient

Osteomyelitis

DEFINITION

- Osteomyelitis is a bone infection resulting from a soft tissue infection that spreads to the bone, open bone fracture, or bone surgery.

KEY ASSESSMENTS

- Pain
- Soft tissue swelling and redness
- Purulent draining
- Fever

History and Examination

- Bone fracture
- Recent acute infection
- Puncture wound
- Vascular insufficiency
- Diabetes mellitus

Diagnostics

- X-ray
- Bone scan

Lab Tests

- Blood cultures
- White blood count (WBC)
- Sedimentation rate (elevated)
- C-reactive protein (CRP)

PLANNING AND IMPLEMENTATION

- Treat pain with analgesics
- Wound care as prescribed
- Monitor wound appearance
- Monitor WBC and wound cultures
- Monitor vital signs
- Elevate affected area
- Administer appropriate antibiotics (expect four-to-six week antibiotic course)
- Monitor for side effects of antibiotic therapy (nephrotoxicity or diarrhea)
- Monitor blood urea nitrogen (BUN) and creatinine (Cr)
- Encourage adequate fluid and nutritional intake
- If diabetic, ensure tight glycemic control
- Meticulous intravenous (IV) site care
- Monitor IV site for redness, drainage, or swelling

NURSING DIAGNOSIS

- Pain, Chronic
- Mobility, Impaired physical
- Skin integrity, Impaired
- Knowledge, Deficient

Osteoporosis

DEFINITION

- Osteoporosis is characterized by low bone mass and strength and is the most frequently diagnosed bone disease.

Risk Factors

- Personal history of fracture as an adult
- Low body weight
- Cigarette smoking
- Use of steroids for more than three months
- Postmenopause
- Lifelong low-calcium intake
- Caucasian
- Female
- Elderly
- Chronic alcohol abuse
- Endocrine abnormalities

KEY ASSESSMENTS

- A silent disease often producing no symptoms until a fracture occurs
- Decrease in height
- Kyphosis (hunchback)
- Back pain

Diagnostics

- Dual energy X-ray absorptiometry (DEXA) scan

Lab Tests

- Calcium, magnesium, vitamin D, and alkaline phosphate (ALP)

PLANNING AND IMPLEMENTATION

- Administer bisphosphonates, selective estrogen receptor modulators, and calcium supplements as prescribed
- Monitor for side effects of medications
- Encourage regular weight-bearing exercise
- Prevent falls

NURSING DIAGNOSIS

- Injury, Potential for
- Nutrition: less than body requirements, Impaired
- Activity intolerance

Otitis Media

DEFINITION

- Otitis media is a middle ear infection and is the most common cause of conductive hearing loss.

KEY ASSESSMENTS

- Ear pain
- Ear inflammation
- Hearing loss

Diagnostics

- Middle ear inflammation on inspection

PLANNING AND IMPLEMENTATION

- Treat pain
- Administer antibiotics as ordered

SPECIAL CONCERNS

- Avoid flying and water sports until the infection is resolved.

NURSING DIAGNOSIS

- Pain, Acute
- Knowledge, Deficient

Ovarian Cyst

DEFINITION

- Ovarian cysts are cysts in the ovaries and are a common finding.

Classifications

- Follicular cysts form in the first half of the menstrual cycle and may become fluid filled, can last up to two months, and then spontaneously resolve. If symptomatic, treatment includes oral contraceptives and, rarely, surgery.
- Corpus luteum cysts form in the last half of the menstrual cycle and are filled with blood and fluid. Persistent cysts are associated with menstrual irregularities and abdominal pain that may radiate to the back, shoulder, legs, or rectum.
- Dermoid cysts are benign complex cysts containing tissue such as fat, hair, and teeth. Symptoms may include pressure and abdominal pain. Surgery is usually indicated to remove the cyst.
- Endometrioma cysts, called chocolate cysts, are formed when endometrial tissue containing old blood attaches to the outside of the ovary. They are typically painful and cause dysmenorrhea and dyspareunia and are removed via laparoscopy.

KEY ASSESSMENTS

- Menstrual abnormalities
- Abdominal pain, pressure
- Dyspareunia (painful intercourse)

Diagnostics

- Ultrasound
- Computed tomography (CT)
- Laparoscopy

Lab Tests

- Pregnancy testing
- Cancer antigen 125 (CA 125)
- Alpha-fetoprotein (AFP) (rule out ovarian cancer)

PLANNING AND IMPLEMENTATION

- Treat pain
- Monitor menstrual cycle
- Anticipate treatment if symptomatic

NURSING DIAGNOSIS

- Pain, Acute
- Fear
- Knowledge, Deficient

Paget's Disease

DEFINITION

- Paget's disease is a chronic bone disease that produces an increase in bone absorption, bone formation, and bone remodeling, resulting in highly vascular and weak bones. Paget's affects long bones, pelvis, lumbar vertebrae, and the skull; it does not have a cure; the cause in unknown; and there is a familial tendency.

KEY ASSESSMENTS

- May be asymptomatic
- Aching pain in the hips and pelvis that worsens with weight bearing
- Bowed legs
- Enlarged skull
- Kyphosis
- Scoliosis

P

Diagnostics

- X-rays
- Bone scan

Lab Tests

- Increase in alkaline phosphatase (ALP)
- Serum calcium
- Urine for calcium, hydroxyproline, N-telopeptide, and deoxypyridinolines

PLANNING AND IMPLEMENTATION

- Monitor calcium levels.
- Monitor for signs of hypercalcemia (hypertension, weakness, or bowel disturbances).
- Promote weight-bearing exercise.
- Monitor for signs of bone fracture.

- Treat pain.
- Administer antiresorptive agents (calcitonin) or biphosphonates as ordered.
- Monitor for side effects of medication therapy.
- Administer biphosphonates on an empty stomach with 6–8 ounces of water and position patient upright for one hour after administration.
- Inform patient that surgery to correct fractures or bone changes may be necessary.

NURSING DIAGNOSIS

- Injury, Risk for
- Falls, Risk for
- Knowledge, Deficient

Paget's Mammary Disease

DEFINITION

- Paget's mammary disease in an uncommon skin cancer characterized by a chronic eczema-like rash of the nipple and adjacent areolar skin. It occurs between 50 and 60 years of age and is more common in women. It is associated with an underlying cancer, either in situ carcinoma of the breast or a more widespread infiltrating cancer.

KEY ASSESSMENTS

- Rash of the nipple and adjacent areolar skin
- Nipple discharge
- Redness
- Scaling
- Inversion, ulceration, or swelling around the nipple

Diagnostics

- Skin biopsy (presence of Paget's cells)
- Mammogram
- Breast magnetic resonance imaging (MRI)
- Extensive diagnostic testing may be necessary to find underlying cancer

Lab Tests

- Complete blood count (CBC)
- Aspartate aminotransferase (AST) and alanine aminotransferase (ALT)

PLANNING AND IMPLEMENTATION

- Provide meticulous skin care for breast area
- Discuss anxiety during testing procedures

NURSING DIAGNOSIS

- Skin integrity, Impaired
- Anxiety
- Knowledge, Deficient

Pancreatitis, Acute

DEFINITION

- Acute pancreatitis is inflammation of the pancreatitis that may be accompanied by life-threatening complications. There are many causes associated with pancreatitis, and 10–30 percent of cases are considered idiopathic.

Clinical Causes

- Gallstone disease
- Alcoholism
- Infections
- Medications (angiotensin-converting enzymes [ACE] inhibitors or salicylates)
- Trauma
- Surgical manipulation
- Duodenal diseases
- Genetic predisposition to cholelithiasis (gallstone formation)

KEY ASSESSMENTS

Acute Pancreatitis

- Acute abdominal pain that radiates to the back
- Nausea and vomiting
- Abdominal distention

- Cullen's sign (periumbicular bruising)
- Turner's sign (bruising noted on the flanks)
- Hypocalcemia
- Fever
- Tachycardia or tachypnea
- Hypotension

Systemic Complications

- Hypoxemia (acute respiratory distress syndrome [ARDS] or pulmonary effusion)
- Decreased urine output (hypovolemia or renal failure)
- Bleeding (disseminated intravascular coagulation)
- Tachycardia, tachypnea, and hypotension (hypovolemia)
- Hyperglycemia
- Metabolic acidosis
- Gastrointestinal (GI) bleeding (stress gastritis)

Diagnostics

- Computed tomography (CT)
- Ultrasound

Lab Tests

- Amylase and lipase
- Alanine aminotransferase (ALT)
- Blood urea nitrogen (BUN) and creatinine (Cr)
- Electrolytes
- Arterial blood gases (ABGs)
- Prothrombin time (PT), partial thromboplastin time (PTT), and international normalized ratio (INR)

PLANNING AND IMPLEMENTATION

- Treat pain. If pain is severe, the patient may require large doses of narcotics (patient-controlled analgesia with Demerol, hydromorphone, and morphine).
- Maintain nothing by mouth (NPO) status.
- Nasogastric tube to low intermittent suction (LIS).
- Maintain adequate hydration with intravenous (IV) fluids.
- Monitor vital signs frequently.
- Monitor pulse oximetry.
- Administer electrolyte replacement.
- Encourage bedrest.
- Administer prophylactic antibiotics intravenously.
- Monitor blood glucose.

- Monitor for complications to renal, GI, respiratory, and cardiovascular systems.
- Monitor intake and output (I & O).
- Monitor for bleeding.
- If patient is NPO for a prolonged period of time, total parenteral nutrition may be required.
- Once patient begins eating, small frequent meals, comprising a bland, low-fat diet, caffeine is restricted and alcohol is encouraged.
- Surgery may be required if the cause is cholelithiasis.

SPECIAL CONCERNS

- If acute pancreatitis is from alcohol use, the patient may need additional resources once discharged to cope with this problem.

NURSING DIAGNOSIS

- Pain, Acute
- Activity intolerance
- Nutrition: less than body requirements, Imbalanced
- Therapeutic regimen management, Ineffective

Pancreatitis, Chronic

DEFINITION

- Chronic pancreatitis is irreversible damage to, and continued irritation of, the pancreas.

Clinical Causes

- Hyperlipidemia
- Hypertriglyceridemia
- Alcoholism
- Trauma
- Cancer of the pancreas
- Congenital abnormalities of the pancreas
- Cystic fibrosis

KEY ASSESSMENTS

- Pain, acute, dull, and constant
- Malabsorption

- Weight loss
- Hyperglycemia
- Steatorrhea

Diagnostics

- Endoscopic retrograde cholangiopancreatography (ERCP)
- Computed tomography (CT)

Lab Tests

- Glucose
- Serum trypsin below 20 mg/dL
- Fecal fat measurement

PLANNING AND IMPLEMENTATION

- Monitor and treat pain
- Monitor intake and output (I & O)
- Take daily weight
- Promote adequate oral and nutritional intake
- Administer digestive enzymes (lipase)
- Monitor glucose and treat
- Adhere to prescribed diet
- Monitor stools for steatorrhea

SPECIAL CONCERNS

Teaching Considerations

- Diet containing moderate fat (30 percent), high protein (24 percent), and low carbohydrates (24 percent)
- Abstain from alcohol
- Adherence of medication schedule
- Monitor weight
- Monitor for complications of diabetes or hyperglycemia if present

NURSING DIAGNOSIS

- Pain, Chronic
- Nutrition: less than body requirements, Imbalanced
- Knowledge, Deficient
- Therapeutic regimen management, Ineffective

Parkinson's Disease

DEFINITION

- Parkinson's disease is a progressive degenerative neurological disorder caused by the loss of nerve cell function in the basal ganglia. The loss of the nerve cells results in reduced dopamine production. The reduction in dopamine, a neurotransmitter essential for functions, such as controlling posture and voluntary motions, causes the clinical symptoms. The cause of Parkinson's disease is unknown, but it does appear to have hereditary links and is associated with aging and exposure to environmental toxins.

KEY ASSESSMENTS

- Tremors
- Rigidity of muscles
- Akinesia (lack of movement)
- Bradykinesia (slow movement)
- Shuffled gait
- Postural disturbances
- Mask-like face
- Difficulty with fine motor activities
- Eating or swallowing difficulties
- Weakness and fatigue
- Cognitive impairments and dementia

Diagnostics

- There are no specific tests to confirm the diagnosis of Parkinson's disease. Diagnosis is based on history, examination, and presence of clinical manifestations of the disease.

PLANNING AND IMPLEMENTATION

- Implement safety measures.
- Monitor the ability to swallow effectively.
- Place patient in high Fowler's position when feeding.
- Monitor fluid and nutritional intake.
- Provide meticulous skin care.
- If restricted to the bed, reposition every two hours.
- Provide oral care every four hours.
- Monitor bowel and bladder function.
- Encourage activity.

- Assist with activities of daily living.
- Anticipate administering dopamine precursors, dopamine receptor antagonists, amantadine, anticholinergic agents, monoamine oxidase (MAO) inhibitors, and catechol-O-methyltransferase (COMT) inhibitors.
- Adhere strictly to medication administration regimens.
- Surgical treatment may include thalamotomy, pallidotomy, insertion of deep-brain stimulator, adrenal tissue, or stem cell transplant.

SPECIAL CONCERNS

Geriatric Considerations

- Parkinson's disease has a peak onset in the sixth decade of life, and 1 percent of the population over 65 is afflicted.

Teaching Considerations

- Teaching should address the physical, emotional, and social aspects of the disease.
- In the early stages of the disease encourage the patient to address long-term issues, such as advanced directives, estate planning, and care options.
- Reinforce medication, nutrition, and safety teaching.

NURSING DIAGNOSIS

- Injury, Risk for
- Thought process, Disturbed
- Fatigue
- Swallowing, Impaired
- Mobility, Impaired physical
- Nutrition, less than body requirements, Imbalanced

Pelvic Inflammatory Disease (PID)

DEFINITION

- PID is an inflammatory condition of the female pelvic organs than can lead to abscess formation, scarring, occlusion of the fallopian tubes, infertility, and an increased risk for ectopic pregnancy.

Clinical Causes

- Untreated sexually transmitted infections
- Sexually active
- Use of intrauterine devices
- Douching

KEY ASSESSMENTS

- Abdominal pain
- Fever
- Cervical discharge
- Dysuria
- Painful intercourse
- Discharge with an abnormal odor

Diagnostics

- Ultrasound
- Laparoscopy
- Pap smear
- Pelvic examination

Lab Tests

- Complete blood count (CBC)
- Pregnancy test
- Urinalysis
- Sexually transmitted infection workup

PLANNING AND IMPLEMENTATION

- Treat fevers with antipyretics
- Administer antibiotics as requested
- Treat abdominal pain
- Discuss infertility fears

NURSING DIAGNOSIS

- Infection
- Pain, Acute
- Knowledge, Deficient

Peptic Ulcer Dyspepsia (PUD)

DEFINITION

- PUD is epigastric pain caused by a loss of the mucosal lining of the stomach or duodenum. If PUD ulcers hemorrhage or perforate, it is an emergent condition.

Clinical Causes

- *Helicobacter pylori* infection
- Side effect of nonsteroidal anti-inflammatory drug (NSAID) use
- Stress

KEY ASSESSMENTS

- Epigastric pain relieved by food or antacids
- Epigastric pain that wakes the patient at night
- Weight loss
- Poor appetite
- Bloating
- Nausea and vomiting
- Signs of ulcer hemorrhage: melena (blood in the feces), hematemesis (vomiting blood), and hemorrhagic shock (low blood pressure, tachycardia)
- Signs of ulcer perforation: melena, hematemesis, hemorrhagic shock, and a rigid, intensely painful abdomen

Diagnostics

- Endoscopy with testing for *H. pylori*
- Barium swallow
- Hemoglobin and hematocrit

PLANNING AND IMPLEMENTATION

- Treat nausea and vomiting.
- Encourage smoking cessation.
- Discontinue NSAIDs.
- Administer antacids, H_2 receptor antagonists, and proton pump inhibitors.
- If *H. pylori* is present, anticipate administering antibiotics (bismuth subsalicylate, metronidazole, and tetracycline).
- Take daily weight.

- Monitor stools for melena.
- Monitor for hematemesis.
- Monitor vital signs for signs of shock.
- Monitor intake and output (I & O).
- Monitor caloric intake.
- Offer small, frequent meals.
- Vagotomy, surgical ligation of the vagus nerve innervating the stomach that decreases acid production by 50–80 percent, may be indicated.
- If the patient experiences hemorrhage, insert two large-bore intravenous (IV) lines, administer 5% albumin or 0.9% normal saline (NS) to maintain blood pressure, notify health care provider, insert an nasogastric tube, and apply low-intermittent suction; administer oxygen therapy, type and cross-match for blood transfusion; and anticipate administering H_2 antagonist IV and packed red blood cells.
- If the patient experiences a perforated ulcer, treat as indicated for hemorrhage and prepare for emergent gastric resection.

SPECIAL CONCERNS

P

- Tobacco smokers are two times more likely to develop PUD.
- If patients are not responsive to PUD therapy, Zollinger-Ellison syndrome (ZES), a gastric acid secreting tumor, should be considered and is diagnosed if fasting gastrin levels are greater that 1,000 pg/mL.

NURSING DIAGNOSIS

- Pain, Acute
- Nutrition: less than body requirements, Imbalanced
- Knowledge, Deficient
- Fluid volume, Risk for deficient

Pericarditis

DEFINITION

- Pericarditis is an inflammation of the pericardium, the membrane that surrounds the heart. Inflammation of the pericardium may exert pressure on heart.

Clinical Causes

- Pericarditis may include infectious, parasitic, drug, or irradiation agents; idiopathic causes; autoimmune diseases; hypothyroidism; renal failure; myocardial infarction; tumors; injury; trauma; or surgery.

KEY ASSESSMENTS

- Pressure-type chest pain
- Fever
- Dyspnea
- Abdominal pain
- Tachypnea
- Tachycardia
- Elevated temperature
- Beck's triad, hypotension, jugular vein distention, and muffled heart sounds
- Pulsus paradoxus, a 10 mm Hg or greater drop in arterial pressure with respiration
- Assess cause

PLANNING AND IMPLEMENTATION

- Treat underlying cause
- Monitor vital signs
- Monitor cardiac status
- Monitor tissue perfusion
- Treat pain
- Avoid stressors
- Teach patient and family about treatments

NURSING DIAGNOSIS

- Hyperthermia
- Tissue perfusion, Ineffective
- Knowledge, Deficient

Peripheral Arterial Disease (PAD)

DEFINITION

- PAD is arterial insufficiency of the peripheral circulation. Atherosclerosis, the formation of plaque deposits causing hardening of the arteries, is the most common cause of PAD. Acute embolic syndrome, loss of arterial blood flow to an extremity, is an emergent condition that must be reported to the health care provider immediately to prevent the loss of a limb.

Clinical Causes

- Smoking
- Hypertension
- Elevated cholesterol
- Smoking
- Diabetes

KEY ASSESSMENTS

- Intermittent claudication (pain occurring during activity that is relieved with rest)
- Nocturnal pain (pain at night when legs are elevated)
- Rest pain (pain when legs are in the dependent position)
- Five P's: pain, pallor, pulse, paresthesia, and paralysis
- Delayed capillary refill
- Absence of leg hair
- Waxy appearance of leg
- Cool to touch
- Arterial ulcers (small, necrotic ulcers with little or no drainage)
- Ankle-brachial index (comparison of perfusion pressure between the lower leg and upper arm) less than 0.95
- Acute embolic syndrome (painful, cold, pulseless extremity with paresthesia and possible paralysis)

Diagnostics

- Arterial Doppler
- Lower extremity angiogram (arterial angiography of the lower extremities)

PLANNING AND IMPLEMENTATION

- Monitor and treat pain.
- Adjust legs to the dependent position.
- Monitor for the development of arterial ulcers.
- If arterial ulcer is present, wound care as ordered.
- Monitor temperature, color, pulse, sensation, and movement.
- If unable to palpate a posterior tibial or dorsalis pedis pulse, use a Doppler to locate the pulse.
- Monitor for the development of acute embolic syndrome.

- If acute embolic syndrome occurs, contact health care provider immediately and prepare the patient for surgical removal of the emboli occluding the artery (embolectomy). Initiate NPO status and a peripheral IV.
- Aorto-femoral bypass may be considered to restore arterial blood flow to the extremity.

SPECIAL CONCERNS

Gender Considerations

- PAD is more common in men than in women.

NURSING DIAGNOSIS

- Tissue perfusion, Impaired
- Pain, Acute
- Pain, Chronic
- Walking, Impaired

Peripheral Nerve Injury

DEFINITION

- A peripheral nerve injury is any injury to a peripheral nerve or a plexus (a network of peripheral nerves) from acute trauma or chronic entrapment. Peripheral nerve injuries can occur from the insertion of intravenous (IV) lines. Immediately remove an IV if a patient complains of numbness or tingling on insertion.

KEY ASSESSMENTS

- Paralysis
- Paresis
- Pain
- Paresthesias
- Muscular atrophy
- Absent deep tendon reflexes
- Sensory loss

Diagnostics

- Computed tomography (CT), magnetic resonance imaging (MRI), or electromyography (EMG)

PLANNING AND IMPLEMENTATION

- Manage pain.
- Implement safety measures.
- Document affected areas for motor strength, color, and temperature.
- Immobilize limb if ordered.
- Prevent injury to affected limb.
- Surgical anastomosis may be required.

NURSING DIAGNOSIS

- Pain, Acute
- Sensory perception, Disturbed

Peripheral Venous Disease (PVD)

DEFINITION

- PVD develops as the valves in the veins in the lower extremities become incompetent, causing venous hypertension, venous stasis, and venous insufficiency. PVD may initiate the development of venous ulcers and increases the risk for developing deep vein thrombosis and cellulitis.

Clinical Causes

- Trauma or surgery on affected leg
- Conditions that increase hydrostatic pressure of the lower extremities, including pregnancy, abdominal tumors, ascites, obesity, prolonged standing, and hypertension

Classifications

- Venous ulcers are skin ulcers that cause venous congestion and poor venous circulation.
- Deep venous thrombosis (DVT) is a thrombus, or blood clot, usually found in the lower extremity. Do not massage a limb with a DVT. If the thrombus breaks loose, it may cause a pulmonary emboli and possible death.
- Cellulitis is an infection of the skin.

KEY ASSESSMENTS

- Peripheral edema
- Hemosiderin staining (skin hyperpigmentation or brownish color)

- Leg pain with dependent positioning
- Varicose veins

Venous Ulcer

- Ulcers or skin breakdown on the lower extremities

DVT

- Unilateral leg swelling
- Warmth and pain to extremity
- Positive Homan's sign (pain in the calf with dorsiflexion)

Cellulitis

- Unilateral leg swelling
- Pain
- Erythema and warmth
- Area of skin breakdown (place where bacteria entered the skin)

Diagnostics

- Venogram
- Venous Doppler (assess for DVT formation)

PLANNING AND IMPLEMENTATION

- Elevate legs.
- Dress affected leg(s) with elastic stocking(s).
- Administer compression boots.
- Monitor for development of DVT.
- Monitor for venous ulcers formation.
- Monitor for development of cellulitis.
- Promote smoking cessation.
- Provide meticulous skin care.
- Document skin assessments.
- Anticipate administering anticoagulant medication to help prevent DVTs.
- Sclerotherapy or vein stripping may be indicated for varicose veins.

Venous Ulcer

- Wound care as ordered
- Document wound size, color, and appearance of drainage
- Elevate leg

Cellulitis

- Elevate leg
- Treat pain

- Apply warm packs
- Administer antibiotic

DVT

- Keep patient on bedrest.
- Do not manipulate or massage affected limb.
- Do not apply compression devices to affected limb.
- Monitor distal pulses.
- Document calf circumference.
- Administer anticoagulants as ordered (heparin, low molecular weight heparin, or Coumadin).
- If the patient cannot tolerate anticoagulants, a venous filter or venous umbrella may be placed in the superior vena cava to trap any thrombus that may become dislodged.
- Monitor for signs of pulmonary emboli (extreme dyspnea, anxiety, chest pain, or low O_2 saturation).

NURSING DIAGNOSIS

- Tissue perfusion, Ineffective
- Knowledge, Deficient
- Infection, Risk for
- Skin integrity, Risk for impaired

Pharyngitis, Acute

DEFINITION

- Acute pharyngitis is an inflammation of the throat caused by either viral or bacterial infection. Group A beta-hemolytic streptococci (GABHS) is the most notable bacteria causing acute pharyngitis and is easily spread from person to person by respiratory droplets. Complications of acute pharyngitis caused by GABHS may include acute rheumatic fever and glomerulonephritis that may lead to kidney or heart failure, and children are especially vulnerable. In the United States, more than 10 million people are diagnosed with acute pharyngitis every year.

KEY ASSESSMENTS

- Sore throat
- Pain with swallowing
- Pharynx and tonsils are red with purulent exudates

- Fever
- Cervical adenopathy

Lab Tests

- Rapid antigen testing or standard throat culture to detect GABHS

PLANNING AND IMPLEMENTATION

- Monitor respiratory status
- Administer analgesics or antipyretics
- Promote warm liquids and adequate intake
- Encourage rest
- Administer antibiotics if bacterial cause

NURSING DIAGNOSIS

- Pain, Acute
- Knowledge, Deficient

Pheochromocytoma

DEFINITION

- Pheochromocytoma is a tumor of the adrenal gland that secretes catecholamines. Pheochromocytomas occur more frequently in men during the fourth or fifth decade of life. One third of pheochromocytomas cause fatal cardiac arrhythmias or stroke before diagnosis.

KEY ASSESSMENTS

- Hypertension
- Headache
- Sweating
- Nausea and vomiting
- Abdominal pain
- Palpitations
- Chest pain
- Severe anxiety

Diagnostics

- Test urine for 24 hours for catecholamines
- Computed tomography (CT) of adrenal glands

PLANNING AND IMPLEMENTATION

Preoperative

- Anticipate surgical removal of tumor
- Monitor vital signs
- Monitor neurological status
- Administer antihypertensive medications (alpha-adrenergic blockers)
- Do not palpate the abdomen

Postoperative

- Monitor for shock
- Fluid resuscitation with saline or colloids
- Monitor glucose
- Treat incisional pain
- Monitor wound for signs of infection

NURSING DIAGNOSIS

- Anxiety
- Injury, Risk for
- Fluid volume, Risk for imbalanced
- Knowledge, Deficient

Plague

DEFINITION

- *Yersinia pestis* cause three forms of plague: bubonic (from infected fleas), septicemic (untreated bubonic plague), and pneumonic (from inhaling bacteria). Pneumonic plague is the form considered most dangerous as a biological weapon, because the bacteria can be aerosolized and spread over large populations quickly. Pneumonic plague has 100 percent mortality if not treated within 24 hours of infection.
- It is spread through the air and from person to person.
- Average incubation is 24 hours to 6 days.

KEY ASSESSMENTS

- Fever
- Chills
- Malaise

- Myalgias
- Headache
- Nausea and vomiting
- Diarrhea
- Abdominal pain
- Bloody sputum

Lab Tests

- Blood and sputum cultures

PLANNING AND IMPLEMENTATION

- Isolate patient.
- Adhere to standard and droplet precautions.
- Wash patient if aerosol contamination expected.
- Initiate antibiotic therapy immediately (streptomycin is the drug of choice, but gentamycin, tetracycline, and chloramphenicol are also effective).
- Exposed health care members must start doxycycline as prophylaxis as soon as possible.
- Initiate intravenous (IV) access.
- Administer oxygen.
- Monitor intake and output (I & O).
- Encourage coughing and deep breathing.
- Anticipate intubation if oxygenation status deteriorates.
- Administer antipyretics for fever.
- Monitor and treat diarrhea.
- Monitor pulse oximetry.
- Monitor respiratory status.
- Monitor vital signs frequently.

NURSING DIAGNOSIS

- Breathing pattern, Ineffective
- Gas exchange, Impaired
- Hyperthermia

Pneumonia

DEFINITION

- Pneumonia is an acute chronic infection of one or both lungs caused by microorganisms (bacterial, viral, or fungal), aspiration of a substance, or chemical irritants. It may also be considered community acquired or hospital acquired based on where the infection took place. It is the fifth leading cause of death in the United States for people 65 years and older.

KEY ASSESSMENTS

- Fever and chills
- Pleuritic chest pain
- Productive cough
- Circumoral cyanosis
- Dyspnea
- Tachycardia and tachypnea
- Hypoxemia
- Confusion
- Dehydration (dry mucous membranes and poor skin turgor)

Lab Tests

- Chest X-ray (CXR)
- Sputum culture
- Complete blood count (CBC)
- Electrolytes

PLANNING AND IMPLEMENTATION

- Monitor respiratory status frequently
- Monitor pulse oximetry continuously
- Anticipate oxygen administration
- Anticipate antibiotic administration
- Monitor fluid status and prevent dehydration
- Elevate head of bed
- Chest physiotherapy
- Encourage incentive spirometry
- Monitor temperature and treat fevers
- Provide frequent rest periods
- Treat pleural pain
- Monitor white blood count (WBC) and chest X-ray (CXR)

SPECIAL CONSIDERATIONS

Gerontological Considerations

- Encourage elderly patients to receive flu and pneumococcal vaccines

NURSING DIAGNOSIS

- Airway clearance, Ineffective
- Breathing pattern, Ineffective
- Infection, Risk for
- Hyperthermia

Pneumothorax

DEFINITION

- A pneumothorax is a collection of air in the pleural cavity, which leads to a partial or full collapse of the lung and interferes with normal oxygenation.

Classifications

- Spontaneous pneumothorax occurs in young men between 20 and 40 years of age without cause.
- Traumatic pneumothorax is a result of trauma and may be from blunt or penetrating trauma.
- Iatrogenic pneumothorax is caused by surgery or invasive line placement.
- Tension pneumothorax is a medical emergency in which the pneumothorax is so large it causes pressure or tension on the heart and the trachea. It is emergently treated with a large-bore needle inserted into the second intercostal space.

KEY ASSESSMENTS

- Dyspnea
- Tachycardia and tachypnea
- Hypotension
- Anxiety
- Tracheal deviation
- Absence of breath sounds over affected area
- Decreased pulse oximetry
- Change in level of consciousness (LOC)

Diagnostics

- Chest X-ray (CXR) confirms diagnosis.
- Arterial blood gases (ABGs) may reflect respiratory alkalosis and hypoxia.

PLANNING AND IMPLEMENTATION

- Position patient in high Fowler's position if blood pressure is stable
- Administer oxygen therapy
- Insert peripheral intravenous (IV) line
- Treat pain and anxiety
- Anticipate chest tube insertion
- Monitor chest tube drainage and notify health care provider if there is an increase in drainage or the presence of an air leak
- Encourage deep breathing
- Encourage mobility if appropriate

SPECIAL CONCERNS

- If the chest tube tubing becomes disconnected from the container, place the open end in a bottle of sterile water to create a water seal.
- If the entire chest tube is accidentally dislodged, place Vaseline gauze over the site and notify the health care provider.

NURSING DIAGNOSIS

- Breathing pattern, Ineffective
- Tissue perfusion, Ineffective
- Anxiety

Polycystic Kidney Disease (PKD)

DEFINITION

- PKD is a genetically inherited kidney disease that causes cysts to form in the renal tubules and ultimately causes renal failure.

KEY ASSESSMENTS

- Family history of PKD
- Hypertension
- Unilateral or bilateral dull to stabbing pain in the lower abdomen
- Hematuria
- Palpable enlargement of the kidneys

Diagnostics

- Renal ultrasound

Lab Tests

- Blood urea nitrogen (BUN) and creatinine (Cr)
- Test urine for 24 hours for Cr clearance
- Urinalysis
- Red blood count
- White blood count

PLANNING AND IMPLEMENTATION

- Take daily weight.
- Monitor intake and output (I & O).
- Avoid nonsteroidal anti-inflammatory medications.
- Treat pain.
- Monitor vital signs, especially blood pressure.
- Administer antihypertensive medications.
- Monitor for signs of a urinary tract infection ([UTI] fever, foul smelling urine, or pain with urination).
- Treat UTI with antibiotics.
- Teach patients signs of UTI and to report symptoms.
- Surgical intervention may be required if cysts cause frequent bleeding, resistant infections, uncontrollable pain, or uncontrollable hypertension.
- Dialysis or kidney transplantation is indicated for renal failure associated with PKD.

SPECIAL CONCERNS

- PKD affects other organs; 75 percent develop cystic liver disease, and 8 percent develop cranial aneurysms.
- See Special Procedures and Treatments for information on Dialysis.

Teaching Considerations

- Signs of UTI
- Promote a low-sodium diet
- Control weight
- Monitor blood pressure at home
- Report gross hematuria
- Report a decreased urine output, peripheral edema, or unexplained weight gain (signs of worsening renal function)

NURSING DIAGNOSIS

- Pain, Acute
- Fluid volume, Risk for imbalanced
- Knowledge, Deficient

Polycystic Ovary Syndrome (PCOS)

DEFINITION

- PCOS is an endocrine disorder affecting 5 to 10 percent of childbearing women. It is characterized by multiple ovarian cysts, oligomenorrhea, hirsutism, acne, obesity, infertility, alopecia, and hypertension. Women with PCOS have insulin resistance and are at higher risk for developing diabetes mellitus and coronary artery disease. The cause is unknown, but genetic mutations are being studied.

KEY ASSESSMENTS

- History of multiple ovarian cysts
- Obesity
- Hypertension
- Menses abnormalities
- Alopecia

Lab Tests

- Glucose
- Lipid profile

PLANNING AND IMPLEMENTATION

- Assist with weight loss planning.
- Encourage aerobic and weight-training exercise.
- Encourage smoking cessation.
- Assist with healthy diet choices.
- Metformin and clomiphene citrate may be administered to induce ovulation if infertility exists.

SPECIAL CONCERNS

Teaching Considerations

- Educate patients about long-term effects, including diabetes mellitus and coronary artery disease
- Teach patients signs of hyperglycemia

NURSING DIAGNOSIS

- Knowledge, Deficient
- Nutrition: more than body requirement, Imbalanced

Polycythemia

DEFINITION

- Polycythemia is an increased amount of red blood cells with a hematocrit level greater than 55 percent in males and 50 percent in females.

Classifications

- Primary polycythemia is a rare neoplastic stem cell disorder that increases the production of red blood cells, white blood cells, and platelets.
- Secondary polycythemia is caused by an elevated erythropoietin level, which increases RBC production, or by chronic reduced amounts of oxygen. Causes include high altitudes, chronic pulmonary disorders, smoking, and renal cell cancer.

KEY ASSESSMENTS

- May be asymptomatic
- Hypertension
- Dizziness
- Fatigue
- Headache or paresthesias
- Ruddy complexion
- Angina
- Claudication
- Dyspnea
- Erythromelalgia, burning sensation in the digits

Lab Tests

- Red blood count, white blood count, and platelet count

PLANNING AND IMPLEMENTATION

- Encourage fluid intake.
- Monitor neurological status.
- Monitor vital signs.
- Chemotherapeutic agents may be ordered to decrease red blood cell levels.
- Phlebotomy, removing blood, to maintain hematocrit within normal levels.

SPECIAL CONCERNS

Cultural Considerations

- Primary polycythemia is more common in European Jewish people between the ages of 40 and 70 years.

Teaching Considerations

- Encourage smoking cessation
- Avoid iron supplements
- Maintain adequate fluid intake
- Explain organ and system effects of untreated polycythemia
- Encourage compliance with phlebotomy and/or chemotherapeutic agents

NURSING DIAGNOSIS

- Tissue perfusion, Ineffective
- Fluid volume, Risk for deficient
- Knowledge, Deficient

Pressure Ulcers

DEFINITION

- Pressure ulcers, also referred to as decubitus ulcers, bedsores, and pressure sores, refer to damage to the skin and underlying tissue from excessive pressure. Many scales are used to identify patients at risk for pressure ulcer development, including the Norton, Gosnell, and Braden scales.

KEY ASSESSMENTS

Determine Risk for Development

- Sensory perception
- Skin moisture
- Activity level
- Ability to move
- Nutritional status
- Incontinence
- Perform and document a thorough skin assessment during each shift

If Present, Determine

- Size, color, and appearance of ulcer
- Presence of drainage
- Ulcer stage (see Figure 2)

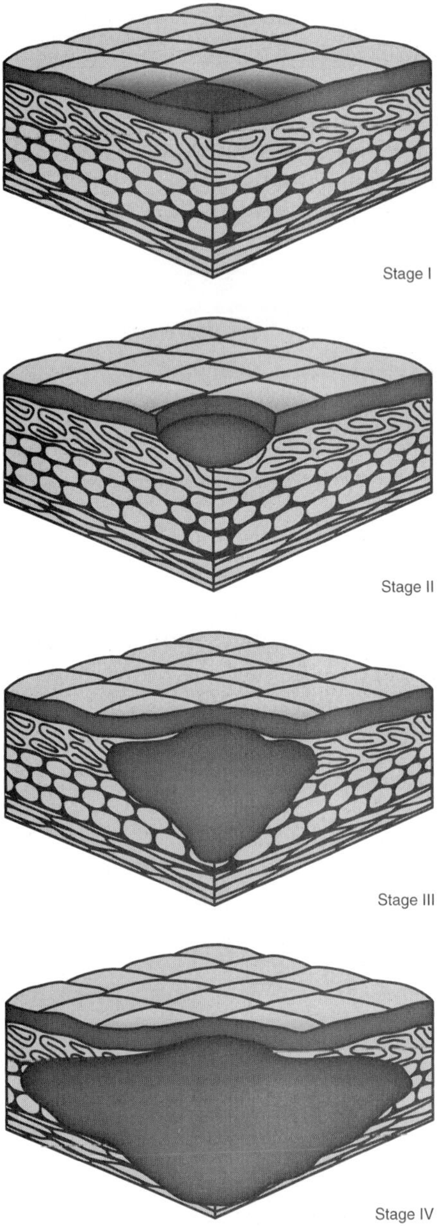

Figure 2 Pressure ulcer staging system.

- Wound considered unstageable if wound depth is obscured by slough (loosely adherent yellow-grey necrotic tissue) or eschar (dried, leathery grey or black necrotic tissue)
- Perform and document a thorough skin assessment during each shift

PLANNING AND IMPLEMENTATION

- Turn patient every two hours
- Use appropriate therapeutic mattress
- If incontinent or involuntary, clean every two hours
- Minimize amount of linens and pads
- Perform skin assessment every shift and document findings
- Dry moist skin
- Apply barrier ointments as ordered
- Promote adequate nutrition and hydration
- Monitor albumin and protein levels
- If a pressure ulcer is present, wound care as ordered by wound care nurse or health care provider

NURSING DIAGNOSIS

- Skin integrity, Risk for impaired
- Skin integrity, Impaired

Primary Aldosteronism

DEFINITION

- Primary aldosteronism is the overproduction of aldosterone from an aldosterone producing adenoma, hyperplasia of the adrenal gland, aldosterone producing carcinoma, or idiopathic hyperaldosteronism.

KEY ASSESSMENTS

- Hypertension
- Weakness
- Loss of energy
- Arrhythmias (hypokalemia)

Diagnostics

- Computed tomography (CT) of adrenal glands

Lab Tests

- Electrolytes (hypokalemia)
- Test urine for 24 hours for aldosterone
- Plasma aldosterone level
- Plasma rennin level

PLANNING AND IMPLEMENTATION

- Monitor cardiac status
- Monitor electrolytes and treat imbalances
- Monitor intake and output (I & O)
- Monitor vital signs frequently
- Take daily weight
- Assist with activities of daily living
- Space activities
- Implement safety measures
- Adrenalectomy indicated if a tumor is present

NURSING DIAGNOSIS

- Fatigue
- Fluid volume, Risk for imbalanced
- Knowledge, Deficient
- Activity intolerance

Primary Biliary Cirrhosis (PBC)

DEFINITION

- PBC is caused by an autoimmune process that results in bile duct inflammation and destruction. Nine out of ten patients with PBC are middle-age women. Liver transplantation is the only definitive treatment for end-stage PBC. Refer to cirrhosis for a more complete discussion on assessments, planning, and evaluation.

SPECIAL CONCERNS

- See Special Procedures and Treatments for information on Liver Transplantation.

NURSING DIAGNOSIS

- Fatigue
- Fluid volume, Risk for imbalanced
- Knowledge, Deficient
- Activity intolerance

Primary Sclerosing Cholangitis (PSC)

DEFINITION

- PSC is an autoimmune disease causing scarring of the bile ducts inside and outside of the liver resulting in bile obstruction. It is associated with ulcerative colitis and Crohn's disease. Liver transplantation is the only cure.

KEY ASSESSMENTS

- Steatorrhea
- Pruritus
- Jaundice

Diagnostics

- Endoscopic retrograde cholangiopancreatography (ERCP)

Lab Tests

- Liver function tests
- Blood urea nitrogen (BUN) and creatinine (Cr)
- Electrolytes

PLANNING AND IMPLEMENTATION

- Prevent infections
- Treat infections if present
- Administer vitamin supplements
- Encourage adequate oral and nutritional intake
- Administer cool baths for pruritus
- Discuss transplantation with patient

NURSING DIAGNOSIS

- Nutrition: less than body requirement, Imbalanced
- Infection, Risk for
- Anxiety

Prostatitis

DEFINITION

- Prostatitis is inflammation of the prostate gland.

Classifications

- Acute bacterial—acute infectious process from bacteria (*Escherichia coli, Enterobacter,* or enterococcus) or a sexually transmitted organism (chlamydia or gonococcus) that invades the prostate by ascending the urethra or extending from the rectum
- Chronic bacterial—recurrent bacterial infections
- Chronic nonbacterial or chronic pelvic pain syndrome—caused by an autoimmune process or the result of neurological damage to tissues surrounding the prostate from bacterial prostatitis
- Asymptomatic inflammatory prostatitis—inflammation of the prostate without symptoms

KEY ASSESSMENTS

- Urinary burning
- Frequency, urgency
- Dysuria
- Fever
- Malaise
- Pain in the testes, rectum, low back, or perineum

History and Examination

- Digital rectal examination to palpate prostate for enlargement and tenderness

Lab Tests

- Culture urethral and prostate secretions
- Urine culture
- Prostate fluid for cytotoxic T cells (autoimmune inflammatory response)

PLANNING AND IMPLEMENTATION

- Administer antibiotics (ciprofloxacin and doxycycline commonly ordered)
- Administer acetaminophen for fever and pain

- Administer nonsteroidal anti-inflammatory drugs (NSAIDs) to decrease inflammation and pain
- Administer sitz baths
- Monitor intake and output (I & O)
- Change positions frequently
- Avoid alcohol, coffee, tea, chocolate, cola, and spices
- Avoid sexual arousal and intercourse until acute infection subsides
- Implement safety measures
- Keep pathway to bathroom clear

NURSING DIAGNOSIS

- Pain, Acute
- Infection
- Urinary elimination, Impaired

Pulmonary Embolism

DEFINITION

- A pulmonary embolism is a thrombus lodged in the pulmonary artery. It may be life-threatening and cause death. The patient is able to ventilate, but perfusion does not occur in the occluded area.

KEY ASSESSMENTS

- Severe shortness of breath
- Tachycardia
- Severe chest pain
- Severe anxiety
- Hypoxia

PLANNING AND IMPLEMENTATION

- Administer oxygen
- Turn patient to left side to encourage embolism to stay in the right side of the heart
- Insert a peripheral intravenous (IV) line
- Treat pain
- Contact primary care provider immediately

- Frequent vital signs including pulse oximetry
- Anticipate spiral computed tomography (CT) of chest
- Anticipate thrombolytic therapy if the patient is a candidate

NURSING DIAGNOSIS

- Breathing pattern, Ineffective
- Anxiety
- Knowledge, Deficient
- Activity intolerance

Pyelonephritis

DEFINITION

- Pyelonephritis is an infection of the upper urinary tract. If untreated, it may cause renal failure.

Clinical Causes

- Untreated urinary tract infection (UTI)
- Drug-resistant UTI
- Any condition causing urinary retention

KEY ASSESSMENTS

- Flank pain at the costovertebral angle
- Fever
- Chills
- Painful urination
- Frequency
- Dysuria
- Nausea and vomiting

Diagnostics

- Computed tomography (CT)

Lab Tests

- Urinalysis
- Urine culture and sensitivity

PLANNING AND IMPLEMENTATION

- Monitor intake and output (I & O)
- Encourage adequate hydration orally and parenterally
- Monitor electrolytes, white blood count, blood urea nitrogen (BUN), and creatinine (Cr)
- Administer urinary antiseptics
- Administer antibiotics

NURSING DIAGNOSIS

- Hyperthermia
- Pain, Acute
- Infection
- Fluid volume, Risk for deficient

Raynaud's Disease

DEFINITION

- Raynaud's disease is the presence of bilateral venospasms of the extremities. The etiology is unknown but is related to other diseases, such as systemic lupus erythematosous, progressive systemic sclerosis, and connective tissue diseases. Episodes of exacerbation can be generated by stress and cold.

KEY ASSESSMENTS

- Pain to extremity
- Cyanosis followed by redness
- Decreased peripheral pulses
- Presence of infection or ulcerations

PLANNING AND IMPLEMENTATION

- Provide warm environment
- Treat pain
- Monitor pulses and capillary refill
- Wound care
- Administer vasodilators

SPECIAL CONSIDERATIONS

Teaching Considerations

- Avoidance of cold temperatures
- Stress management
- Medication compliance
- Safety with sharp objects
- Smoking cessation
- Monitor skin for infections or ulcers

NURSING DIAGNOSIS

- Tissue Perfusion, Ineffective
- Knowledge, Deficient

Reactive Arthritis

DEFINITION

- Reactive arthritis, or Reiter's syndrome, is associated with an infectious process (chlamydia or enteritis) with symptoms occurring one to four weeks after infection and persisting from five days to five months.

KEY ASSESSMENTS

- Urethritis
- Conjunctivitis
- Arthritis pain to low back pain
- "Sausage toe," red, swollen, painful toe
- Heel pain

PLANNING AND IMPLEMENTATION

- Administer nonsteroidal anti-inflammatory drugs (NSAIDs)
- Treat initial infection

NURSING DIAGNOSIS

- Pain, Acute
- Infection
- Knowledge, Deficient

Renal Artery Stenosis

DEFINITION

- Renal artery stenosis is the partial blockage of the renal artery.

Clinical Causes

- Atherosclerosis
- Fibromuscular hyperplasia

KEY ASSESSMENTS

- Hypertension

Diagnostics

- Renal angiogram
- Intravenous pyelogram (IVP)

PLANNING AND IMPLEMENTATION

- Monitor blood pressure
- Anticipate renal angioplasty

NURSING DIAGNOSIS

- Knowledge, Deficient

Renal Failure, Acute (ARF)

DEFINITION

- ARF is a rapid decline in renal function and may be effectively treated or may progress to chronic renal failure; 30 percent of intensive care unit patients develop ARF.

Classifications

- Prerenal—injury to the kidneys from hypoperfusion. Causes include hypotension, fluid volume deficit, decreased cardiac output, and heart failure.
- Intrarenal—tubular necrosis of the kidneys, or acute tubular necrosis (ATN). Usually occurs from medications and infections (drugs and bugs). Causes include nonsteroidal anti-inflammatory

drugs (NSAIDs), antibiotic therapy, glomerulonephritis, renal artery stenosis or thrombosis, hemolytic uremic syndrome, multiple myeloma, and contrast-induced nephropathy.
- Postrenal—injury to the kidney occurs from an obstruction. Causes include benign prostatic hyperplasia (BPH) and tumors.

Phases of Renal Failure

- Onset phase begins with the insult to the kidney and ends with oliguria phase.
- Oliguric phase begins with a decrease in urine output, usually less than 30 mL/hr and ends with an increase in urine output. Many patients progress to chronic renal failure from this phase. The serum creatinine is elevated and electrolyte imbalances may occur.
- Diuretic phase begins with an increase in urine output and ends with resolution of renal function. The serum creatinine decreases, and electrolyte imbalances may occur.
- Recovery phase is the period after ARF in which healing occurs. This phase may last six months.

KEY ASSESSMENTS

Oliguric Phase

- Review recent history, medication list, and fluid volume status to determine cause of ARF
- Cardiac arrhythmias (hyperkalemia)
- Fluid volume overload—peripheral edema, hypertension, shortness of breath (SOB), crackles, and acute weight gain
- Fluid volume deficit—thirst, poor skin turgor, dry mucous membranes hypotension, weight loss, and tachycardia
- Decrease in urine output
- Dark urine
- Anorexia
- Nausea or vomiting
- Diarrhea
- Metabolic acidosis
- Lethargy

Diuretic Phase

- Fluid volume deficit—thirst, poor skin turgor, dry mucous membranes hypotension, weight loss, and tachycardia
- Cardiac arrhythmias (hypokalemia)

Diagnostics

- X-ray of kidney, ureters, and bladder (KUB)
- Renal ultrasound
- Bladder scan

Lab Tests

- Blood urea nitrogen (BUN), creatinine (Cr), and glomerular filtration rate (GFR)
- Complete blood count (CBC)
- Electrolytes

PLANNING AND IMPLEMENTATION

Oliguric Phase

- Treat underlying cause (i.e., if medication induced, discontinue offending agent).
- Monitor for hyperkalemia and treat.
- Monitor cardiac status if hyperkalemia is present.
- Monitor electrolytes and renal labs.
- Maintain a patient intravenous (IV) line.
- Restrict fluids.
- Restrict potassium.
- Monitor intake and output (I & O).
- Take daily weight.
- Monitor for pulmonary congestion.
- Elevate head of bed to 30 degrees.
- Institute safety precautions.
- Administer frequent oral care.
- Encourage low-protein, low-sodium, low-potassium, and low-phosphorus diet.
- Monitor neurological function.
- Provide frequent rest periods.
- Monitor medications for potential nephrotoxicity.
- Anticipate renal adjustment of mediations metabolized in the kidney.
- Administer diuretics (furosemide and mannitol).
- If contrast induced tyrosinase-negative oculocutaneous albinism (ATN), administer *N*-acetylcysteine (Mucomyst).
- Administer bicarbonate for acidosis.
- Administer low-dose dopamine to increase renal perfusion.
- Dialysis may be indicated.

Diuretic Phase

- Monitor for hypokalemia and treat with potassium replacements
- Monitor cardiac status if hypokalemia is present
- Monitor electrolytes and renal labs
- Maintain a patient intravenous (IV) line
- Monitor intake and output (I & O)
- Take daily weight
- Elevate head of bed to 30 degrees
- Administer frequent oral care
- Anticipate increasing IV fluids

SPECIAL CONCERNS

- See Special Procedures and Treatments for information on Dialysis.
- Acute renal failure (ARF) may occur unexpectedly in the hospitalized patients and often evokes anxiety. Reassure, educate, and involve patients in their ARF care.

NURSING DIAGNOSIS

- Fluid volume, Risk for imbalanced
- Injury, Risk for
- Knowledge, Deficient

Renal Failure, Chronic (CRF)

DEFINITION

- CRF is the progressive and irreversible decline in renal function ranging from mild dysfunction to end-stage renal disease (ESRD) requiring dialysis or transplantation.

Clinical Causes

- Diabetes
- Hypertension
- Unresolved ARF
- Proteinuria
- Metabolic disorders
- Infections
- Immune diseases
- Nonmodifiable risk factors (male, African American, family history of CRF, and elderly)

KEY ASSESSMENTS

- Hypertension
- Peripheral edema
- Pallor
- Shortness of breath
- Crackles
- Dry skin with azotemia (powder-like substance on the skin from metabolic wastes)
- Pruritus
- Anorexia
- Nausea
- Vomiting
- Constipation
- Loss of secondary sexual characteristics
- Uremic encephalopathy (cognitive changes ranging from mild cognitive changes to coma)

Diagnostics

- Chest X-ray (CXR)
- Test urine for 24 hours for creatinine clearance
- Electrocardiogram (ECG), if hyperkalemia is present

Lab Tests

- Complete blood count ([CBC], anemia)
- Urinalysis
- Blood urea nitrogen (BUN), creatinine (Cr), and glomerular filtration rate (GFR)
- Electrolytes
- Glucose

PLANNING AND IMPLEMENTATION

- Monitor cardiac status.
- Monitor vital signs frequently.
- Monitor respiratory status.
- Auscultate breath sound for crackles.
- Encourage deep breathing.
- Monitor peripheral edema.
- Monitor intake and output (I & O).
- Take daily weight.
- Implement safety features.
- Implement fluid restriction.
- Administer frequent oral care.

- Monitor bowel sounds and record bowel movements.
- Administer stool softeners to prevent constipation.
- Administer cool baths and apply lotion for pruritus.
- Encourage nail trimming to prevent skin scratching from pruritus.
- Monitor medications for potential nephrotoxicity.
- Observe for signs of hyperkalemia, hypocalcemia, and hyperphosphatemia.
- Monitor electrolytes, renal labs, CBC, white blood count (WBC), and glucose.
- Administer phosphate binders (Amphojel) vitamin supplements, bicarbonate tablets, and Epogen.
- Monitor for infection.
- Monitor and treat nausea and vomiting.
- Provide low-protein, low-potassium, low-sodium, and low-phosphorus diet.
- Maintain glucose control in diabetics.
- Dialysis may be indicated.

SPECIAL CONCERNS

- See Special Procedures and Treatments for information on Dialysis.

NURSING DIAGNOSIS

- Nutrition: less than body requirements, Imbalanced
- Fluid volume, Excess
- Nausea
- Breathing pattern, Ineffective
- Knowledge, Deficient

Renal Trauma

DEFINITION

- Renal trauma is a kidney injury caused by a blunt or penetrating injury. The classification of the renal injury is based on the extent and depth of parenchymal damage.

KEY ASSESSMENTS

- Hemorrhage
- Hypovolemic shock (hypotension, tachycardia, or tachypnea)

- Bowel sounds (paralytic ileus)
- Decreased urine output
- Pain
- Hematuria
- Nausea and vomiting
- Abdominal rigidity

Diagnostics

- Computed tomography (CT)
- Intravenous pyelogram (IVP)

Lab Tests

- Complete blood count (CBC)
- Blood urea nitrogen (BUN) and creatinine (Cr)

PLANNING AND IMPLEMENTATION

- Wound care (if laceration is present)
- Monitor vital signs for shock
- Monitor urine output for amount and color
- Monitor intake and output (I & O)
- Treat pain
- Monitor labs for renal failure
- Monitor bowel sounds
- Monitor for signs of infection
- Monitor for retroperineal hemorrhage
- Maintain fluid balance with intravenous (IV) fluids
- Surgery—may be indicated for major injuries

NURSING DIAGNOSIS

- Pain, Acute
- Fluid volume, Risk for deficient
- Infection, Risk for

Renal Vein Thrombosis

DEFINITION

- Renal vein thrombosis is a thrombus or clot in the renal vein, which increases the venous pressure in the kidney.

Clinical Causes

- Renal cancer
- Renal trauma
- Nephrotic syndrome

KEY ASSESSMENTS

- Hematuria
- Flank pain
- Fever
- Shortness of breath (SOB), low pulse oximetry reading, and chest pain (signs of a pulmonary emboli if the thrombus dislodges)

Diagnostics

- Renal ultrasound
- Computed tomography (CT) of kidney

Lab Tests

- Prothrombin time (PT), partial thromboplastin time (PTT), and international normalized ratio (INR)
- Blood urea nitrogen (BUN) and creatinine (Cr)

PLANNING AND IMPLEMENTATION

- Monitor and treat pain
- Anticipate administering anticoagulants
- Monitor PT, PTT, and INR
- Monitor for signs of pulmonary emboli (SOB, decrease in pulse oximetry reading, and chest pain)
- Implement bleeding precautions
- Monitor intake and output (I & O)
- Monitor temperature
- Administer antipyretics

NURSING DIAGNOSIS

- Hyperthermia
- Pain, Acute

Respiratory Acidosis

DEFINITION

- Respiratory acidosis is a metabolic state in which the body retains too much CO_2. Regardless of cause, ineffective respirations result in the retention of CO_2, which leads to an increased acid load in the body. Excessive acid acts as a central nervous system (CNS) depressant. Guidelines to determine respiratory acidosis: pH less than 7.35, $PaCO_2$ greater than 45, and HCO_3 greater than 28.

Clinical Causes

- Narcotic use
- Chronic obstructive pulmonary disease (COPD)
- Rib fractures
- Patients that had thoracic or abdominal surgery
- Patients with severe pain
- Guillain-Barre syndrome
- Amyotrophic lateral sclerosis (ALS)

KEY ASSESSMENTS

- Confusion
- Lethargy
- Coma
- Shallow respirations
- Apnea
- Arrhythmias

PLANNING AND IMPLEMENTATION

- Monitor respiratory status
- Monitor cardiac status
- High Fowler's position, if possible
- Treat pain
- Monitor arterial blood gases (ABGs)
- Increase activity
- Deep-breathing exercises
- Bronchodilators

SPECIAL CONCERNS

- If other efforts not successful, mechanical ventilation may be necessary

NURSING DIAGNOSIS

- Ventilation, Impaired spontaneous
- Tissue perfusion, Ineffective

Respiratory Alkalosis

DEFINITION

- Respiratory alkalosis is a respiratory state in which the lungs excrete too much CO_2. Regardless of cause, the decreased CO_2 level reduces the acid load in the body causing alkalosis. Alkalosis acts as a central nervous system (CNS) irritant. Alkalosis decreases the amount of calcium available in the blood stream and can cause hypocalcemia. Guidelines to determine respiratory alkalosis are pH greater than 7.45, $PaCO_2$ less than 35, and HCO_3 of 22–26.

Clinical Causes

- Anxiety
- Pain
- Fever
- Hypoxia
- Hyperventilation

KEY ASSESSMENTS

- Hypoxia
- Respiratory rate
- Anxiety
- Pain
- Seizures
- Fever
- Trousseau's sign—inflate blood pressure cuff on the arm and hand will spasm
- Chvostek's sign—tapping on the facial nerve and spasm of facial muscle on tapped side
- Tingling of lips and fingers

PLANNING AND IMPLEMENTATION

- Administer oxygen
- Manage pain
- Reduce fever

- Relieve anxiety
- Have patient breathe into a paper bag, forcing rebreathing of CO_2

NURSING DIAGNOSIS

- Anxiety
- Pain
- Tissue perfusion, Ineffective

Retinal Detachment

DEFINITION

- Retinal detachment occurs as the retina detaches from its normal position and if not promptly treated, may cause permanent vision loss.

KEY ASSESSMENTS

- Floaters or specks that float in the visual field
- Shadow in the visual field
- Side vision impairment

Diagnostics

- Ophthalmoscope examination reveals a hole or tear at the edge of detachment.

PLANNING AND IMPLEMENTATION

Presurgical

- Cover affected eye
- Prepare the patient for surgery to correct the tear

Postsurgical

- Monitor for redness and swelling
- Treat pain
- Notify health care provider if visual impairment worsens

NURSING DIAGNOSIS

- Pain, Acute
- Knowledge, Deficient
- Sensory perception, Disturbed

Rhabdomyolysis

DEFINITION

- Rhabdomyolysis is a condition of massive muscle tissue destruction with the release of myoglobin causing acute renal failure.

Clinical Causes

- Severe burns
- Crush injuries
- Tetanus
- Gas gangrene
- Excessive exercise
- Diabetic ketoacidosis
- Hypothermia
- Polymyositis
- Ischemia causing muscular death

KEY ASSESSMENTS

- History of patient's recent activities
- Visible muscle injury or ischemia
- Burns
- Hypertension or hypotension
- Dark urine
- Reduced urine output

Lab Tests

- Blood urea nitrogen (BUN) and creatinine (Cr)
- Positive urine for myoglobin
- Hyperkalemia
- Elevated creatine phosphokinase skeletal muscle (CPK-MM)
- Hyperphosphatemia
- Hypocalcemia
- Elevated uric acid levels

PLANNING AND IMPLEMENTATION

- Refer to Renal Failure, Acute
- Treat initial injury causing rhabdomyolysis
- Monitor intake and output (I & O)
- Cardiac monitoring

- Observe for signs of hyperkalemia (tented T waves and arrhythmias)
- Treat hyperkalemia if present; see Hyperkalemia
- Insert peripheral intravenous (IV) line
- Fluid administration if hypotension is present
- Treat pain caused by initial injury

SPECIAL CONCERNS

- See Special Procedures and Treatments for information on Dialysis, Hemodialysis.

NURSING DIAGNOSIS

- Fluid volume, Risk for Imbalanced
- Tissue perfusion, Ineffective

Rheumatic Heart Disease

DEFINITION

- Rheumatic heart disease originates from a type of bacterial endocarditis caused by group A beta-hemolytic streptococcal pharyngitis, a common cause of a sore throat, called rheumatic fever. Untreated rheumatic fever may cause rheumatic heart disease that destroys the valves of the heart.

KEY ASSESSMENTS

- Malaise
- Anorexia or weight loss
- Back and joint pain
- Janeway lesions—flat red-bluish spots on the palms and soles
- Roth's spots—retinal hemorrhages with a central area of clearing
- Petechiae in the conjunctiva
- Clubbing of fingers
- Transient ischemic attacks due to emboli
- History of untreated sore throat

PLANNING AND IMPLEMENTATION

- Blood cultures
- Echocardiogram
- Administer antibiotic therapy

- Monitor vital signs
- Monitor cardiac status
- Monitor for emboli
- Teach patient and family about treatments
- Murmur
- Surgical valve replacement—may be necessary

NURSING DIAGNOSIS

- Cardiac output, Decreased
- Fatigue
- Knowledge, Deficient

Rheumatoid Arthritis (RA)

DEFINITION

- RA is a chronic, debilitating autoimmune disease that causes inflammation in the connective tissue in the joints and results in joint deformity. The exact cause of RA is not understood, and there is no cure.

Phases of Joint Deformity

- Initiation—beginning changes in the synovial lining are evident.
- Immune response phase—CD4 cells stimulate the immune response resulting in a release of immunoglobulin M (IgM) antibodies measured in the serum rheumatoid factor (RF).
- Inflammatory phase—increased inflammation and thickening of the synovial lining.
- Destruction phase—scar tissue forms and adheres to the surface of the cartilage fusing joints and permanent deformity.

KEY ASSESSMENTS

- Musculoskeletal pain
- Decreased joint mobility
- Reports of stiffness on waking
- Anorexia
- Joint swelling
- Joint deformity
- Presence of rheumatoid nodules in the subcutaneous tissue
- Raynaud phenomenon (painful, transient lack of circulation affecting fingers and toes exacerbated by cold temperatures)

- Systemic symptoms (fever, malaise, rash, lymph node, or spleen enlargement)
- Sjögren's syndrome (decreased tear and saliva production causing dry mouth and irritated, dry eyes)
- Pulmonary fibrosis
- Pericarditis

Lab Tests

- Positive RA factor (80 percent with positive RA test)
- Positive antimitochondrial antibodies (AMA), antinuclear antibodies (ANA), arteriosclerosis obliterans (ASO), and lupus erythematosus (LE) prep
- X-rays of joints reveal joint changes
- Synovial fluid has fibrin present and elevated white blood count (WBC)

PLANNING AND IMPLEMENTATION

- Encourage participation in activities of daily living
- Balance rest and activity
- Observe for signs of infection (medications increase susceptibility for infection)
- Social support
- Monitor for depression
- Monitor joint mobility
- Use orthotic equipment to promote self-care and feeding
- Take daily weight
- Monitor oral and nutrition intake
- Muscle strengthening activities
- Implement safety measures
- Apply heat for stiffness
- Implement complimentary therapies (yoga or guided imagery)
- Surgical procedures (tendon transfer, joint replacement, or arthroplasty)
- Administer medications as prescribed and observe for side effects (see Table 13)

SPECIAL CONCERNS

- See Special Procedures and Treatments for information on Joint Replacement.

Gender Considerations

- Women are three times more likely than men to develop RA.

TABLE 13

Examples of Drugs Used for Rheumatoid Arthritis (RA) Therapy

Drug Classification	Characteristics	Side Effects	Precautions or Interventions
Nonselective NSAIDs Motrin, Advil (ibuprofen) Aleve (naproxen) Indocin (indomethacin) Relafen (nabumetone) Feldene (piroxicam)	Provide pain and stiffness relief Inhibit the cyclooxygenase pathways, which produce prostaglandins during inflammation cascade	Esophagitis, gastritis, and gastroduodenal ulceration	Misoprostol (Cytotec) a prostaglandin analogue to protect gastric mucosa *Caution:* not to be used in pregnant women, nursing mothers, and women planning pregnancy Prilosec (omeprazole) and other proton pump inhibitors to protect gastric mucosa
Selective NSAIDs COX-2 inhibitors	Reduce pain and inflammation. Most effective in combination with disease modifying antirheumatic drugs (DMARDs)	Gastric irritation (reduced in comparison to NSAIDs)	Proton pump inhibitors to reduce gastric side effects Some removed from market due to cardiovascular problems
Synthetic DMARDs Methotrexate (MTX) Infliximab Adalimumab	Diminish progression of RA	Bone marrow suppression, hepatoxicity, pulmonary fibrosis, pneumonitis Hypersensitivity reactions	Vigilant monitoring of liver and renal function and symptoms of immunosuppression. CBC and CXRs *Caution:* not for pregnant women or women planning pregnancy Alcohol abstinence

continued

TABLE 13

Examples of Drugs Used for Rheumatoid Arthritis (RA) Therapy—cont'd

Drug Classification	Characteristics	Side Effects	Precautions or Interventions
Biologic DMARDs Tumor necrotizing factor (TNF)-alpha antagonists Enbrel (etanercept) Remicade (infliximab) Humira (adalimumab) Adalimumab	Diminish cytokine response to inflammation; reduces damaging effects (erosion of bone) Safe for children over 4 years old with juvenile RA	Immunosuppression Infliximab: greater chance for developing lymphoma	Discontinue drug if infection occurs Pregnancy safety is unknown Children to have immunizations up to date
Costimulatory Blockers Abatacept (CTLA4Ig)	Inhibits stimulation of antigen-presenting cells in activation of T lymphocytes Best results in combination with MTX	Upper respiratory infection, GI distress, rash, and dizziness	Monitor for adverse side effects
Interleukin antagonists Kinerel (anakinra)	Reduces erosive damage due to cytokines released by monocytes and macrophages	Injection site reactions, headache, and GI distress	Not be used in combination with TNF antagonists—increased risk of infection Contraindicated for people with active or chronic infections No live vaccines to be given Has not been tested in children or for pregnancy safety
Drugs under investigation Rituxan (rituximab) Genetically engineered monoclonal antibody	Targets specific surface antigens on circulating B lymphocytes Shows promise alone and in combination with MTX to reduce progress of RA	Immunosuppressant	Not known

R

Teaching Considerations

- Explain medication regimens and side effects
- Promote participation in social activities
- Home safety
- Monitor disease progress

NURSING DIAGNOSIS

- Pain, Acute
- Pain, Chronic
- Mobility, Impaired physical
- Activity intolerance
- Self-care deficient, Dressing/grooming

Rotator Cuff Injury

DEFINITION

- Rotator cuff injury results from trauma to or overuse of the shoulder and can range from mild straining to tears.

KEY ASSESSMENTS

- Pain
- Limited range of motion

Diagnostics

- Magnetic resonance imaging (MRI)

PLANNING AND IMPLEMENTATION

- Administer nonsteroidal anti-inflammatory drugs (NSAIDs)
- Ice shoulder
- Limit movement of shoulder
- Surgical correction—may be required

NURSING DIAGNOSIS

- Pain, Acute
- Mobility, Impaired physical

Scleroderma

DEFINITION

- Scleroderma, or progressive systemic sclerosis (PSS), is a connective tissue disease causing excessive collagen deposits and changes in immunity. It may affect the skin and internal organs. The etiology is unknown, and there is no cure.

KEY ASSESSMENTS

- Calcinosis (hard, oval white skin lesions surrounded by a purple ring)
- Raynaud's phenomenon (painful, transient lack of circulation affecting fingers and toes exacerbated by cold temperatures)
- Swollen, waxy appearance of hands
- Stiffness and pain in the extremities
- Difficulty swallowing
- Organ dysfunction

Diagnostics

- Antimitochondrial antibodies (AMA) and antinuclear antibodies (ANA)
- The presence of another autoimmune disease, such as rheumatoid arthritis or systemic lupus erythematosis
- Specific testing for organ involvement

PLANNING AND IMPLEMENTATION

- Treat pain
- Assist with activities of daily living
- Meticulous skin care
- Avoid temperature extremes
- Monitor extremities' temperature and pulse
- Observe for organ dysfunction
- Mechanical soft diet
- Upright position for feeding
- Provide emotional support
- Anticipate administering steroid and immunosuppressant medications
- Monitor for infections (risk is increased from medications)

NURSING DIAGNOSIS

- Pain, Chronic
- Tissue perfusion, Ineffective

Seizure

DEFINITION

- A seizure is a sudden, uncontrolled discharge of electricity in the brain. A convulsion is the abnormal motor response that may occur during a seizure. Epilepsy is recurring seizure activity. Approximately 3 percent of the population receives the diagnosis of epilepsy in their lifetime. If seizures continue, the patient may experience status epilepticus and require airway support.
- Phases of a seizure include prodromal, before a seizure; aural, the sensation experienced by a patient before a seizure; ictal, the seizure itself; and postictal, the period after a seizure.

Clinical Causes

- Metabolic causes include hypoglycemia, hypoxia, uremia, hepatic encephalopathy, electrolyte disturbance, acid-base disturbance, and hyperthermia.
- Structural causes include stroke, brain injury, brain tumors, and postcraniotomy.
- Medication-induced causes include side effects of medication (prescribed or illicit), withdrawal of medication (prescribed or illicit), or alcohol withdrawal.

Classifications

- Partial seizures originate in one hemisphere.
  - Simple partial seizures originate in one hemisphere and occur without an impairment of consciousness.
  - Complex partial seizures originate in one hemisphere and occur with an impairment of consciousness.
- Generalized seizures involve both hemispheres and occur with an impairment of consciousness; many partial seizures evolve into generalized seizures.
- Status epilepticus is defined as continuous seizures lasting more than five minutes. The most common cause is abruptly stopping antiepileptic medications. It is considered a medical emergency, because it is accompanied by respiratory distress. Treatment includes intravenous (IV) Ativan to relax airway muscles, airway

support with the administration of oxygen, and antiepileptic medications.

- Types of seizures include:
  - Absence seizures usually arise in childhood and may occur frequently, but last only 5–10 seconds with a brief loss of consciousness (mistaken for "spacing out" in class).
  - Myoclonic seizures are characterized by sudden, brief muscle jerking.
  - Tonic seizures are characterized by sudden brief muscle stiffening.
  - Tonic-clonic seizures, formerly called grand mal seizures, involve bilateral stiffness and jerking of the limbs with an impaired consciousness and may last two to three minutes.
  - Atonic seizures are characterized by sudden loss of muscle control and loss of consciousness. Serious injury may occur as a result of falls associated with the seizure.
  - Unclassified seizures are seizures that are not characterized by any other seizure type description.

KEY ASSESSMENTS

- Aura
- Onset of seizure activity
- Duration of seizure
- Type of seizure
- Loss of consciousness
- Pulse oximetry
- Respiratory status

Diagnostics

- Diagnostics are used to rule of structural cause and include computed tomography (CT), magnetic resonance imaging (MRI), and positron emission tomography (PET).
- Electroencephalogram (EEG) helps diagnose seizure type and identify the area of origin for the seizure.

Lab Tests

- Lab tests to help rule out metabolic causes include complete blood count (CBC), glucose, electrolytes, and toxicology.
- Determine if antiepileptic medication levels are therapeutic.

PLANNING AND IMPLEMENTATION

- Monitor respiratory status
- Maintain a safe environment

- Stay with the patient during the entire seizure episode
- Do not restrain the patient or put anything in the mouth
- Maintain a patent IV
- Anticipate administering Ativan intravenously for seizures causing respiratory distress
- Anticipate administering antiepileptic medications
- Place the patient in the recovery position after a seizure
- Monitor antiepileptic medication levels
- Seizure precautions—may be instituted

SPECIAL CONCERNS

Teaching Considerations

- Explain about actions, side effects, and the importance of medication compliance. A safe home environment is essential.

NURSING DIAGNOSIS

- Airway clearance, Ineffective
- Injury, Risk for
- Knowledge, Deficient
- Home maintenance, Impaired

Severe Acute Respiratory Syndrome (SARS)

DEFINITION

- SARS results from a coronavirus that leads to severe upper respiratory infection and has a high mortality rate. It is a new disease that was first recognized in 2002.
- Spread is person to person, droplet, from touching contaminated objects, and it is hypothesized to be airborne.
- Average incubation is 1 to 10 days.

KEY ASSESSMENTS

Prodrome Phase

- Fever
- Chills
- Rigors

- Myalgia
- Headache

Three to Seven Days Later

- Development of acute respiratory distress syndrome (ARDS) and accumulation of the interstitial space of the lungs making oxygenation difficult
- Hypoxia
- Nonproductive cough

History and Examination

- Recent travel to China, Hong Kong, or Taiwan

Diagnostics

- Chest X-ray (CXR)

Lab Tests

- Coronavirus antibodies in the blood
- Fluid or tissue culture for coronavirus

PLANNING AND IMPLEMENTATION

- Isolate patient
- Standard, airborne, and droplet precautions
- Disposable equipment only
- Anticipate intubation and mechanical ventilation
- Supportive care; no effective treatment regimen known to date
- Administer antiviral medications
- Monitor respiratory status
- Monitor vital signs
- Initiate two large-bore peripheral intravenous (IV) lines
- Fluid resuscitation with 0.9% normal saline (NS)
- Monitor intake and output (I & O)
- Antipyretics to reduce fever
- Sedate patient if required

NURSING DIAGNOSIS

- Tissue perfusion, Ineffective
- Airway clearance, Ineffective
- Fluid volume, Risk for deficient
- Breathing pattern, Ineffective

Sexually Transmitted Diseases (STDs)

DEFINITION

- STDs are infections contracted through sexual contact and include gonorrhea, chlamydia, syphilis, human papillomavirus (HPV), herpes infection, hepatitis B, and human immunodeficiency virus (HIV).

Classifications

- Gonorrhea is a bacterial infection that infects the cervix, anus, and throat. Symptoms include purulent vaginal or cervical discharge, dysuria, and abdominal pain. Treatment consists of oral antibiotic therapies.
- Chlamydia is a bacterial infection caused by *Chlamydia trachomatis,* which infects the cervix, urethra, anus, and pharynx. Symptoms include pain with urination and vaginal discharge. It is treated with oral antibiotics.
- Syphilis is caused by the bacteria *Treponema pallidum* and may be contracted through sexual contact, contact with a primary syphilis genital ulcer, or syphilis-infected blood. It is often asymptomatic, but it may produce a genital ulcer that heals. If not treated with antibiotics, it can progress to a secondary stage with a rash on the hands and feet or to tertiary syphilis with brain and nervous system involvement.
- HPV is a family of viruses that are associated with genital warts (condyloma) and cervical cancer. HPV is usually asymptomatic, and routine Pap smears show abnormal results and appropriate treatment.
- Herpes infection is a sexually transmitted virus. Both forms (herpes 1 and herpes 2) may cause a genital herpes infection producing small, painful, transient, fluid-filled blisters. Treatment is an oral antiviral medication.
- Hepatitis B—see Hepatitis.
- HIV—see Human immunodeficiency virus.

KEY ASSESSMENTS

- Unprotected sexual contact
- Dysuria
- Vaginal, cervical, penile, or anal discharge
- Vaginal, cervical, penile, or anal lesions
- Abdominal pain

Diagnostics

- Pap smear
- Culture of discharge

Lab Tests

- Complete blood count (CBC)

PLANNING AND IMPLEMENTATION

- Implement appropriate treatments
- Prevent spread

NURSING DIAGNOSIS

- Knowledge, Deficient

Shock Syndrome

DEFINITION

- Shock syndrome is a condition in which blood flow is insufficient for normal heart function and for the transportation of oxygen to organs and tissue. Any factor that affects blood volume, blood pressure, or cardiac function can initiate shock.

Clinical Causes

- Hemorrhage
- Drug reaction
- Trauma
- Pulmonary embolism
- Myocardial infarction
- Dehydration
- Heat stroke
- Infection

Classifications

Etiological

- Hypovolemic—loss of intravascular volume from profound dehydration or massive blood loss
- Anaphylactic—a hypersensitivity reaction causing loss of vascular tone

- Cardiogenic—diminished cardiac output from ischemia, decreased pumping ability, or an irregular heart beat
- Neurogenic—loss of sympathetic tone from a neurological injury
- Septic—caused by an infectious process

Functional

- Hypovolemic—loss of intravascular volume from profound dehydration or massive blood loss
- Transport—loss of sympathetic tone
- Obstructive—barriers to flow are present (pulmonary embolism or tension pneumothorax)
- Cardiogenic—diminished cardiac output from ischemia, decreased pumping ability, or an irregular heart beat

Four Phases of Shock

- Initial—marked by a decrease in cardiac output and impaired tissue perfusion and clinically noted with hypotension. Cellular metabolism switches to anaerobic metabolism and lactic acid forms.
- Compensatory—the body initiates compensatory mechanisms (activation of the sympathetic nervous system and shunting of blood to internal organs).
- Progressive—as shock progresses, cellular damage prevents cells from functioning, and every body system is affected. Referred to as multiple organ dysfunction syndrome (MODS) or multiple organ failure (MOF).
- Refractory—the body is unable to compensate, cellular death occurs, and death is eminent.

KEY ASSESSMENTS

- Systolic blood pressure less than 90 mm Hg
- Narrowed pulse pressure
- Change in level of consciousness (LOC)
- Anxiety
- Muscle weakness
- Slow capillary refill to extremities
- Hypothermia
- Tachycardia (or bradycardia if in refractory phase)
- Thready pulse
- Extremities cool to the touch
- Cyanosis
- Decreased or absent urine output
- Dyspnea
- Decreased bowel sounds

Diagnostics

- X-ray
- Computed tomography (CT)

Lab Tests

- Complete blood count (CBC)
- Glucose
- Electrolytes
- Prothrombin time (PT), partial thromboplastin time (PTT), international normalized ratio (INR), and platelets
- Blood cultures

PLANNING AND IMPLEMENTATION

- Initiate two large-bore peripheral intravenous (IV) lines
- Start fluid resuscitation with 0.9% normal saline (NS)
- Monitor vital signs frequently
- Monitor pulse oximetry
- Monitor neurological status
- Assess for injury that may be cause for shock
- Apply pressure to site if massive bleeding is present
- Administer oxygen
- Position flat or with feet elevated
- Monitor breath sounds
- Maintain blood glucose less than 150 mg/dL
- Monitor arterial blood gases (ABGs)
- Anticipate intubation and mechanical ventilation for respiratory compromise
- Administer blood products as requested, keeping hemoglobin above 7 g/dL
- Administer broad spectrum antibiotics and steroid therapy for septic shock
- Consider use of recombinant activated protein C for septic shock
- Anticipate vasopressor medications (vasopressin, dopamine, or norepinephrine)
- Anticipate administering medications to increase cardiac output (dobutamine or milrinone)
- Monitor fluid and electrolyte status
- Prepare patient for surgery if trauma or injury is the cause
- Maintain a safe environment
- Use intra-aortic balloon pump or ventricular assist device in cardiogenic shock

NURSING DIAGNOSIS

- Tissue perfusion, Ineffective
- Cardiac output, Decreased
- Fluid volume, Deficient
- Infection, Risk for

Sjögren's Syndrome

DEFINITION

- Sjögren's syndrome is a chronic inflammatory disorder that obstructs the secretory ducts causing dryness and is associated with autoimmune diseases.

KEY ASSESSMENTS

- Keratoconjunctivitis sicca (dry eyes)
- Xerostomia (dry mouth)
- Dysphagia
- Vaginal dryness

PLANNING AND IMPLEMENTATION

- Monitor for mouth ulcerations
- Monitor dysphagia
- Monitor for corneal abrasions
- Administer lubricants (artificial tears, artificial saliva, vaginal lubricants)

NURSING DIAGNOSIS

- Oral mucous membrane, Impaired
- Knowledge, Deficient

Sleep Apnea, Obstructive

DEFINITION

- Obstructive sleep apnea is episodes of apnea or not breathing that occurs during the night. The obstruction occurs at the level of nasopharynx or oropharynx. Risk factors include a family history of sleep apnea, hypothyroidism, recessed chin, and large, thick neck.

KEY ASSESSMENTS

- Reports of apnea or loud snoring by bed partners
- Daytime somnolence
- Morning headaches
- Memory problems

Diagnostics

- Polysomnography is used to diagnose sleep apnea.

PLANNING AND IMPLEMENTATION

- Encourage obese individuals to lose weight.
- Encourage refraining from alcohol or sedatives.
- Continuous positive airway pressure (CPAP) via mask at night is the standard treatment. CPAP allows air to be delivered with pressure through a mask to prevent the soft tissues from collapsing during sleep.
- Rarely, tonsillectomy or uvulopalatopharyngoplasty may be performed for patients with enlarged tissue causing obstruction.

SPECIAL CONCERNS

- Patients must understand the importance of treatment, because over time sleep apnea may cause life-threatening complications, such as hypertension, arrhythmias, myocardial infarction, stroke, hypoxia, hypercapnia, pulmonary hypertension, or right-sided heart failure.

NURSING DIAGNOSIS

- Ventilation, Impaired spontaneous
- Tissue perfusion, Ineffective
- Fatigue
- Sleep pattern, disturbed

Smallpox

DEFINITION

- Smallpox is caused by two forms of the virus orthopox: variola major (most common and deadly) and variola minor. In 1980, smallpox was declared eradicated worldwide, and the current population has not been vaccinated against the virus.
- Spreads through face-to-face contact or direct contact with contaminated objects.
- Average incubation is between 7 and 19 days.

KEY ASSESSMENTS

Prodrome Phase (2–4 Days)

- Malaise
- Rigors
- Vomiting
- Headache
- Backache
- High fever

Macular Rash Stage (14–19 Days)

- Macular rash (flat, red spots) is on tongue and mouth and spreads to extremities.
- Four days into the rash, it raises into fluid-filled lesions.
- Scabs begin to form at 10 days.
- Scabs fall off at 14–19 days. Once the scabs are gone, the patient is not contagious.

Diagnostics

- Culture of fluid from rash (only a few labs can diagnose the orthopox virus)

PLANNING AND IMPLEMENTATION

- Isolate patient
- Standard, airborne, and droplet precautions
- Vaccinate all persons in contact with the patient
- Treatment of the patient is supportive
- Monitor vital signs
- Administer oxygen
- Administer antipyretics

- Meticulous skin and mouth care
- Monitor intake and output (I & O)
- Provide intravenous (IV) fluids to maintain fluid balance

NURSING DIAGNOSIS

- Infection, Risk for
- Skin integrity, Impaired

Spinal Cord Injury

DEFINITION

- Spinal cord injury is any injury or process that leads to the interruption of the normal structure and functioning of the spinal cord at any level. High cervical injuries above C3 result in loss of respiratory function and death if ventilatory support is not provided immediately. Spinal shock and autonomic dysreflexia are life-threatening complications of spinal cord injury.

Clinical Causes

- Injury from degenerative spine changes, trauma, tumors, and gunshot wounds

Classifications

- Complete spinal cord injury is a complete transaction of the spinal cord resulting in total loss of motor and sensory function below the level of injury.
- Incomplete spinal cord injury occurs when a portion of the spinal cord is disrupted leaving partial sensory or motor defects (see Table 14).

Key assessments for complete spinal injury

- Levels of injury
    - Cervical injuries may result in quadriplegia or loss of movement of the arms and legs. If injury is above C3, ventilatory support is required. Bowel and bladder dysfunction may be present.
    - Thoracic injuries may result in paraplegia or loss of movement of the legs. Bowel and bladder dysfunction may be present.

S

TABLE 14

Syndromes of Incomplete Cord Injury

Syndrome	Type of Injury	Functional Deficit
Anterior Cord Syndrome	Flexion injury to cervical spinal cord	Motor paralysis below level to injury; decreased sensation, pain, and temperature secretion below level of injury
Brown Séquard Syndrome	Penetrating injury (gunshot wound or knife wound) causes hemisection of the spinal cord	Ipsilateral motor paralysis and loss of vibration and position sense; contralateral loss of pain and temperature
Central Cord Syndrome	Hyperextension-hyperflexion injury damages cervical central cord; anterior horn is damaged	Weakness in upper extremities greater than weakness in lower extremities
Posterior Cord Syndrome	Cervical hypertension injury damages posterior cervical spinal cord	Loss of sense of position

KEY ASSESSMENTS

Emergent

- Airway, breathing
- Level of consciousness (LOC)
- Pain
- Assess for spinal shock or neurogenic shock—bradycardia, hypotension, or flaccidity
- Sensation and movement of extremities
- Deep tendon reflexes
- Loss of bowel or bladder control
- Presence of other injuries

Poststabilization

- Airway support for high cervical injuries
- Assess for autonomic dysreflexia or hyperreflexia in patients with injuries above the T6 level
    - Hypertension (blood pressure greater than 200/100 mm Hg)
    - Pounding headache
    - Flushed warm skin above level of injury
    - Bradycardia

  - Visual disturbances
  - Anxiety
  - Cool, pale skin below the level of injury
- Skin for signs of breakdown
- Bowel and bladder function
- Spasticity
- Pain
- Presence of deep venous thrombosis (DVT)

Diagnostics

- X-rays
- Computed tomography (CT)
- Magnetic resonance imaging (MRI)

PLANNING AND IMPLEMENTATION

Emergent

- Provide airway support
- Immobilize patient
- Insert two large-bore peripheral intravenous (IV) lines
- Monitor blood pressure
- Monitor deep tendon reflexes
- Anticipate administering high-dose steroids
- Anticipate possible surgical stabilization
- Treat spinal shock with IV fluids and antiembolism stockings (to prevent venous pooling)
- Treat pain
- Provide emotional support

S

Poststabilization

- Treat autonomic dysfunction immediately
  - Raise head of bed
  - Remove antiembolic stockings
  - Assess for cause and treat bladder distention or bowel impaction
  - Monitor vital signs frequently
  - Report incident to the health care provider
  - Anticipate administering short-acting antihypertensive agents
- Encourage deep breathing and coughing
- Monitor sputum production for signs of pulmonary infections
- Monitor for complications of immobility, including DVTs, skin breakdown, and contracture formation
- Encourage adequate fluid and nutritional intake

- Bladder care including intermittent catheterization and monitoring for urinary retention; if in-dwelling catheter is necessary, monitor for presence of urinary tract infection
- Institute a bowel elimination program, including stool softeners
- Promote safe mobility
- Meticulous skin care
- Turn patient every two hours
- Document skin assessments every shift
- Monitor and treat spasticity
- Monitor for signs of depression and report to the health care provider
- Establish trust with the patients

Discharge Planning

- Patients often need major changes to their home environment before discharge. Health care providers assist patients and their families in locating resources to help implement these changes (such as building a wheelchair ramp to gain access to the home).

SPECIAL CONCERNS

- Sexuality is affected in all spinal cord injury patients. Patients need to speak with health care providers who can openly discuss the effects of the injury on sexuality and options available to improve sexual function.
- Families will experience a transformation in role patterns and expectations and should be encouraged to talk about these changes.

Teaching Considerations

- Patients and their families have a great deal to learn to adequately take care of the patient at home. Encourage patients and families to participate in care and ask questions. Stress safety and the prevention of complications.

NURSING DIAGNOSIS

- Skin integrity, Risk for impaired
- Autonomic dysreflexia, Risk for
- Self-care deficit, Toileting

Sprain

DEFINITION

- A sprain occurs when the ligaments of the ankle are stretched beyond normal capacity. A sprain may be mild, moderate, or severe.

KEY ASSESSMENTS

- History of injury
- Swelling
- Pain

Diagnostics

- X-ray
- Magnetic resonance imaging (MRI)

PLANNING AND IMPLEMENTATION

- Rest extremity
- Apply ice
- Compress joint with an elastic wrap
- Elevate extremity above level of the heart
- Administer analgesics
- Use of crutches

NURSING DIAGNOSIS

- Pain, Acute
- Mobility, Impaired physical

Stroke

DEFINITION

- Stroke or cerebrovascular accident (CVA) occurs when a portion of the brain is damaged from a lack of blood flow to brain tissue. Stroke is the third leading cause of death and the leading cause of long-term disability in the United States. Transient ischemic attacks (TIA), also known as ministrokes, are a temporary loss of

blood to part of the brain and are a strong predictor of an impending stroke.
- Modifiable stroke risk factors include hypertension, hypercholesterolemia, atherosclerosis, atrial fibrillation, obesity, drug and alcohol abuse, and smoking.
- Nonmodifiable stroke risk factors include increased age, male, family history, and history of previous stroke.

Classifications

- Ischemic stroke causes a lack of blood flow due to a thrombus (a blood clot) or emboli (plaque or clot) that occlude a cerebral vessel; 88 percent of strokes are ischemic.
- Hemorrhagic stroke causes lack of blood flow from burst cerebral vessel that causes bleeding into surrounding brain tissue.

KEY ASSESSMENTS

- Exact time of onset of symptoms
- Unilateral weakness or paralysis
- Slurred speech
- Unilateral facial drooping
- Ptosis
- Headache
- Double vision
- Incontinence
- Change in level of consciousness (LOC)
- Anisocoria (unequal pupils)
- Hypertension

Diagnostics

- Computed tomography (CT) of the head is the gold standard for stroke diagnosis and should be performed as soon as possible.
- Magnetic resonance imaging (MRI), magnetic resonance angiography (MRA), cerebral angiography, positron emission tomography (PET) scan, carotid ultrasound, and transcranial Doppler studies may be ordered after emergent care is rendered.

Lab Tests

- Completed blood count(CBC)
- Prothrombin time (PT), partial thromboplastin time (PTT), and international normalized ratio (INR)
- Electrolytes and glucose

PLANNING AND IMPLEMENTATION

Emergent Care

- Monitor LOC.
- Administer frequent, complete neurological checks.
- Insert two large-bore peripheral intravenous (IV) lines.
- Treat excessive hypertension (higher than180 mm Hg systolic).
- Monitor airway and breathing.
- Institute safety measures.
- Administer oxygen and continual pulse oximetry.
- Monitor vital signs frequently.
- Report any change in neurological status immediately to the health care provider.
- If the diagnosis of ischemic stroke is made and the patient is a candidate, tissue plasminogen activator (tPA) or "clot-buster" may be ordered and administered, ideally within three hours of onset of symptoms.
- If bleeding or neurological deterioration occurs during tPA therapy, immediately discontinue therapy and notify health care provider.
- If diagnosis of hemorrhagic stroke is made, treatment will be supportive to control increased intracranial pressure.

Long-Term Care

- Institute safety measures.
- Monitor vital signs and neurological signs.
- Prevent skin breakdown.
- Prevent contractures.
- Provide bowel and bladder training.
- Provide a means of communication.
- Monitor gag and cough reflex.
- Carefully feed to prevent food aspiration.
- Encourage range-of-motion exercises.
- Assist with activities of daily living.
- Encourage physical, occupational, and speech therapy.
- Implement seizure precautions.
- Carotid endarterectomy is a surgical procedure to remove plaque formation in a carotid artery. This procedure may prevent a stroke or prevent another from occurring.
- Carotid stenting involves introducing a catheter into the carotid artery and leaving a mesh tube in place to maintain the patency of the carotid artery. This procedure may prevent a stroke or prevent another from occurring.

Discharge Planning

- If the patient has significant neurological impairment, he or she may be unable to be discharged to the home setting. Long-term placement may be necessary to provide adequate care for the patient.

SPECIAL CONCERNS

- The change in a patient's physical and cognitive function is devastating for families. There are rapid role changes that affect every aspect of the family's life from financial changes to changes in sexuality.

NURSING DIAGNOSIS

- Neglect, Unilateral
- Mobility, Impaired
- Transfer ability, Impaired
- Swallowing, Impaired

Subclavian Steal Syndrome

DEFINITION

- Subclavian steal syndrome occurs when the subclavian artery is occluded and blood flow is diminished to the upper extremity.

KEY ASSESSMENTS

- Reports of upper extremity pain, weakness, and paresthesia
- Blood pressure difference of 20 mm Hg or greater on arms
- Subclavian bruit
- Diminished brachial and radial pulses
- Cyanosis of the extremity

PLANNING AND IMPLEMENTATION

- Monitor bilateral blood pressures.
- Treat pain.
- Document extremity color and pulse strength.
- Treatment is usually surgical intervention with subclavian artery enterectomy, carotid to subclavian graft bypass, or subclavian artery angioplasty with stent placement.

NURSING DIAGNOSIS

- Pain, Acute
- Tissue perfusion, Ineffective

Syndrome of Inappropriate Antidiuretic Hormone (SIADH)

DEFINITION

- SIADH is hypersecretion of antidiuretic hormone from the posterior pituitary gland.

Clinical Causes

- Malignant lung disease
- Lymphoma
- Sarcoma
- Infections
- Medications (thiazides or vincristine)
- Adrenal insufficiency
- Hypopituitarism

KEY ASSESSMENTS

- Headache
- Seizure
- Fatigue
- Nausea and vomiting
- Fluid volume overload (edema, weight gain, or pulmonary congestion)
- Sluggish or absent deep tendon reflexes

Lab Tests

- Electrolytes (hyponatremia)
- Osmolality (high)

PLANNING AND IMPLEMENTATION

- Monitor neurological status
- Implement seizure precautions
- Implement safety precautions
- Monitor electrolytes frequently

- Take daily weight
- Monitor intake and output (I & O)
- Monitor for fluid volume overload
- Request fluid restriction if necessary
- Replace sodium judiciously with 3% NaCl (do not exceed 50 mL/hr)

NURSING DIAGNOSIS

- Fluid volume, Excess
- Injury, Risk for
- Confusion, Acute

Systemic Inflammatory Response Syndrome (SIRS)

DEFINITION

- SIRS is an acute inflammatory response of multiple organs resulting from an original inflammatory insult (see causes). SIRS is an activation of neutrophils, macrophages, and lymphocytes, which damages the vascular endothelium, affects the transportation of nutrients to organs, and may lead to multiple organ dysfunctions. Transition from SIRS to the dysfunction of multiple organs occurs with failure to control the inflammation or infection, persistent hypoperfusion, the presence of necrotic tissue, and altered cellular oxygen consumption.

Clinical Causes

- Infection
- Pancreatitis
- Ischemia
- Multiple trauma
- Hemorrhagic shock
- Massive transfusions

KEY ASSESSMENTS

- Tachycardia
- Tachypnea
- Fever

Diagnostics

- SIRS is diagnosed when a patient has two or more of the following symptoms.
  - Fever greater than 38° C (98.6° F) or less than 36° C (100.4° F)
  - Tachycardia—greater than 90 beats per minute
  - Tachypnea—a respiratory rate greater than 20 per minute or a $PaCo_2$ less than 32 mm Hg
  - Elevated white blood count greater that 12,000 cells/μL
  - Inability to create white blood cells (count less than 4,000 cells/μL)
  - More than 10 percent immature white blood cells

PLANNING AND IMPLEMENTATION

- Monitor oxygen status
- Administer supplemental oxygen to maintain O_2 saturation above 90 percent
- Monitor intake and output (I & O)
- Maintain patent intravenous (IV) line
- Monitor white blood count
- Monitor for signs of infection
- Monitor vital signs
- Monitor neurological status
- If hypotension occurs, promptly treat with fluid administration
- Administer antibiotics if fever is present
- Anticipate blood, urine, sputum and wound cultures
- Monitor for signs of organ dysfunction (i.e., kidneys, decreased urine output, and increased creatinine)

S

NURSING DIAGNOSIS

- Tissue perfusion, Ineffective
- Fluid volume, Risk for deficient
- Infection, Risk for

Systemic Lupus Erythematosus (SLE)

DEFINITION

- SLE is an autoimmune disorder in which autoantibodies (ANAs) develop and trigger inflammation in connective tissue causing tissue damage. The etiology in unknown, and it is characterized by exacerbations and remissions. Women with SLE are prone to spontaneous abortions and premature delivery. Discoid lupus erythematosus (DLE) is a milder form that affects the skin of the face and upper chest.

KEY ASSESSMENTS

Neurological

- Lethargy, malaise
- Delirium
- Seizures
- Psychosis
- Coma

Integument

- Red, raised, butterfly-shaped rash across the bridge of the nose extending to the cheeks
- Polyarthritis
- Joint pain
- Raynaud's phenomenon
- Joint swelling
- Hair loss

Respiratory

- Pleural effusions
- Shortness of breath

Cardiovascular

- Tachycardia
- Cardiomyopathy
- Vasculitis
- Pericarditis
- Anemia

Gastrointestinal (GI)/Genitourinary (GU)

- Renal dysfunction (glomerulonephritis is the most common cause of death)
- Nausea
- Vomiting
- Bloody stools
- Hepatic dysfunction
- Gastric ulcers

Immunological

- Generalized lymphadenopathy
- Fever
- Weight loss
- Splenomegaly

Lab Tests

- No single test confirms the diagnosis of SLE. The clinical picture, lab testing, and presence of organ dysfunction from SLE aids the health care provider in making the diagnosis of SLE.
  - Positive ANA titer
  - Positive Sm nuclear antigen
  - Decreased C3 and C4 complement factors
  - Testing for organ dysfunction (creatinine [Cr] and aspartate aminotransferase [AST])
  - Magnetic resonance imaging (MRI)

PLANNING AND IMPLEMENTATION

- Prevent progressive organ dysfunction
- Monitor renal function and urine output
- Treat pain
- Meticulous skin care
- Document and monitor rashes or skin breakdown
- Monitor and treat nausea and vomiting
- Monitor hemoglobin and hematocrit (H & H)
- Contact health care provider if urine output is less than 30 mL/hr
- Elevate head of bed
- Take daily weight
- Promote rest
- Implement safety measures
- Provide psychological support
- Implement stress-reducing techniques
- Monitor neurological status and report changes to the health care provider
- Monitor and document distal pulses and skin temperature
- Monitor for infections
- Provide additional resources for knowledge and support
- Administer nonsteroidal anti-inflammatory drugs (NSAIDs) for pain and fever; antimalarials, corticosteroids, and immunosuppressives for systemic effects

SPECIAL CONCERNS

Cultural Considerations

- SLE affects 1 in 250 African American women.

Gender Considerations

- SLE predominately affects women.
- DLE predominately affects men.

Teaching Considerations

- Consider pregnancy counseling
- Implement stress-reducing techniques
- Medication use and side effects
- Monitor temperature
- Use of sunscreen while outdoors
- Avoid the sun

NURSING DIAGNOSIS

- Pain, Chronic
- Mobility, Impaired physical
- Activity intolerance
- Tissue perfusion, Ineffective

Thrombocytopenia

DEFINITION

- Thrombocytopenia is defined as a platelet count less than 100,000 per mL of blood. The lack of platelets may result in spontaneous bleeding (when platelet count is less than 20,000) or prolonged bleeding because the lack of platelet aggregation.

Classifications

- Immune thrombocytopenia purpura (ITP), also known as idiopathic thrombocytopenia purpura, is an autoimmune disorder with platelet destruction.
    - Proteins on the platelet cell stimulate the production of autoantibodies, which then adhere to the platelet membrane. The spleen sees these platelets as foreign bodies and destroys them.
    - ITP can be acute (more common in children) or chronic (common in those 20–40 years of age).

- Thrombotic thrombocytopenia purpura (TTP) is a rare disease in which thrombi form and occlude arterioles and capillaries. It affects much of the body and may be fatal. The cause is unknown.
- Secondary thrombocytopenia is a thrombocytopenia with a known cause. Causes include aplastic anemia, bone cancer, radiation therapy, disseminated intravascular coagulation, or drug therapy. Treatment includes withdrawal of the offending agent and platelet transfusion.

KEY ASSESSMENTS

- Bruising without trauma
- Bleeding gums
- Black or tarry stools
- Hematemesis
- Headache
- Nosebleed
- Change in neurological status

Lab Tests

- Platelet count
- Complete blood count (CBC)
- Antinuclear antibodies (ANA)
- Cytomegalovirus (CMV)
- Possible bone marrow aspiration (to confirm aplastic anemia)

PLANNING AND IMPLEMENTATION

- Monitor level of consciousness (LOC)
- Observe for signs of bleeding (cerebral bleeding)
- Obtain consents for blood or platelet administration
- Bleeding precautions
- Implement safety precautions
- No intramuscular (IM) injections
- Explain cause and treatments associated with thrombocytopenia
- Platelet transfusion (with secondary thrombocytopenia)
- Corticosteroids
- Immunosuppressive drugs (i.e., azathioprine or cyclosporine)
- Plasmapheresis (the patient's plasma is removed and replaced)

SPECIAL CONCERNS

Gender Considerations

- Chronic ITP is more common in females between the ages of 20 and 40 years.

NURSING DIAGNOSIS

- Injury, Risk for
- Fluid volume, Risk for deficient
- Knowledge, Deficient

Thrombophlebitis

DEFINITION

- Thrombophlebitis is the inflammation of a vein accompanied by the formation of a blood clot or thrombus and is referred to as a deep venous thrombosis (DVT). DVTs occur most often in the deep veins of the lower extremities and if dislodged may lead to pulmonary emboli.

Clinical Causes

- Increased risks include postsurgical procedures, pregnancy, ulcerative colitis, fractures, heart failure, immobility, paralysis, intravenous (IV) therapy, infections, and trauma.
- Virchow's triad includes venous stasis, vessel injury, and altered blood coagulation.

KEY ASSESSMENTS

- Pain, warmth, redness, and swelling at thrombus site
- Fever or malaise
- Fatigue
- Edema

PLANNING AND IMPLEMENTATION

- Doppler flow or impedance plethysmography
- Treat pain
- Bed rest
- Anticoagulation therapy
- Monitor distal pulses
- Monitor for pulmonary embolism

SPECIAL CONCERNS

Teaching Considerations

- DVT prevention is vital. Educate patients on the need for early ambulation after surgery and about the importance of using thromboembolic elastic stockings and pneumatic pulsation devices to prevent DVT formation.

NURSING DIAGNOSIS

- Pain, Acute
- Tissue perfusion, Ineffective
- Mobility, Impaired

Tonsillitis

DEFINITION

- Tonsillitis is the inflammation of the tonsils caused by either bacterial or viral infection. The adenoids may become inflamed as well. Recurrent tonsillitis is diagnosed when the patient has at least seven episodes in one year.

KEY ASSESSMENTS

- Change or loss in voice
- Painful swallowing
- Foul breath
- Red, swollen tonsils
- Fever

PLANNING AND IMPLEMENTATION

- Viral tonsillitis is treated with supportive care of analgesics, rest, and encouragement of warm fluid intake.
- Bacterial tonsillitis, in addition to supportive care, is treated with appropriate antibiotics.
- Recurrent tonsillitis may be treated with surgical excision of the tonsils, or tonsillectomy. Postoperative care after a tonsillectomy includes:
  - Pain relief with an ice collar to the neck and cold liquids (once gag reflex has returned)
  - Analgesic administration
  - Monitoring for hemorrhage (drop in blood pressure, tachycardia, or emesis of blood)

NURSING DIAGNOSIS

- Pain, Acute
- Swallowing, Impaired

Toxic Shock Syndrome (TSS)

DEFINITION

- TSS is an acute illness caused by toxin-producing *Staphylococcus aureus* bacteria, which is present in 2 percent of women. It is highly associated with menstruation and tampon use, but it may occur postpartum, postoperative, and with diaphragm use. There is 3 percent mortality despite aggressive care.

KEY ASSESSMENTS

- High fever (greater than 102° F [39° C])
- Diffuse rash
- Hypotension
- Nausea and vomiting
- Diarrhea
- Myalgias
- Confusion

Lab Tests

- Blood urea nitrogen (BUN) and elevated creatinine (Cr)
- Elevated aspartate aminotransferase (AST) and alanine aminotransferase (ALT)
- Low platelet count
- Complete blood count (CBC)
- Electrolytes
- Platelets, international normalized ratio (INR), prothrombin time (PT), and partial thromboplastin time (PTT)

PLANNING AND IMPLEMENTATION

- Remove tampon or diaphragm if present
- Insert two large-bore peripheral intravenous (IV) lines
- Initiate fluid with 0.9% normal saline (NS) to maintain blood pressure
- Administer oxygen
- Anticipate intubation if oxygenation status deteriorates

- Administer vasopressor agents (hospital policy may require a central line for administration)
- Administer antibiotics
- Monitor vitals signs closely
- Monitor level of consciousness (LOC)
- Insert Foley catheter
- Monitor intake and output (I & O)
- Anticipate administering blood and platelets
- Monitor for signs of external and internal bleeding
- Administer antipyretics

NURSING DIAGNOSIS

- Infection
- Hyperthermia
- Fluid volume, Deficient
- Tissue perfusion, Ineffective
- Injury, Risk for

Trigeminal Neuralgia

DEFINITION

- Trigeminal neuralgia is intense pain affecting one or more branches of cranial nerve (CN) V. It is believed to be caused by pressure exerted by blood vessels on the nerve. The pain associated with trigeminal neuralgia may result in severe activity restriction.

KEY ASSESSMENTS

- Intense, sharp, burning pain to one or more branches of CN V (forehead, cheek, and jaw areas)
- Pain increases with chewing, touching, and movement
- Facial tic on affected side
- Weight loss
- Poor oral care

Diagnostics

- Diagnosis is usually based on patient report
- Computed tomography (CT) to rule out other causes
- Magnetic resonance imaging (MRI)

PLANNING AND IMPLEMENTATION

- Treat pain
- Encourage fluid and nutritional intake
- Assist patient in identifying and avoiding aggravating factors
- Anticipate pharmacological interventions (Tegretol or Dilantin)
- Surgical intervention may be necessary

NURSING DIAGNOSIS

- Pain, Acute
- Nutrition: less than body requirements, Imbalanced

Tuberculosis (TB)

DEFINITION

- TB is a chronic infection of the lungs caused by a mycobacterium infection and resulting in the development of tubercles in the lungs. Tubercles are the nodules seen on a chest X-ray (CXR). They consist of lymphocytes and epithelioid cells. Mycobacterium enters the body through inhaled droplets.

Clinical Causes

Conditions that may precipitate TB infection

- Human immunodeficiency virus (HIV) infection
- Silicosis
- Cancer
- Renal disease
- Chronic malabsorption syndromes
- Living in a long-term facility
- Socioeconomic factors, such as being poor, being medically underserved, and living in crowed quarters

KEY ASSESSMENTS

- Cough and hemoptysis
- Fever and chills
- Weight loss
- Night sweats
- Weakness
- CXR with granulomas present

- Sputum positive for mycobacterium
- Positive Mantoux skin test

PLANNING AND IMPLEMENTATION

- Place patient in a negative flow room
- Monitor airway
- Chest physiotherapy
- Administer oxygen
- Keep head of bed elevated
- Administer treatment regimes for TB
- Monitor for side effects of therapy, including neuropathy and hepatotoxicity
- Encourage adequate nutritional and fluid intake
- Encourage frequent rest periods
- Treat fevers with antipyretics

Discharge Planning

- Encourage other household or family members to be tested for TB
- Discuss financial concerns and if the patient can afford the medication regimen
- Emphasize the importance of strictly adhering to medication regimens
- Explain the side effects of medications and when to contact the health care provider

NURSING DIAGNOSIS

- Airway clearance, Ineffective
- Fatigue
- Therapeutic regimen management, Ineffective family
- Knowledge, Deficient

Tuberculosis, Renal

DEFINITION

- Renal tuberculosis is tubercle bacilli infection of the kidney. The kidney is the most common site of extrapulmonary tuberculosis.

KEY ASSESSMENTS

- Frequency
- Dysuria
- Urgency
- Hematuria
- Groin pain

History and Examination

- Family history of pulmonary tuberculosis
- Exposure to a patient with pulmonary tuberculosis

Diagnostics

- Chest X-ray (CXR)
- Abdominal X-ray
- Intravenous pyelogram (IVP)
- Computed tomography (CT) of abdomen

Lab Tests

- Urine acid-fast bacillus (AFB) culture
- AFB sputum cultures
- Blood urea nitrogen (BUN) and creatinine (Cr)

PLANNING AND IMPLEMENTATION

- Monitor intake and output (I & O)
- Monitor kidney function tests
- Administer antituberculin medications
- Monitor for side effects of medication therapy

NURSING DIAGNOSIS

- Pain, Acute
- Infection
- Urinary elimination, Impaired
- Knowledge, Deficient

Tumors, Spinal Cord

DEFINITION

- A spinal cord tumor is an abnormal growth in the spine that exerts pressure and causes spinal dysfunction.

Classifications

- Benign tumors include meningiomas and neurofibromas.
- Metastatic tumors are metastasis to the spine from primary cancers, including breast, kidney, prostate, colon lymphomas, and myelomas.

KEY ASSESSMENTS

- Specific sites of pain and motor and sensory disturbance depend on tumor location and size
- Back pain
- Reports of bowel or bladder dysfunction
- Muscle wasting
- Unilateral or bilateral weakness
- Deep tendon reflexes

Diagnostics

- Computed tomography (CT)
- Magnetic resonance imaging (MRI)
- Positron emission tomography (PET)
- Myelogram
- Cerebral spinal tap

PLANNING AND IMPLEMENTATION

- Implement safety measures
- Monitor gait, muscle strength, and sensory function
- Treat pain
- Assist with activities of daily living
- Encourage adequate fluid and nutritional intake
- Monitor bowel and bladder dysfunction
- Meticulous pericare
- If paralysis is present, ROM to affected limb
- Report any sudden loss of function to the health care provider immediately
- Anticipate steroid administration
- Anticipate surgical excision of tumor, chemotherapy, and radiation

SPECIAL CONCERNS

- See Special Procedures and Treatments for information on Cancer.

NURSING DIAGNOSIS

- Pain, Acute
- Mobility, Impaired
- Injury, Risk for

Ulcerative Colitis

DEFINITION

- Ulcerative colitis is a chronic inflammatory bowel disease (IBD) causing inflammation of the mucosa and submucosa of the colon and rectum. The etiology is unknown, but it is postulated to be autoimmune in nature. Ulcerative colitis has exacerbations and remissions ultimately causing the bowel to narrow, shorten, and thicken from inflammation.

KEY ASSESSMENTS

- Diarrhea
- Abdominal pain in the left lower quadrant (LLQ)
- Rectal bleeding
- Fatigue
- Dehydration
- Anorexia
- Weight loss
- Weakness
- Tachycardia
- Hypotension

Diagnostics

- Proctosigmoidoscopy (inflammation)
- Barium study

Lab Tests

- Complete blood count (CBC)
- IBD serology panel (antineutrophilic cytoplasmic antibodies [ANCA], immunoglobulin G [IgG], anitsaccharomyces cerevisiae mannan antibodies [ASCA], immunoglobulin A [IgA], alpha outer membrane protein C immunoglobin antibodies [OmpC IgA])

PLANNING AND IMPLEMENTATION

- Treatment depends on the severity of symptoms
- Monitor vital signs
- Monitor intake and output (I & O)
- Calorie count
- Encourage fluid and nutritional intake
- Administer vitamins and nutritional supplements
- Take daily weight
- Administer anti-inflammatory, immunomodulator, and antidiarrhea medications

NURSING DIAGNOSIS

- Pain, Chronic
- Diarrhea
- Nutrition: less than body requirements, Imbalanced
- Skin, Impaired integrity
- Fluid volume, Risk for deficient

Urethral Stricture

DEFINITION

- Urethral stricture is the narrowing of the urethra from inflammation or subsequent fibrotic scar tissue.

Clinical Causes

- Self-catheterization
- Recent urethral instrumentation
- Sexually transmitted infections (gonorrhea or chlamydia)
- Benign prostatic hyperplasia (BPH)

KEY ASSESSMENTS

- Difficulty voiding
- Dysuria
- Pelvic pain
- Urinary frequency and urgency

Diagnostics

- Cystoscopy
- Retrograde urethrogram

Lab Tests

- Urinalysis
- Urine culture
- Test for presence of sexually transmitted disease

PLANNING AND IMPLEMENTATION

- Treat infections with appropriate antibiotics
- Monitor intake and output (I & O)
- Encourage adequate fluid intake
- Treat pain and inflammation with nonsteroidal anti-inflammatory drugs (NSAIDs)
- Provide clear path to the bathroom
- Implement safety measures
- Urethral dilation
- Urethral stent
- Urethrotomy (direct visualization of the urethra through an endoscope and the creation of small longitudinal incisions through scar tissue)
- Urethroplasty (remove diseased portion of the urethra and insert a newly constructed urethra)

NURSING DIAGNOSIS

- Urinary elimination, Impaired
- Knowledge, Deficient
- Pain, Acute

Urethritis

DEFINITION

- Urethritis is inflammation of the urethra commonly occurring with genitourinary tract infections (UTIs) or trauma, including self-catheterization.

KEY ASSESSMENTS

- Dysuria
- Penile discharge
- Erythema

History and Examination

- Trauma
- Self-catheterization
- Recent unprotected sex
- Recent UTI

Lab Tests

- Urine culture

PLANNING AND IMPLEMENTATION

- Treat with appropriate antibiotics for infection
- Administer nonsteroidal anti-inflammatory drugs (NSAIDs) for pain and inflammation

NURSING DIAGNOSIS

- Pain, Acute
- Urinary elimination, Impaired
- Knowledge, Deficient
- Infection

Urinary Incontinence (UI)

DEFINITION

- UI is the complete or partial loss of bladder control causing the involuntary passage of urine. UI commonly affects women and the elderly.

Clinical Causes

- Urinary tract infections (UTIs)
- Prostate infection
- Stool impaction
- Side effects of medications
- Diabetes mellitus
- Pregnancy
- Weight gain
- Spinal injuries
- Cerebral vascular accident
- Benign prostatic hyperplasia

- Pelvic prolapse
- Bladder cancer
- Weak pelvic muscles

Classifications

- Stress incontinence is loss of urine with increased intra-abdominal pressure (coughing, sneezing, laughing, or pregnancy).
- Urge incontinence is loss of urine preceded by a strong, urgent need to void.
- Overflow incontinence is the loss of urine due to chronic urinary retention or a flaccid bladder.
- Functional incontinence is the loss of urine in those with normal bladder control who unable to get to the bathroom in time to void (patients with arthritis or mobility issues).

KEY ASSESSMENTS

- Assess type of UI
- Assess for history of underlying medical problem causing UI

Diagnostics

- Bladder scan

Lab Tests

- Urinalysis
- Urine culture

PLANNING AND IMPLEMENTATION

- Encourage bladder training (urinating on a schedule).
- Explain use of Kegel exercise (voluntary contraction of pelvic floor muscles).
- Regulate bowel to avoid constipation.
- Encourage smoking cessation (reduce coughing and bladder irritation).
- Avoid alcohol and caffeinated beverages.
- Administer medications to treat incontinence, including anticholinergics and antidepressants.
- Monitor intake and output (I & O).
- Encourage adequate fluid intake.
- Treat with appropriate antibiotics if UTI is present.
- Use incontinence pads.
- Do not call incontinence pads diapers; it is demeaning to the patient.

- Surgical intervention may be required to correct the urethra.
- Pelvic or uterine suspension operations may be required in women.

NURSING DIAGNOSIS

- Urinary elimination, Impaired
- Knowledge, Deficient

Urinary Retention

DEFINITION

- Urinary retention is the presence of some urine in the bladder after attempting to empty it. The condition may be acute or chronic.

Clinical Causes

- Renal calculi
- Fecal impaction
- Prostatitis
- Prostatic carcinoma
- Benign prostatic hyperplasia
- Retroverted gravid uterus
- Postoperatively
- Tumor or clot in the bladder
- Any medication with anticholinergic or alpha adrenergic effect
- Spinal cord lesions or injuries
- Multiple sclerosis
- Genital herpes

U

KEY ASSESSMENTS

- Large palpable bladder
- Urge to void
- Dull, lower abdominal pain
- Urinary frequency with voiding small amounts

Diagnostics

- Bladder scan
- Intravenous pyelogram (IVP)

Lab Tests

- Urinalysis
- Prostate-specific antigen (PSA)

PLANNING AND IMPLEMENTATION

- Monitor intake and output (I & O)
- Bladder scan to document volume retained
- Straight catheterize patient as needed
- Encourage adequate fluid intake
- Monitor for urinary tract infection (fever, painful urination, or foul smelling urine)

NURSING DIAGNOSIS

- Urinary retention
- Pain, Acute
- Infection, Risk for

Urinary Tract Infection (UTI)

DEFINITION

- A UTI, or cystitis, is an infection that may involve the kidneys, ureters, bladder, or urethra. UTI covers a range of conditions from asymptomatic infection to severe kidney infection and systemic sepsis. Early diagnosis and treatment are important.

Classifications

- Lower UTI affects urethra, bladder, or prostate.
- Upper UTI affects the ureters or kidney(s).

KEY ASSESSMENTS

- Painful urination
- Fever
- Cloudy, bloody, or foul smelling urine
- Frequency
- Urgency
- Hesitation
- Lower abdominal pain
- Nausea and vomiting

- Chills
- Flank pain

Diagnostics

- Urinalysis
- Urine culture and sensitivity

PLANNING AND IMPLEMENTATION

- Encourage oral intake
- Treat pain
- Administer antipyretics
- Administer antibiotics

SPECIAL CONCERNS

- In the hospital setting, in-dwelling urinary catheters are a common cause of UTIs and should be removed as soon as the condition allows.

Gender Considerations

- UTIs are more common in females because of a shorter urethra.

Teaching Considerations

- Urinate after intercourse.
- Drink six to eight glasses of water daily.
- Cranberry juice may help prevent UTIs.

NURSING DIAGNOSIS

- Pain, Acute
- Infection
- Urinary elimination, Impaired

Urolithiasis

DEFINITION

- Urolithiasis, or calculi, refers to a kidney stone in the urinary tract. Continued symptoms are referred to as nephrolithiasis (kidney stone disease). Although there appear to be dietary factors involved in calculi formation, the etiology is unclear.

KEY ASSESSMENTS

- Sudden, severe unilateral flank pain
- Nausea and vomiting
- Hematuria
- Fever

Diagnostics

- Helical computed tomography (CT)
- Intravenous pyelogram (IVP) CT

Lab Tests

- Leukocytosis
- Urinalysis (red blood count, white blood count, or presence of crystals)

PLANNING AND IMPLEMENTATION

- Treat pain with narcotics
- Initiate intravenous (IV) therapy and fluid replacement therapy
- Strain all urine for presence of calculi
- Observe for ureteral or urethral strictures (narrowing of the ureters and urethra respectively) for a decrease in stream spray and incomplete bladder emptying
- Anticipate cystoscopic stone removal if calculi does not pass spontaneously
- Other therapy (extracorporeal shock wave lithotripsy and percutaneous nephrostolithotomy)

Gender Considerations

- Urolithiasis affects women three times more frequently than it does men.

Teaching Considerations

- Increase fluid intake to 2–3 liters/day
- Limit calcium intake
- Limit ingestion of animal protein
- Encourage alkaline foods, such as fruits, green vegetables, and legumes
- Encourage vitamin B_6 supplements

NURSING DIAGNOSIS

- Pain, Acute
- Urinary elimination, Impaired
- Infection, Risk for

Uterine Fibroids

DEFINITION

- Uterine fibroids, or leiomyomata, are benign, estrogen-dependent growths originating from the smooth muscle of the uterus. Fibroids may be single, multiple, small or large, and within or external to the uterus and are the most common reason for hysterectomy.

KEY ASSESSMENTS

- Often asymptomatic
- Excessive menstrual bleeding
- Pelvic pressure
- Constipation
- Increased abdominal girth
- Urinary retention

Diagnostics

- Ultrasound
- Complete blood count (CBC)

PLANNING AND IMPLEMENTATION

- Notify health care provider, insert peripheral IV, and anticipate surgical intervention if fibroids hemorrhage
- Myomectomy (remove fibroids and preserve uterus)
- Uterine artery embolization (eliminates blood supply)
- Medical therapy with hormones
- Hysterectomy
- No treatment is indicated if no symptoms are present

NURSING DIAGNOSIS

- Knowledge, Deficient
- Constipation

Uterine Prolapse

DEFINITION

- Uterine prolapse is the relaxation of the support structures holding up the uterus resulting in the descent of the uterus into the vagina. Risks for pelvic relaxation include obesity, family history, and parity.

Other Pelvic Relaxation Conditions

- Urethrocele is the prolapse of the urethra into the vagina.
- Cystocele is the prolapse of the bladder into the vagina.
- Rectocele is the prolapse of the rectum into the vagina.

KEY ASSESSMENTS

- Feeling of something falling out of the vagina
- Protruding cervix outside of vagina

PLANNING AND IMPLEMENTATION

- Surgical repair to hold up uterus or hysterectomy may be indicated.

NURSING DIAGNOSIS

- Knowledge, Deficient
- Skin integrity, Risk for impaired

Vaginitis

DEFINITION

- Vaginitis is inflammation of the vagina regardless of the cause.

Clinical Causes

- Candida is a vaginal yeast infection commonly caused by *Candida albicans*. The infection can be caused by a shift in vaginal flora (antibiotic administration) in the presence of high blood sugar or suppressed immune system (diabetes mellitus or human immunodeficiency virus [HIV]). It is treated with oral or vaginal antifungal products.

- Bacterial vaginosis is an overgrowth of the bacteria normally found in the vagina and is associated with douching and being sexually active. Women require treatment with oral or vaginal antibiotics (metronidazole or clindamycin).
- Trichomoniasis is an infection caused by a small parasite, *Trichomonas vaginalis,* through sexual contact. Men are often asymptomatic, yet both partners need treatment with oral metronidazole.
- Herpes virus is a sexually transmitted virus that produces small transient fluid filled blisters and is treated with oral antiviral medication.

KEY ASSESSMENTS

- Pain
- Inflammation
- Dysuria
- Abnormal vaginal discharge or odor
- Itching

Lab Tests

- Pelvic examination with microscopic examination of vaginal secretions

PLANNING AND IMPLEMENTATION

- Explain treatment and how to prevent spread

NURSING DIAGNOSIS

- Knowledge, Deficient
- Body image, Disturbed

Varicocele

DEFINITION

- Varicocele is a group of varicose veins within the scrotum. Varicocele may enlarge with increased intra-abdominal pressure (sneezing or straining for a bowel movement).

KEY ASSESSMENTS

- Testicle feels like a bag of worms when palpated
- Scrotal pain and tenderness

Diagnostics

- Scrotal ultrasonography

PLANNING AND IMPLEMENTATION

- Treat pain.
- If experiencing pain, surgical removal of the varicocele may be performed (varicocelectomy).
- Discourage patient from straining for bowel movements.

SPECIAL CONCERNS

- Infertility may occur in conjunction with varicocele because the increased blood flow raises scrotal temperature.

NURSING DIAGNOSIS

- Knowledge, Deficient
- Pain, Acute
- Fear

Varicose Veins

DEFINITION

- Varicose veins are dilated veins that lack surrounding muscle support. The saphenous veins of the legs are commonly affected, but hemorrhoids and esophageal varices are varicosities as well. There is a familial tendency. Thrombophlebitis, obesity, prolonged standing, and pregnancy are risk factors.

KEY ASSESSMENTS

- Distended, torturous bluish veins
- Pain of the legs
- Prolonged capillary refill

PLANNING AND IMPLEMENTATION

- Weight loss
- Exercise
- Use of support hose
- Avoid prolonged standing
- Treatment—may include chemical sclerosing or surgical intervention with vein ligation and stripping

NURSING DIAGNOSIS

- Pain, Chronic
- Activity intolerance

Venous Stasis Ulcers

DEFINITION

- A venous stasis ulcer is an erosion of the skin that may lead to skin necrosis, open wounds, and eschar formation. Approximately 75 percent of venous stasis ulcers are caused by chronic venous insufficiency. Other risks include diabetes, arterial insufficiency, neuropathy, burns, being elderly, and certain blood disorders.

KEY ASSESSMENTS

- Pain at ulcer site
- Edema of affected foot and ankle
- Open wound with or without the presence of infection

PLANNING AND IMPLEMENTATION

- Routine wound care.
- Antibiotics if infection is present.
- Provide adequate nutrition.
- Treat pain.
- Document wound assessment.
- Debridement, a mechanical method of eliminating necrotic tissue, may be performed to promote healing.

NURSING DIAGNOSIS

- Skin integrity, Impaired
- Tissue integrity, Impaired

Wegener Granulomatosis

DEFINITION

- Wegener granulomatosis is a multisystem disease that causes small vessel vasculitis with inflammation. The etiology is not clear, but autoimmune responses are implicated. There is no cure, and it is often lethal.

KEY ASSESSMENTS

- Shortness of breath (SOB)
- Hemoptysis
- Hearing loss
- Vision loss
- Weakness
- Fever
- Hypertension
- Reports of decreased urine output
- Pain over facial sinuses

Diagnostics

- Computed tomography (CT) of lungs
- Bronchoscopy with lung biopsy
- Renal biopsy

Lab Tests

- Complete blood count (CBC)
- Urinalysis
- Antineutrophil cytoplasmic antibodies

PLANNING AND IMPLEMENTATION

- Position patient in high Fowler's position
- Monitor oxygenation status including pulse oximetery
- Encourage deep breathing
- Take daily weight
- Encourage low-sodium diet
- Monitor intake and output (I & O)
- Monitor laboratory reports
- Administer antipyretics, antihypertensives, steroids, and cyclophosphamide
- Monitor for side effects of medications

NURSING DIAGNOSIS

- Airway clearance, Ineffective
- Fatigue
- Hyperthermia

West Nile Virus

DEFINITION

- West Nile virus is a flaviviridae virus transmitted from an infected mosquito, which results in an illness that ranges from mild symptoms to death.
- Spread is from a bite from an infected mosquito and can be passed from contaminated organs and blood.
- Average incubation period is 3 to 14 days.

KEY ASSESSMENTS

- Headache
- Myalgias
- Backache
- Anorexia
- Gastrointestinal (GI) disturbance
- Swollen lymph nodes
- Less than 1 percent of those infected develop life-threatening symptoms including:
  - High fever
  - Nuchal rigidity (stiff neck)
  - Severe headache
  - Decreased level of consciousness (LOC)
  - Seizures
  - Paralysis
  - Coma

History and Examination

- Recent mosquito bites

Diagnostics

- Lumbar puncture (check for virus in cerebral spinal fluid)

Lab Tests

- West Nile virus antibodies in the blood

PLANNING AND IMPLEMENTATION

- Implement standard precautions.
- Treatment is supportive.
- Treat pain.
- Implement safety precautions.
- Administer antipyretics for fever.
- Monitor LOC.
- Monitor for signs of increased intracranial pressure (change in LOC, increased headache, and anisocoria).
- Monitor vital signs frequently.
- Initiate intravenous (IV) lines.
- Monitor intake & output (I & O).
- Elevate head of bed to 30 degrees.

SPECIAL CONCERNS

- Prevention of West Nile virus is vital.
- Wear mosquito repellant with N,N-diethyl-meta-toluamide (DEET).
- Wear long-sleeved shirts and long pants during evening hours.
- Remove any stagnant water.
- Cover infant strollers with mosquito netting.

NURSING DIAGNOSIS

- Hyperthermia
- Thought process, Disturbed
- Pain, Acute
- Injury, Risk for
- Confusion, Acute

Wilson's Disease

DEFINITION

- Wilson's disease is an autosomal recessive disorder characterized by the inability to secrete copper. The excess copper accumulates over years, damaging many organs including the liver.

KEY ASSESSMENTS

- Tremors
- Rigidity
- Inappropriate behavior
- Difficulty with speech
- Kayser-Fleischer rings (brown, ring-shaped pigmentation in the cornea)
- Ascites
- Clay-colored stool
- Dark urine
- Abdominal pain

Diagnostics

- Serum ceruloplasmin (low in Wilson's disease)
- Liver biopsy

PLANNING AND IMPLEMENTATION

- Avoid foods high in copper.
- Administer chelating agents.
- Liver transplantation may be indicated.
- Avoid alcohol consumption.

SPECIAL CONCERNS

Teaching Considerations

- Avoid foods high in copper, including liver, shellfish, mushrooms, nuts, chocolate, dried fruit, dried peas, beans, lentils, soy products, avocados, barley, bran products, and nectarines
- Test tap water for copper
- Avoid vitamins with copper
- Avoid alcohol use

NURSING DIAGNOSIS

- Knowledge, Deficient
- Thought process, Disturbed

SECTION

2

Special Procedures and Treatments

Bariatric Surgery

DEFINITION

- Bariatric surgery is surgery that causes weight loss and is recommended for severely obese patients (body mass index [BMI] greater than 40) and obese patients with comorbid diseases (i.e., diabetes, heart disease, or sleep apnea).

Classifications

Types of bariatric surgeries

- Adjustable gastric banding—a silicon rubber band is placed around the upper part of the stomach creating a small pouch and a narrow passage into the remainder of the stomach.
- Vertical banded gastroplasty—the stomach is stapled, and a band is placed below the esophagus creating a small pouch and narrowed opening to the remainder of the stomach.
- Roux-enY gastric bypass—a stomach pouch is created and connected to the small intestine allowing food to bypass the majority of the stomach and the upper small intestine. The remnant stomach is attached to the jejunum.
- Complications of all bariatric surgeries include dumping syndrome (after a high carbohydrate meal the patient experiences nausea, abdominal pain, bloating, weakness, and diarrhea), vomiting, and long-term nutritional deficiencies.

KEY ASSESSMENTS

Postsurgery

- Pain
- Incision site
- Return of gag and cough reflex
- Nausea and vomiting
- Diarrhea

PLANNING AND IMPLEMENTATION

Postsurgery

- Use medical equipment that is safe for the bariatric patient. (Medical equipment, such as wheelchairs and beds, usually has a weight load limit of 250 lbs.)

- Limit fluid intake to 4 ounces per hour of noncarbonated beverages.
- Monitor for nausea and vomiting.
- Treat incisional pain.
- Monitor intake and output (I & O).
- Take daily weight.
- Monitor electrolytes.
- Administer nutritional supplements as ordered.

NURSING DIAGNOSIS

- Nausea
- Pain, Acute

Cancer

DEFINITION

- Cancer is a group of diseases characterized by abnormal growth and spread of cells. Metastasis is the spread of cancer from the original site to other locations in the body. Three known factors that contribute to cancer development are heredity, environment, and lifestyle.

Classifications

Staging describes the extent or spread of the tumor within the body from the original site. Tumor-nodes-metastasis (TNM) system for staging solid tumors:

- T—describes the primary tumor
  - Tx cannot be assessed
  - T0 no evidence of tumor
  - Tis tumor in situ
  - T1, T2, T3, or T4 tumor size from small to large
- N—nodal involvement
  - Nx cannot be assessed
  - N0 no evidence of regional lymph node metastasis
  - N1, N2, or N3 lymph node involvement from some to extensive
- M—presence or absence of metastasis
  - Mx unable to assess
  - M0 no presence of metastasis
  - M1 presence of metastasis

Grading describes the degree of malignancy or cell differentiation of the tumor cells.

- G1 or I, G2 or II, G3 or III, G4 or IV from highly differentiated cells (more resembles normal cells) to no specific differentiation (highly aggressive and rapidly multiplying tumors); Gx grade cannot be assessed.

Treatments

Goals of treatment are to cure the cancer, control the spread, or palliative care.

- Surgical resection—see Pre- and Postoperative Care.
- Radiation uses high-energy ionizing rays to damage or kill cancer cells by preventing them from growing and dividing.
  - External radiation delivers high-energy rays directly to the tumor site from a linear accelerator.
  - Internal radiation, or brachytherapy, involves the implantation of a small amount of radioactive material in or near the cancer.
  - Internal radiation general guidelines include assigning the patient to a private room, posting radiation precaution signs, limiting the amount of time in the room, observing a distance of six feet when possible, wearing a dosimeter badge when in the room, restricting visitation from pregnant women and children, and properly disposing of all secretions and excreta, which are considered radioactive.
- Chemotherapy is the use of antineoplastic agents (a drug that prevents, kills, or blocks the growth and spread of cancer cells) to disrupt the cellular growth and replication of cancer cells to kill them. Neoadjuvant chemotherapy reduces the tumor size prior to surgery or radiation. Adjuvant chemotherapy is given after a primary treatment (surgery or radiation) to eliminate any cancer cells remaining.
  - Chemotherapy is administered by specially trained registered nurses following strict administration protocols, is dosed by the body surface area of the patient, and is usually given in cycles.
  - Chemotherapeutic agents are potentially toxic; avoid spills, wear protective equipments, and dispose of in white chemotherapy waste containers.
  - Many chemotherapy agents are vesicants posing risk for tissue necrosis. Make frequent assessments of the intravenous (IV) line for patency and skin for signs of infiltration paramount.
  - Patient body fluids are considered hazardous for 48 hours after treatment and should be disposed of properly.

- Hormone therapy is used to limit hormones that stimulate the growth of certain cancers, including breast and prostate.
- Biological therapy uses naturally produced substances by the immune system to fight cancer directly or lessened the effects caused by some cancer treatments.
- Bone marrow transplantation is a process in which bone marrow is harvested, and implanted stem cells will produce healthy blood cells and may cure certain leukemias and lymphomas. The bone marrow may be autologous (from the patient) or allogenic (from a carefully matched donor). Patients usually receive chemotherapy and immune suppression prior to the transplant making patients at high risk for infection and graft-versus-host disease (GVHD).

KEY ASSESSMENTS

- Fatigue
- Radiation enteritis nausea, vomiting, abdominal cramping, or diarrhea
- Shortness of breath
- Peripheral neuropathy (tingling, numbness of extremities)
- Skin irritation
- IV site for signs of infiltration (redness or burning at site)
- Weight
- Hair loss
- Stomatitis (mouth sores)

PLANNING AND IMPLEMENTATION

- Monitor and treat pain with narcotics
- Maintain adequate oral fluid and nutritional intake
- Monitor vital signs
- Monitor oxygenation status and provide oxygen if necessary
- Monitor intake and output (I & O)
- Take daily weight
- Provide small frequent meals, avoiding foods with strong odors
- Administer antidiarrheal medications (Lomotil)
- Administer antinausea medications (Compazine or Zofran)
- Meticulous skin care
- Assist with activities of daily living
- Encourage the patient to change positions slowly
- Meticulous oral care
- Viscous lidocaine for stomatitis
- Monitor for signs of infection (fever or tachycardia)

- Monitor complete blood count (CBC) for anemia, neutropenia, and infection
- Monitor platelets for thrombocytopenia
- Monitor electrolytes and glucose
- Administer blood products as requested
- Administer colony stimulating factors (erythropoietin or filgrastim)
- Administer cannabis mediations to promote appetite as prescribed
- Monitor for bleeding and bruising
- Document skin assessment
- Maintain a regular sleep schedule
- Encourage visitation with friends and family
- Implement safety measures
- Monitor level of consciousness
- Monitor for evidence of organ dysfunction or distant metastasis

SPECIAL CONCERNS

- Pain, postoperative care

Teaching Considerations

- External radiation markers should not be removed; skin should be washed with gently; do not apply lotion or powders unless prescribed; avoid sunlight.
- Infection control measures include frequent hand washing, brushing teeth with a soft toothbrush, protecting skin, washing fresh fruits and vegetables and removing skins, avoiding crowds, thoroughly cooking food, not keeping fresh-cut flowers, wiping from front to back when toileting, avoiding sick people, checking temperature daily, and calling if temperature is greater than 38° C or 100° F.
- Side effects from chemotherapy include fatigue, anemia, thrombocytopenia, neutropenia, hair loss, nausea, vomiting, risk for infection, weight loss, changes in taste, poor concentration, and memory loss.
- Complementary therapy, including aromatherapy, art therapy, biofeedback, massage therapy, meditation, music therapy, acupuncture, prayer, spiritual practices, tai chi, and yoga, may reduce physical symptoms, increase quality of life, and lessen or prevent depression.

NURSING DIAGNOSIS

- Fatigue
- Diarrhea

- Fluid volume, Risk for imbalanced
- Injury, risk for
- Activity intolerance
- Hopelessness
- Pain, Acute
- Pain, Chronic
- Nausea
- Skin integrity, Risk for impaired
- Spiritual distress
- Nutrition: less than body requirements, Imbalanced
- Body image, Disturbed
- Infection, Risk for
- Knowledge, Deficient
- Fear
- Sleep pattern, Disturbed

Coronary Angiography

DEFINITION

- Coronary angiogram, or heart catheterization, involves puncturing an artery, advancing a catheter toward the heart, and injecting a radiopaque contrast to visualize coronary arteries. This invasive procedure is considered the gold standard for the diagnosis of coronary artery disease (CAD).

KEY ASSESSMENTS

Preangiography

- Allergies (shellfish and iodine allergies must be reported)
- Presence of renal disease (contrast is nephrotoxic)
- Consents
- Nothing by mouth (NPO) after midnight
- Assess and document pulses

Postangiography

- Assess puncture site for bleeding or hematoma formation
- Vital signs for shock related to reaction or hemorrhaging frequently as ordered
- Assess and document pulses frequently as ordered
- Assess for angina

PLANNING AND IMPLEMENTATION

- Do not move the punctured limb for four to six hours or as prescribed by physician
- Monitor vital signs for signs of shock related to hemorrhage
- Monitor neurological status, and call health care provider if changes occur
- Encourage fluids
- Monitor for intense back pain (retroperineal bleed)
- Monitor intake and output (I & O)
- Monitor site for evidence of bleeding or hematoma formation
- If site bleeds, use personal protective devices, including eyewear, and hold pressure over site
- Monitor distal pulses
- If pulses are absent, contact the health care provider immediately and anticipate emergency embolectomy
- Monitor and treat pain
- Monitor blood urea nitrogen (BUN) and creatinine (Cr)
- Monitor for evidence of chest pain and if present, obtain 12-lead electrocardiogram (ECG), and administer nitroglycerin as prescribed
- Head of bed at prescribed degree (less than 30) until bedrest is completed

NURSING DIAGNOSIS

- Fluid volume, Risk for deficient
- Mobility, Impaired
- Knowledge, Deficient
- Tissue perfusion, Ineffective

Coronary Angioplasty

DEFINITION

- Coronary angioplasty, or percutaneous transluminal coronary angioplasty (PTCA), involves puncturing an artery, advancing a catheter toward the heart, and inflating a balloon in a stenosed coronary artery(s) to restore blood flow. Stents (small tubular devices that maintain the patency of the coronary arteries) may be placed at this time. This invasive procedure is used emergently with acute coronary syndromes or electively in patients with known coronary artery disease (CAD).

KEY ASSESSMENTS

Preangioplasty

- Allergies (shellfish and iodine allergies must be reported)
- Presence of renal disease (contrast is nephrotoxic)
- Consents
- Nothing by mouth (NPO) after midnight
- If emergent, initiate NPO on admission
- Assess and document pulses

Postangioplasty

- Assess puncture site for bleeding or hematoma formation
- Vital signs for shock related to reaction or hemorrhaging frequently as ordered
- Assess and document pulses frequently as ordered
- Assess for angina
- Assess for arrhythmias
- Assess for ST segment changes

PLANNING AND IMPLEMENTATION

- Arterial sheaths may be left in place or removed.
- If arterial sheaths are in place, attach to pressure monitor system to monitor blood pressure and place alarms on.
- If removed, do not move the punctured limb for four to six hours or as prescribed by the health care provider.
- Monitor vital signs for signs of shock related to hemorrhage (hypotension or tachycardia).
- Monitor neurological status, and call health care provider if changes occur.
- Encourage fluids.
- Monitor for intense back pain (retroperineal bleed).
- Monitor heart rate and rhythm.
- Treat arrhythmias per protocol. Arrhythmias may be signs of reperfusion (restored blood flow) or of occlusion (coronary vessel spasm).
- Monitor ST segments, and report changes.
- Monitor for diaphoresis and nausea (signs of coronary occlusion).
- If the patient is experiencing signs of coronary occlusion, anticipate emergent return to cardiac catheterization unit for subsequent angioplasty to open the occlusion.
- Monitor intake and output (I & O), and call health care provider for urine output less than 30 mL/hour.
- Monitor site for evidence of bleeding or hematoma formation.

- If site bleeds, don personal protective devices, including eyewear, and hold pressure over site.
- Monitor distal pulses.
- If pulses are absent, contact the health care provider immediately and anticipate emergency embolectomy.
- Monitor and treat pain.
- Monitor blood urea nitrogen (BUN) and creatinine (Cr).
- Monitor cardiac enzymes.
- Monitor electrolytes.
- Monitor for evidence of chest pain, and if present, obtain 12-lead electrocardiogram (ECG) and administer nitroglycerin as prescribed.
- Head of bed at prescribed degree (less than 30) until bedrest is completed or sheaths are removed.

NURSING DIAGNOSIS

- Fluid volume, Risk for deficient
- Mobility, Impaired bed
- Knowledge, Deficient
- Tissue perfusion, Ineffective

Coronary Artery Bypass Grafting (CABG)

DEFINITION

- CABG is a surgical procedure that uses veins and arteries to bypass coronary artery stenosis.
- CABG is indicated for patients with significant coronary artery disease (CAD) lesions, especially when the CAD affects more than one coronary artery.
- Postoperatively monitor for, prevent, and treat complications such as bleeding, cardiac tamponade, arrhythmias, and death.

Classifications

- Traditional coronary artery bypass grafting—the heart is approached through a sternotomy incision, and the patient is placed on cardiopulmonary bypass.
- Off pump coronary artery bypass (OPCAB)—the heart is approached by a sternotomy incision, the surgery is performed on

a beating heart (no cardiopulmonary bypass), and the heart is stabilized with a cage-type device.

- Thoracotomy approach—the heart is approached by a thoracotomy approach, and the surgery is performed on a beating heart.
- Minimally invasive direct coronary bypass (MIDCAB)—the heart is approached by a small incision (keyhole bypass), and no sternotomy is required.

Grafts

Grafting materials

- Saphenous vein—the vein is harvested from the saphenous veins in the leg.
- Radial artery—the radial artery is harvested. Allen's test needs to be performed preoperatively to ensure adequate blood flow to the extremity.
- Internal mammary artery—the internal mammary artery is harvested, and no incision is apparent.
- Xenographs—arterial grafts harvested from pigs may be used if the patient does not have adequate vasculature to harvest.
- Cadaver grafts—arterial grafts harvested from cadavers may be used if the patient does not have adequate vasculature to harvest.
- Synthetic grafts—grafts made from synthetic materials may be used if the patient does not have adequate vasculature to harvest.

KEY ASSESSMENTS

Postoperative

- Goals may be different based on the individual patient or preference of the health care provider.
  - Respirations—goal is to wean the patient quickly from the ventilator keeping O_2 saturations above 95 percent, the arterial blood gases (ABGs) within normal limits, and the patient alert and spontaneously breathing.
  - Blood pressure—goal is to keep the systolic blood pressure between 100 and 140 systolic.
  - Temperature—maintain normothermia.
  - Heart rate—goal is between 80 and 110 beats per minute without arrhythmias.
  - Cardiac output—a swan Ganz catheter is present to maintain a cardiac output of 4 mm Hg.
  - Peripheral pulses and temperature—goal is moderate to strong (+2 or +3) peripheral pulses and extremity warmth (indicators of adequate cardiac output).

  - Neurological status—goal is to have the patient alert, moving all four extremities to command, and breathing spontaneously.
  - Urine output—goal is to have urine output at least 30 mL/hour and is an indicator of adequate cardiac output, adequate renal function, and adequate fluid status.
  - Chest tube output—goal is less than 100 mL/hour output.
  - Pain—goal is for the patient to have a pain score less than 4 out of 10.
  - Wounds—goal is for sternotomy, if present, and surgical incisions to be free of infection.

Diagnostics

- Chest X-ray (CXR)

Lab Tests

- Electrolytes
- Glucose
- Complete blood count (CBC)
- ABGs
- Blood urea nitrogen (BUN) and creatinine (Cr)
- Liver panel
- Coagulation studies

PLANNING AND IMPLEMENTATION

- Monitor for complications (in addition to standard postoperative care).
  - Cardiac tamponade—bleeding within the pericardial sac and is noted in the patient with hypotension, muffled heart tones, pulsus paradoxus, and tachycardia and is verified with CXR showing a widened mediastinum. Death will occur if not treated immediately. The nurse should anticipate chest reentry at the bedside or immediate return to surgery. Support the patient with adequate fluids, blood, and vasopressor medications to maintain a blood pressure over 90 mm Hg and maintain airway.
  - Excessive chest tube output—notify the health care provider for a chest tube output greater than 100 mL/hour. Anticipate administering blood products and autotransfuse blood if less than 4 hours postoperatively to maintain blood pressure above 90 mm Hg. The patient may have to return to surgery for repair of the cause of bleeding.
  - Oxygenation problems—if the pulse oximetry is less than 95 percent or ABGs are abnormal, notify the health care

provider. Anticipate increasing ventilatory settings, obtaining a CXR, and albuterol nebulizer treatments. Auscultate breath sound; absence may indicate hemo- or pneumothorax and another chest tube may have to be inserted. Suction the endotracheal tube as necessary.

- Inadequate cardiac output—noted by weak peripheral pulses, cool extremities, inability to maintain an adequate blood pressure, urine output less than 30 mL/hour, and a cardiac output less than 4 mm Hg. Anticipate administering fluid volume (0.9% normal saline [NS], albumin, or blood products) to correct any fluid volume deficit and administering vasspressor medications (including dopamine, levophed, vasopressin, and epinephrine).
- Hypertension—should be avoided because the high pressure puts strain on the new grafts and may cause bleeding. Assess the patient for pain and anxiety and treat (propofol or morphine), if hypertension still exists, anticipate administering medications to lower blood pressure quickly (Nipride).
- Cardiac arrhythmias—common in the postoperative setting, yet need prompt treatment. Monitor and correct all electrolyte imbalances, which are a common cause of arrhythmias (hypokalemia or hypomagnesia). Anticipate antiarrhythmic medications (lidocaine or amiodarone). Ventricular tachycardia and atrial fibrillations and flutter may be treated with synchronized cardioversion, ventricular fibrillation with defibrillation. If the patient has pacemaker wires, pacing may be indicated for bradycardia.
- Neurological problems—a patient who is not waking from surgery, is unable to move extremities to command, or has unequal pupils may have had an ischemic or hemorrhagic stroke during surgery. Notify the health care provider, and anticipate computed tomography (CT) scan of the head and treatment according to the cause.
- Pain—monitor patient for pain and medicate as appropriate.

NURSING DIAGNOSIS

- Cardiac output, Decreased
- Fluid volume, Risk for imbalanced
- Breathing pattern, Ineffective
- Infection, Risk for
- Pain, Acute
- Injury, Risk for

Craniotomy

DEFINITION

- A craniotomy is a surgical procedure in which a piece of the skull is removed to allow access to the brain. It is performed for numerous brain problems.

Clinical Causes

- Brain tumors
- Arterial venous malformations
- Aneurysms
- Hemorrhagic stroke
- Epidural hematoma
- Subdural hematoma
- Hydrocephalus
- Large-volume ischemic strokes

KEY ASSESSMENTS

- Oxygenation status
- Vital signs
- Level of consciousness (LOC)
- Cranial nerve function
- Motor strength and sensation
- Urine output
- Fluid status
- Intracranial pressure (ICP)
- Cerebral perfusion pressure
- Wound appearance
- Cerebrospinal fluid color and amount
- Pain level

Diagnostics

- Computed tomography (CT) of head
- Chest X-ray (CXR)

Lab Tests

- Arterial blood gases (ABGs)
- Electrolytes
- Glucose
- Blood urea nitrogen (BUN) and creatinine (Cr)

PLANNING AND IMPLEMENTATION

Postoperative

- In addition to standard postoperative care
  - Neurological status—monitor LOC, cranial nerve function, pupil size and reactivity, motor strength, extremity sensation, Glasgow Coma Scale (GCS) score, and ability to speak. Any change in status should be reported to the health care provider immediately. If changes are acute, anticipate intubation, administering mannitol and CT of the head. Confused or combative patients may require sedation and restraints for protection. Monitor glucose levels, and hyper- and hypoglycemia may cause neurological changes.
  - Oxygenation—monitor ability to have spontaneous respirations, respiratory patterns (changes in respiratory patterns may occur with increased ICP), presence of pneumonia (aspiration pneumonia may occur when patients lack adequate gag or cough reflex), monitor CO_2 levels (hypercarbnia cause vasodilatation and may increase ICP; hypocarbia may cause vasoconstriction and cerebral ischemia), maintain pulse oximetry above 93 percent. Patients with GCS less than 9 usually require intubation to protect the airway.
  - Seizures—see Seizures. Anticipate administering Dilantin for seizure prophylaxis. Monitor sodium levels.
  - Safety—implement safety measures, including seizure precautions, and if restraints are necessary, obtain an order for restraints prior to placing them. If extremity weakness or altered LOC is present, obtain assistance when transferring or mobilizing patients. If a bone flap removed, do not turn patient on affected side.
  - Vital signs—monitor for signs of Cushing's Triad (a sign of increased ICP) including systolic hypertension, bradycardia, and bradypnea. Maintain adequate blood pressure for cerebral perfusion. Excessive hypertension may put the patient at risk for cerebral hemorrhage. Hyperthermia is avoided and if present, treated with acetaminophen and cooling devices. Monitor electrolytes to prevent electrolyte induced arrhythmias.
  - ICP—monitor with neurological status and vital signs. If the patient has an ICP monitoring device, document readings hourly and call the health care provider when greater than ordered limit; level at the tragus, and do not attach to a pressure bag; use sterile technique and document insertion

site appearance; do not inject or withdraw anything into device; if ordered to drain, clarify and closely follow orders. Anticipate draining cerebrospinal fluid (CSF) if monitor is present and mannitol for acute increases in ICP.

- Avoid activities that increase ICP—clustering activities, frequent endotracheal suctioning, positioning flat, neck flexion, excessive stimulation, vomiting, coughing, and straining for bowel movements.
- Activities to help reduce ICP—space nursing activities, avoid straining for bowel movements, prevent nausea, maintain neck in the neutral position, avoid excess stimulation, minimize anxiety, and treat pain.
- Pain—monitor and treat pain. Excessive pain medication may alter neurological examination.
- Mobility—monitor for complications associated with mobility. Turn every two hours, prevent foot drop, eye care if eyes do not close completely. Deep venous thrombosis (DVT) prophylaxis, including pneumatic devices and elastic stockings, meticulous skin care, oral care, and encourage mobility when appropriate. Maintain head of bed at least 30 degrees.
- Nutrition—monitor ability to swallow. If unable to swallow without difficulty, request speech and swallow studies. Follow feeding directions as requested by speech pathologist. Monitor patient for aspiration pneumonia (fever or cough). If patient is unable to obtain nutrition orally, anticipate nasogastric tube or dobhoff tube feedings. Check for placement before feeding and maintain head of bed at least 30 degrees.
- Wound care—assess craniotomy wound for redness, swelling, purulent drainage. Assess for CSF drainage by observing for halo (clear fluid with tan ring around drainage) on the pillowcase. Contact health care provider if any abnormalities exist. If bone flap is out, do not turn toward affected side, and report excessive bulging at the site.

Discharge Planning

- Patients may require additional rehabilitation and be discharged to rehabilitation centers instead of home.

NURSING DIAGNOSIS

- Thought process, Disturbed
- Fluid volume, Risk for imbalanced
- Breathing pattern, Ineffective
- Infection, Risk for

- Pain, Acute
- Injury, Risk for
- Skin integrity, Impaired
- Activity intolerance
- Falls, Risk for
- Self-care deficit, Feeding
- Swallowing, Impaired

Dialysis, Hemodialysis (HD)

DEFINITION

- HD is the removal of metabolic wastes and fluid by pumping the patient's blood through a semipermeable membrane, which bathes the blood with dialysate fluid (a solution containing a premixed concentrate of electrolytes and components) and draws metabolic wastes and fluid out of the blood. The cleansed blood is returned to the patient.
- Patients with acute renal failure may have hemodialysis performed via temporary vascular catheters.
- Patients with chronic renal failure (CRF) have dialysis performed via permanent catheters three times a week.
- Duration of HD is usually three to four hours but depends on the amount of fluid and waste to be removed.
- Hemodialysis requires the use of anticoagulants.
- Patients with poor vascular access or the inability to tolerate rapid fluid shifts (patients with severe heart failure) are not HD candidates.

Temporary Access

- A dual lumen catheter is inserted in large veins (i.e., subclavian vein) and is for patients with acute renal failure (ARF) or those with CRF until a permanent catheter is placed. The catheters should not be used except for dialysis and maintain sterile dressing per hospital protocol.

Permanent Access

- This is a surgically created anastomosis of an artery and a vein in the nondominate lower arm, refered to as an arteriovenous (AV) fistula.
- Complications include thrombosis, infection, and steal syndrome (inadequate blood flow to the distal extremity noted by pain, coolness, and paresthesias).

- To confirm and document patency of the AV fistula, the turbulence of the arterial and venous blood flow are noted by ausculating a bruit (turbulent blood flow ausculated over AV fistula) and palpating a thrill (feeling a turbulent blood flow noted by a vibratory hum). Document both findings every shift. If they are not present, notify the health care provider.
- Nephrology precautions in patients with AV fistula, including no blood pressure measurement, no intravenous (IV) access, or lab draws on affected arm.

KEY ASSESSMENTS

During Dialysis

- Monitor vital signs for cardiac arrhythmias and hypotension

Postdialysis

- Assess dry weight (the ideal patient weight after excess fluid has been removed)
- Headache, nausea, muscle twitching, and confusion (signs of disequilibrium syndrome—the rapid change in fluids and electrolytes that occurs during HD may cause a transient increase in intracranial pressure causing headache, nausea, muscle twitching, and confusion)
- AV fistula site for active bleeding
- Presence of thrill and bruit

PLANNING AND IMPLEMENTATION

Before Dialysis

- Hold any medications that may be dialyzed out during dialysis

During Dialysis

- Monitor blood pressure and observe for arrhythmias
- Observe site for active bleeding

Postdialysis

- Document dry weight
- Frequent vital signs
- Administer any medications held prior to dialysis (evaluate blood pressure before administering antihypertensives)
- Disequilibrium syndrome—the rapid change in fluids and electrolytes that occurs during HD may cause a transient increase

in intracranial pressure causing headache, nausea, muscle twitching and confusion

- AV fistula site for active bleeding
- Presence of thrill and bruit
- Monitor site for infection
- Monitor for arterial steal syndrome

SPECIAL CONCERNS

Teaching Considerations

- Patients with AV fistula—do not wear restrictive clothing, sleep on arm, or lift heavy objects with affected arm
- Palpate thrill twice a day, and notify health care provider if not present
- Nephrology precautions—no blood pressure measurement, IV access, or lab draws on affected arm

NURSING DIAGNOSIS

- Fluid volume, Risk for imbalanced
- Infection, Potential for
- Thought process, Disturbed
- Skin integrity, Impaired
- Knowledge, Deficient

Dialysis, Peritoneal (PD)

DEFINITION

- PD is the process of removing metabolic wastes and fluid using the peritoneal cavity to instill dialysate solution and using an osmotic gradient to draw excess fluid and waste into the peritoneum where is it removed.
- Peritoneal dialysis is performed via a peritoneal catheter tunneled from the skin of the abdomen into the peritoneal cavity.
- Peritoneal dialysis is a sterile procedure in the hospital and a clean procedure in the home setting.
- Less dietary and fluid restrictions are required with PD because of the continuous process.
- Patients and families must be knowledgeable and able to perform PD at home.

Steps of PD

- Connect—prescribed dialysate to PD catheter
- Inflow—allow dialysate bag to empty into the peritoneum
- Dwell—allow the dialysate to dwell in the peritoneum for the prescribed time
- Outflow—connect the PD catheter to a bag allowing the effluent (waste material) flow out of the peritoneum
- Repeat above steps

KEY ASSESSMENTS

- Assess for signs of peritonitis (infection in the peritoneal lining)
- Fever
- Malaise
- Abdominal tenderness
- Cloudy outflow

Lab Tests

- Culture effluent sample
- Blood urea nitrogen (BUN) and creatinine (Cr)

PLANNING AND IMPLEMENTATION

- Sterile technique while performing PD in the hospital setting
- Monitor for signs of peritonitis (fever, cloudy outflow, abdominal tenderness, and malaise)
- Take daily weight
- Monitor intake and output (I & O)
- Monitor complete blood count (CBC), white blood count (WBC), and electrolytes
- If peritonitis is present, administer antibiotics in PD dialysate as ordered

SPECIAL CONCERNS

Teaching Considerations

- Describe signs of peritonitis.
- Stress catheter care.
- Ensure effluent is clear by placing a newspaper under effluent bag. If unable to read the paper through the effluent, contact the health care provider.
- Keep dialysate solution at room temperature. If the solution is cold it can cause cramping during inflow and dwelling periods of PD.

NURSING DIAGNOSIS

- Knowledge, Deficient
- Infection, Risk for

Endotracheal Intubation and Mechanical Ventilation

DEFINITION

- Endotracheal intubation is the planned or emergent passage of a tube into the trachea through either the mouth or nare to maintain an open airway and aid ventilation. Physicians, nurse anesthestists, and paramedics typically perform intubation.

Necessary Equipment

- Suction equipment
- Personal protective equipment including eyewear
- Intubation tray (usually consists of laryngeal scope, lubricant, stylet, syringe, oral airway, and endotracheal tubes)
- AMBU bag attached to supplemental oxygen
- Ventilator
- End tidal CO_2 monitor

KEY ASSESSMENTS

Once Intubation Is Complete

- Auscultate breath sounds for bilateral breath sounds and rate
- Pulse oximetry
- End tidal CO_2 device
- Secretion color and amount
- Vital signs
- Anxiety
- Chest X-ray (CXR) to verify tube placement
- Assess endotracheal tube holder for secure ness of airway

PLANNING AND IMPLEMENTATION

(See Table 15)

SPECIAL CONCERNS

- Keep emergency equipment near by when caring for the ventilated patient in case of accidental tube removal and subsequent reintubation.

NURSING DIAGNOSIS

- Ventilation, Impaired spontaneous
- Swallowing, Impaired

TABLE 15

Nursing Management of Patients Requiring Mechanical Ventilation

1. Secure artifical airway and monitor for tube movement.	This action helps to prevent unplanned extubation.
2. Auscultate lung field at least every hour hours and as needed.	This action will help monitor for effectiveness of intervention.
3. Suction artificial airway as needed; hyperoxygenate before, during, and after procedure.	This action helps to prevent desaturation during suctioning of the patient.
4. Position patient in semi-Fowler's or high Fowler's position if possible.	This position helps to facilitate lung expansion. This position helps to prevent aspiration of secretions.
5. Administer antibiotics and bronchodilators as ordered.	The bronchodilators help to promote secretion removal. Antibiotics will be appropriate for the patient with infection.
6. Monitor the patient's volume status and hydrate as appropriate.	This action will help promote thinner secretions and aid in their removal.
7. Turn the patient every two hours and as appropriate.	This helps to facilitate secretion removal.
8. Maintain constant monitoring of pulse oximetry values. Document values on flow sheet.	Pulse oximetry monitoring helps to detect decreases in oxygen saturation. Documentation helps to identify changes in saturations in accordance with treatments and interventions.

TABLE 15

Nursing Management of Patients Requiring Mechanical Ventilation—cont'd

9. Titrate FiO_2 according to SpO_2 values.	This action helps to prevent hypoxemia or oxygen toxicity.
10. Monitor arterial blood gas (ABG) results and adjust ventilator settings accordingly.	This helps to maximize therapeutic effects of adjusted settings.
11. If necessary, apply soft wrist restraints to patient.	This helps to prevent unplanned extubation.
12. If the patient is orally intubated, secure tube on alternating sides of the mouth daily. For example, left side on Day 1, then right side on Day 2.	This action helps to prevent ulcer generation and tissue necrosis from the pressure of the endotracheal (ET) tube.
13. Monitor ET tube cuff pressure at least once per shift.	This action helps to prevent overinflation of the ET tube cuff and possible tissue necrosis.
14. Provide oral care at least every two hours as needed.	This helps to prevent dryness and ulcer formation in the mouth.
15. Ensure appropriate ventilator alarm settings. Review meanings of high- and low-pressure alarms. Respond to ventilator alarms promptly.	These actions help to prevent further injury to the patient when complications occur or the patient becomes disconnected from life support.
16. Monitor ET tub and ventilator circuits turning and repositioning patient.	Careful monitoring of tubing and ET tube helps to prevent unplanned extubation.
17. Wash hands before and after any patient care activities.	This helps to prevent ventilator-associated pneumonia.
18. Explain all procedures to patient and family.	This helps to ensure compliance with ventilator.
19. Administer anti-anxiety medication as ordered and required by the patient.	This action helps to promote ventilator compliance.
20. Provide alternative methods of communication.	This action helps to lessen feelings or powerlessness in the patient and helps to reduce anxiety.

Intraoperative Patient Care

DEFINITION

- Intraoperative care is the period of care from entry into the surgical suite until the completion of the surgery.

Surgical Team

- Surgeon and anesthesiologist (both medical doctors with specialized training)
- Nurses—including certified registered nurse anesthetist, operating room nurses (circulator, scrub, and registered nurse first assistant), operating room educator, and director of surgical services
- Surgical technologists (an allied health professional)

Surgical Specialties

- Cardiothoracic, cardiovascular
- General
- Neurosurgery
- Obstetrics and gynecology
- Ophthalmology
- Oral and maxillofacial
- Orthopedic
- Otolaryngology
- Plastic and reconstructive
- Genitourinary, urology

Types of Anesthesia

- Local
- Regional
- Spinal
- Epidural
- General

Levels of Sedation

- Conscious sedation—drug-induced depression of consciousness, but patient still responds to verbal command.
- Deep sedation—drug-induced depression of consciousness in which patient responds only to painful stimulation.
- Full sedation—drug-induced depression of consciousness in which patient does not respond to any stimulus. The airway must be fully supported.

KEY ASSESSMENTS

- Preoperative assessments are complete.
- Patient is correctly identified.
- Surgical site is correctly identified and verified.

PLANNING AND IMPLEMENTATION

- Maintain the sterile field
- Position patient
- Implement protective measures to prevent injury due to thermal, chemical, or mechanical sources
- Implements protective measures to prevent injury due to electrical, laser, or radiation sources
- Perform skin preparations
- Manage patient temperature
- Pass instruments and supplies
- Assess and anticipate needs of the patient and surgeon
- Count items
- Specimen care
- Dressing applications

SPECIAL CONCERNS

- Do not resuscitate (DNR) status is usually suspended when a patient goes to surgery. This should be discussed with the patient and the family when there is a DNR order prior to surgery.
- Retained objects are a preventable occurrence, and the entire surgical team may be held liable.

Genetic Considerations

- Malignant hyperthermia is a life-threatening, acute pharmacogenetic disorder that develops during or after general anesthesia. It is an autosomal-dominant inherited disorder. The incidence is 1 in 10,000. Hyperthermia, tachycardia, hypoxia, and rigor of muscles are all signs of malignant hyperthermia.

NURSING DIAGNOSIS

- Injury, Risk for perioperative-positioning
- Skin integrity, Risk for impaired

Joint Replacement

DEFINITION

- Joint replacement surgery, or arthroplasty, is the surgical removal of the affected joint and replacement with prosthetic joint (see Boxes 1–3). Joint replacement is a common surgical procedure for the elderly patient and can greatly enhance quality of life.

BOX 1

Care of the Patient with a Total Joint Arthroplasty (Preoperative)

Assessment

- History and physical: Gather information on past medical and surgical history. Is there any medical condition(s) that may cause postoperative concerns (e.g., hypertension, chronic obstructive pulmonary disease [COPD], or bleeding disorders)? What are the current medications taken (prescribed, over-the-counter, and herbal or natural)? If the patient has had surgery in the past, was there any reaction to anesthesia? Assess patient's gait and use of any mobility devices. What is the patient's preoperative range of motion in the affected extremity?
- Social history: Gather information regarding with whom the patient lives. If the patient lives alone, will he or she have a support individual to assist him or her in the home after surgery, will he or she go to a family member's residence after surgery, or does the patient anticipate needing to go to an extended care facility (ECF) for a short while to recover? Does the home have a first-floor restroom? How many steps will the patient need to negotiate in order to get into the home? Does the patient have access to the necessary equipment for assistance with activities of daily living (e.g., walker, elevated toilet seat, or reachers)?
- Financial information: Are there any referrals that are needed by the insurance company? Is a social work consult necessary to assist with payment for the surgery?

Planning and Implementation

- History and physical: Assure patients that any medical conditions that they currently have will be addressed by the surgeon, anesthetist, and nursing staff so that their other conditions will not adversely affect their recovery from surgery. Patient teaching should include what

continued

BOX 1

Care of the Patient with a Total Joint Arthroplasty (Preoperative)—cont'd

medications the patient should stop taking before surgery and when he or she should stop taking them. Explain the operative procedure (preoperative room, what happens during surgery, and postanesthesia care unit). If available, provide written or video material that explains the surgical experience and postoperative recovery requirements that the patient can take home with him or her and will reinforce teaching already completed.

- Social history: Help the patient explore options about posthospital recovery regarding where he or she will be staying and equipment needed. Usually the hospital can provide resources for equipment for the patient. However, the patient may have relatives or friends who have had to use this type of equipment and might be able to loan or give it to the patient. Also, some churches keep such equipment that can be borrowed. If the patient anticipates going to an ECF after being discharged from the hospital, does he or she know which facility he or she would like to use? Also, consider involving social workers now or early on during the hospital stay.
- Financial information: Make the appropriate referrals and contact the insurance company if preauthorization is necessary.

Evaluation

- History and physical: Patient verbalizes an understanding of the basics of what will happen on the day of surgery and the general course during the hospital stay. He or she will verbalize what medications to stop taking before surgery.
- Social history: Patient verbalizes where he or she will be staying after discharge from the hospital and who will be available to assist him or her. The patient will verbalize where equipment can be obtained.
- Financial information: Patient verbalizes any financial concerns.

BOX 2

In-Hospital Postoperative Recovery

Assessment

- Routine physical assessment consists of neurological, pulmonary, cardiac, gastrointestinal, psychological, and neurovascular assessments as well as assessing the operative site. Pain will need to be assessed. Arthroplasties tend to be painful (a different pain than experienced

continued

BOX 2

In-Hospital Postoperative Recovery—cont'd

preoperatively). Adequate pain assessment and control will enhance the patient's recovery.

- Potential complications (most common) include deep vein thrombosis (DVT), wound infection, hematoma at the surgical site, neurovascular compromise, and dislocation (hip).
- Also assess any patient or family concerns regarding the patient's progress.
- Assess the patient's learning of correct mobility techniques and precautions related to the specific surgery (e.g., patient verbalizes that he should not cross his legs after a total hip arthroplasty).

Planning and Implementation

- Administering pain medications, antibiotics, and anticoagulants as ordered. Emphasize to the patient that keeping pain under control will assist in the recovery process by making it easier to ambulate and rest more comfortably.
- Report any questionable assessments to the physician immediately to minimize adverse effects from complications.
- Generally physical therapy (PT) is the first to instruct a patient in how to get out of bed and to ambulate. Nursing is capable of doing the initial teaching but most generally reinforces the teaching of PT. Encourage the patient to gradually increase mobility, without pushing him or herself too far.
- Encourage patient and family to verbalize concerns and questions to you and any member of the nursing or medical staff.

Evaluation of Outcomes

Potential outcomes for the patient following surgery include:

- Patient verbalizes adequate pain control and willingly participates in therapy.
- Patient does not suffer from any postoperative complications.
- Patient's mobility steadily increases.
- Patient and family are freely able to express concerns and have concerns and questions addressed promptly.

BOX 3

After Discharge from the Hospital

Assessment

- Medications: Assess patient's understanding of prescribed postoperative medications and what preoperative medications the patient should continue taking after discharge.
- Mobility and exercise: Assess patient's need to obtain and maintain prescribed postoperative mobility and therapy. Does the person have a walker, crutches, or cane for home use?
- Wound care: Assess patient's knowledge of appropriate wound care postoperatively.
- Home environment: If being discharged to a private residence, assess physical layout of the unit by asking questions. How many steps? Are there throw rugs? Are there chairs high enough to sit on (for "hip patients")?
- Follow-up care: Does the patient or caregiver understand when to see the surgeon for a follow-up appointment?

Planning and Implementation

- Medications: Teach patient which medications should be taken at home and continued. Often, antibiotics and anticoagulants are sent home with the patient. If the patient is sent home on warfarin (Coumadin), arrangements will need to be made to draw weekly or biweekly international normalized ratio (INR) levels with a home health agency, a local clinic, or a health care provider's office. Encourage the patient to take all the prescribed antibiotics and to take the warfarin as prescribed. Caution the patient that the health care provider may change the warfarin prescription after blood tests are drawn to prevent excessive bleeding. Pain medication prescriptions are most always sent home with the patient. Encourage the patient to take the pain medication about 30 minutes before exercising to keep pain to a minimum. Teach the patient about not driving when on this medication because it can cause drowsiness. Also, caution the patient not to share his or her medications with others. Tell the patient to flush any unused pain medication down the toilet.
- Mobility and exercise: If formal therapy is prescribed, contact a home health agency to arrange this. Reinforce the necessity to increase amount of mobility each day to strengthen the muscles in the affected extremity.
- Wound care: Teach the patient appropriate wound care at home.

continued

BOX 3

After Discharge from the Hospital—cont'd

- Home environment: Encourage the caregiver to remove any throw rugs in the home. The health care provider will recommend how many times a patient can go up and down stairs. The rule of thumb is up and down stairs once a day for the first two weeks, then increase as the patient tolerates after that.
- Follow-up care: Tell the patient when the surgeon wants to schedule a follow-up appointment. You may make the appointment or allow the patient to do so.

Evaluation

- The patient recovers and returns to normal activities of daily living without complications.

NURSING DIAGNOSIS

- Pain, Acute
- Mobility, Impaired physical
- Infection, Risk for

Pain

DEFINITION

- Pain is an unpleasant sensory and emotional experience arising from actual or potential tissue damage or described in terms related to the damage. Pain is defined subjectively based on a person's experience. Simply, pain is what the person says it is and exists when the person says it does. Pain is currently considered the fifth vital sign and should be included in patient assessment.

Terms Associated with Pain Medication Use

- Physical dependence is an involuntary altered physiological state produced by repeated administration of a medication. Medication should be gradually withdrawn to avoid symptoms.
- Addiction is a compulsive disorder in which a person focuses on obtaining and using a substance even though it results in a decreased quality of life.
- Tolerance is when higher doses of a drug are required to achieve the desired effect.

KEY ASSESSMENTS

(See Table 16)

- Pain history
- Description

TABLE 16

Pain Descriptions

Nociceptive Pain

Nociceptive pain involves stimulation by chemical, mechanical, or noxious stimuli (heat or cold). The pain occurs when there is normal processing of the pain impulse over intact nerves, and no injury or malfunction of the neuronal transmission process.

- Cutaneous or superficial pain can be readily localized, and the person can indicate where the pain is located.
- Somatic pain (from body wall muscles and bone) is less localized and can be described as aching or throbbing. It may be accompanied by nausea, sweating, bradycardia, and hypotension due to the autonomic nervous system response. Pain may radiate from the primary site as seen in lumbar disc pain that radiates down the sciatic nerve. Arthritis is a type of chronic somatic pain.
- Visceral, or splanchnic, pain is poorly localized and is described as dull, colic-like, or cramping. It is often accompanied by diarrhea, sweating, and hypertension because the pain is transmitted by small unmyelinated fibers that travel along with the sympathetic nerves to the spinal cord. Cancer pain and chrome pancreatitis are examples.
- Referred pain can be severe at the body surface although there is minimal or no pain at the primary site of injury because both the body surface area and the deeper tissues are innervated by the same spinal nerve segment.

Pathologic Pain Syndromes

Neuropathic pain occurs as result of damage at any point in the pain pathway to peripheral nerves, the spinal cord, brain stem, thalamus, or cerebral areas. It is described as a burning or severe shooting electrical pain sensation, which frequently travels down a nerve to the dermatome associated with the peripheral nerve. It is also referred to as stabbing pain or a “pins and needles” sensation. Examples include diabetic neuropathy, postherpetic neuralgia, and phantom limb pain.

- Bone and muscular pain (includes ligaments, joint capsules, fascia, and tendons) usually occurs following stretching, ischemia, or forceful or sustained contractile activity. Injury causes a release of lactic acid and other substances that increase pain intensity. Pain often radiates into surrounding tissues. Tension headaches are often due to tense neck and scalp muscles. Muscle ischemia due to intermittent claudication (a spasm in the extremities during walking) as result of occlusive vascular disease; the pain of coronary occlusion is due to ischemia also.
- Vascular pain may be due to a pathological condition of the vessels or surrounding tissues, such as mixed vascular and neuropathic complications related to chronic diabetes mellitus. Other examples include migraine headaches and headaches associated with hypertension, brain tumors, and increased cranial pressure.
- Pain due to inflammation occurs from infection or as the result of trauma and the subsequent release of acidic chemicals and distension of tissues.

continued

TABLE 16

Pain Descriptions—cont'd

Pathologic Pain Syndromes—cont'd

- Central pain results from injury to the central nervous system (CNS) due to tumors, disease, stroke, or damage to the spinal cord. Pain can be severe and constant. Brain masses can involve the cerebral cortex and elicit central pain in the opposite side of the body.
- Thalamic pain is the perception of pain in one half of body following injury to thalamus. This type of pain is rare.
- Back pain is common and usually occurs in the cervical or lumbar regions. It is commonly due to spinal disc injury or herniation of the nucleus pulposus, the cushioning substance between the intervertebral discs. Sensory and motor nerve damage may occur.

Peripheral and Mixed Central or Peripheral Pathologic Pain

- Causalgia from peripheral nerve injury, such as the brachial plexus, median, and sciatic nerves. Pain is severe and persistent (intractable pain that is resistant to treatment) can lead to depression and suicide. Any stimulus can initiate paroxysms of excruciating pain.
- Trigeminal neuralgia (Tic Douloureux) pain occurs along the mixed trigeminal cranial nerve. Severe facial pain results from minimal stimuli including brushing teeth, chewing, or talking, draft of cold air, and so on.
- Phantom pain following amputation of a body part consists of sensations that the part is still present. More severe pain is described as throbbing, burning, stabbing, or vise-like. Stump, or residual limb, pain may be caused by a neuroma at the amputation site.
- Intracranial headache has many causes including changes in intracranial pressure, hypertension, hypoxia, medications, infection, and hemorrhage. The most common is the migraine. Headaches due to extracranial origin also have many causes. The most common problems include muscle tension; temporomandibular joint syndrome; and problems related to the eye, sinus, dental, and ear.
- Cancer, or malignant, pain is commonly due to pressure or displacement of nerves by the tumor growth, interference with blood supply, muscle spasms, pathological bone fracture, and the result of treatments.
- Pain associated with human immunodeficiency virus (HIV) frequently occurs in the gastrointestinal tract, from herpes and cytomegalovirus infections, peripheral neuropathy, headache, and Kaposi's sarcoma lesions that obstruct the lymph system.
- Psychogenic pain refers to the pain that is primarily due to emotional factors. The pain begins with a physiological basis and is exacerbated by stress, anxiety, and fear or anger. This type of pain is real to the patient. Chronic muscle tension can lead to tension headache, backache, or visceral changes. It is often referred to as somatoform disorder and necessitates identification of the cause and appropriate treatment.
- Pain of psychological origin is defined as seeking treatment for pain when no actual pain exists. Some patients are aware that they are using this strategy as an excuse to avoid a responsibility, to obtain drugs, to gain sympathy or attention, or to claim an injury to receive compensation. This is also referred to as malingering or pretending; however, it should never be assumed that pain does not exist; a thorough assessment and accurate diagnosis are needed to rule out an actual problem.

- Onset
- Frequency
- Duration
- Exacerbating factors
- Alleviating factors
- Impact on activities of daily living
- Medications
- Nonpharmacological treatments
- Spiritual, social, and cultural influences on pain experience

Physiological Effects

- Complementary therapy
- Blood pressure
- Heart rate
- Respirations
- Pupil dilatation
- Nausea and vomiting
- Diaphoresis
- Weakness
- Sleep changes

Pain Scales

- Numerical Rating Scale—pain intensity on a 0 to10 scale
- Wong-Baker Faces Scale—uses faces to assist in describing pain (particularly useful in pediatric and language-challenged patients)
- Verbal Graphic Rating Scale—words are used to describe intensity of pain
- PAINAD Scale—uses breathing and facial expressions to assess pain, especially useful in patients with dementia

PLANNING AND IMPLEMENTATION

- Administer analgesic medications.
- Opioids (narcotics), morphine, fentanyl, and hydromorphone.
- Non-opioids, acetaminophen, and nonsteroidal anti-inflammatory drugs (NSAIDs).
- Adjuvants, anticonvulsants, tricyclic antidepressants, antidepressants, and benzodiazepines.
- Side effects of each category of drug should be monitored.
- All pain therapy is best when used around the clock and administered before pain is severe.
- Often a combination of pain medications provides the best relief.
- Reassess pain frequently.

SPECIAL CONCERNS

- Responses to pain are affected by social-cultural influences and gender differences.
- Side effects of opioids include respiratory depression, and this should be monitored for closely.
- Educate patients on how to medicate their pain before discharge and about the side effects of each medication prescribed.
- Pain medications should be kept out of the reach of children.
- Pain medications may potentially be abused by other family members.

NURSING DIAGNOSIS

- Pain, Acute
- Pain, Chronic
- Knowledge, Deficient

Palliative Care

DEFINITION

- Palliative care involves the active total care of patients whose disease is not responding to curative treatments.

KEY ASSESSMENTS

- Pain frequently
- Dyspnea
- Loss of appetite
- Nausea
- Vomiting
- Constipation
- Urinary incontinence
- Anxiety
- Depression

PLANNING AND IMPLEMENTATION

(See Table 17)

- Emphasis is attainment of highest possible quality of life and symptom control

TABLE 17

Physiology of Dying

Cardiovascular System

- The heart fails to pump, resulting in insufficient blood flow and ischemia.
- Insufficient peripheral blood flows results in a decrease in skin temperature and changes in skin color, such as pallor or mottling, beginning at the distal extremities and moving toward the torso.
- A decrease in circulation time between the lungs and the brain results in Cheyne-Stokes respirations.
- Signs of cardiac decompensation including decreasing blood pressure, tachycardia, irregular pulse, decreased mentation, cool extremities, reduced urinary output, pulmonary congestion, and hepatic distention. Symptoms include chest pain and dyspnea.

Pulmonary System

- Respiratory failure begins as hypoxia leads to high carbon dioxide levels; this results in confusion and restlessness and can lead to coma.
- Underlying causes of respiratory failure include pneumonia, pulmonary embolism, and pulmonary edema.
- Respiratory systems can begin with dyspnea on exertion with increased respiratory rate and depth and progress to dyspnea at rest.
- Early signs of hypoxia include confusion, orthopnea, irregular breathing, tachycardia, and use of accessory muscles to breathe. Symptoms of hypoxia include restlessness, irritability, and anxiety.

Central Nervous System

- Changes in level of consciousness are manifest by periods of confusion, disorientation, and lethargy progressing to stupor.
- Periods of sleep increase, and periods of wakefulness decrease.
- Sluggish pupil constriction progresses to dilation in a fixed position as brain hypoxia increases.

Renal System

- Urine volume decreases and concentration increases as fluid intake decreases and kidney function and renal blood flow diminishes.

Managing Pain

- Give medications around the clock
- Use simplest dosing schedule and the least invasive route
- Do not undertreat pain

Managing Dyspnea

- Place patient in semi-Fowler's position
- Use a bedside fan and keep the room cool
- Antianxiety and diuretic medications (may be helpful)

Managing Loss of Appetite, Constipation, Incontinence, Nausea, and Vomiting

- Eliminate strong odors or foods with odors
- Supply an emesis container within reach
- Administer antiemetics as ordered
- Offer frequent oral care
- Provide small frequent meals
- Routinely administer stool softeners (opioid medications cause constipation)
- Do not hesitate to place an in-dwelling catheter if requested by the patient

Managing Anxiety and Depression

- Encourage the patients to discuss their concerns
- Help patients explore and use coping strategies that have been helpful in the past
- Antianxiety or antidepressant medications (may be helpful)
- Provide spiritual support

NURSING DIAGNOSIS

- Anxiety, Death
- Pain, Acute
- Incontinence, Total urinary
- Breathing pattern, Ineffective
- Grieving, Anticipatory
- Skin integrity, Risk for impaired
- Self care deficit, Toileting

Postoperative Patient Care

DEFINITION

- Postoperative care begins when the surgery ends. Some patients recover from surgery in a postanesthesia care unit until they are completely awake and their vital signs are stable; others go directly to an intensive care unit.

KEY ASSESSMENTS

- Respirations
- Blood pressure and heart rate

- Temperature
- Pulse oximetry
- Level of consciousness (LOC)
- Pain
- Surgical site
- Nausea and vomiting
- Urinary retention
- Paralytic illeus

PLANNING AND IMPLEMENTATION

- Monitor vital signs frequently
- Oxygen administration
- Encourage deep breathing
- Splint incision when patient coughs
- Treat pain
- Monitor LOC
- Monitor wound status
- Thermoregulation
- Keep head of bed elevated unless contraindicated
- Report to the nurse receiving the patient on the floor and include the following information:
    - Operative procedure
    - Complications, if any
    - Time and type of anesthesia
    - Time of completion of surgery
    - Estimated blood loss
    - Fluid replacement
    - Location of lines, tubes, and dressings
    - Vital signs
    - Positioning during surgery
    - Comparison of preoperative and current status

SPECIAL CONCERNS

- Provide postoperative reports to a floor nurse over secure phone lines.
- Information shared among perioperative health care providers is on a need-to-know basis only.

NURSING DIAGNOSIS

- Fluid volume, Risk for deficient
- Pain, Acute

- Skin integrity, Impaired
- Infection, Risk for
- Fluid volume, Risk for imbalanced

Preoperative Patient Care

DEFINITION

- Preoperative care is the period of care prior to the intraoperative period or events leading up to the entry into the surgical suite.

Types of Surgery

- Elective surgery—a planned surgery that allows time to prepare and fully plan for the surgical experience.
- Emergency surgery—an unexpected surgery. The need for surgery is immediate, and there is little time to plan for the surgical experience.
- Short-stay surgery—a surgery in which the patient is discharged within 23 hours of admission.
- Major surgery—involves a greater risk to life and involves a longer time in surgery or surgery to major organs or systems.
- Minor surgery—involves a minimal risk to life and a short time in surgery and does not involve multiple body systems.

KEY ASSESSMENTS

- Medical history
- Surgical history
- Head-to-toe assessment
- Prior blood transfusions
- Any previous family or personal complications to anesthesia
- Medication history
  - Prescribed medication—what and when taken last
  - Over-the-counter medications—what and when taken last
  - Herbal or dietary supplements—what and when taken last
  - Alcohol, tobacco, and street drug use—what and when taken last
- Allergy history to medications and foods and what type of reaction
- Social, cultural, or religious requests
- Verify patient's understanding of the surgical procedure
- Consents for surgery and blood (if necessary) signed
- Verify any preparations have been completed
- Verify with the patient and mark the site to confirm location of the operative site

PLANNING AND IMPLEMENTATION

- Recent laboratory results
- History and physical is on the chart
- Nail polish removed
- Jewelry and person items secured
- Dental or body prosthesis removed
- Identifying band intact
- Nothing by mouth (NPO) time documented
- Vital signs performed
- Verify family or significant others know where to wait for patient
- Assist patient in voiding prior to surgery
- Administer any preoperative medications as ordered

SPECIAL CONCERNS

- If a patient cannot verbalize what type of surgery he or she is having or why it is being performed, even if the consents are signed, the surgeon must visit to reexplain and obtain consent before the patient goes to surgery.
- Report any abnormal lab or finding to the surgeon before sending the patient to surgery.

NURSING DIAGNOSIS

- Anxiety
- Knowledge, Deficient

Transplantation, Renal

DEFINITION

- Renal transplantation is the transplantation of a single kidney into a patient with end-stage renal disease. Pretransplantation counseling and testing is performed before the patient is eligible for kidney transplant.

Classifications

- Cadaveric renal transplant—kidney is donated from a brain-dead patient.
- Live donor renal transplant—kidney is donated by a living family member or other compatible person.

KEY ASSESSMENTS

- Hemodynamic status (monitor for hypovolemia-hypotension or tachycardia)
- Oxygenation status
- Bleeding
- Acute graft rejection (nausea, pain, fever, or jaundice)
- Level of consciousness (LOC)
- Urine output and color (in-dwelling urinary catheter is left in place to allow utereral implant healing without bladder filling)
- Wound appearance

Diagnostics

- Renal ultrasound

Lab Tests

- Blood urea nitrogen (BUN), creatinine (Cr), and glomerular filtration rate (GFR)
- Electrolytes
- Complete blood count (CBC)

PLANNING AND IMPLEMENTATION

- Take vital signs hourly.
- Check urine output hourly (immediate postoperative urine output results in large amounts of dilute urine and gradually decreases to normal as the patient is able to concentrate the urine).
- Call health care provider for drastic changes in urine output.
- Administer replacement fluid.
- Administer electrolytes to correct imbalances.
- Encourage deep breathing.
- Administer sterile wound care.
- Treat incisional pain.
- Strict hand washing.
- Monitor cardiac status continuously.
- Monitor labs (BUN, Cr, CBC, white blood count [WBC], or electrolytes).
- Monitor for signs of rejection (pain over site, fever, tachycardia, or decrease in urine output).
- Monitor for signs of infection (pain over site, fever, or tachycardia).
- Monitor for signs of renal artery thrombosis (acute cessation of urine output, acute abdominal pain, and rapid increase in creatinine).

- Monitor for signs of ureteral anastomosis failure (fluid collection around the kidney, increased wound drainage, and rise in Cr).
- Administer immunosuppressive medications, including corticosteroids, cyclosporine, FK-506, tacrolimus, sirolimus, Imuran, and mycophenolate mofetil.
- Monitor for side effects of immunosuppressive therapy.
- Patient may experience acute renal failure postoperatively. (See Diseases and Disorders, Renal Failure, Acute.)

SPECIAL CONCERNS

- Patients are at risk for infection and rejection for the rest of their lives and must understand the medication therapy, side effects, signs of infection, signs of rejection, and the importance of taking only prescribed medications.

Teaching Considerations

- Signs of infection
- Signs of rejection
- Call health care provider before taking over-the-counter medications
- Take medications as prescribed
- Monitor for side effects of medication therapy
- Do not eat raw fish
- Do not empty cat litter boxes
- Wash bagged, prepared salads before eating
- Flu and pneumococal vaccines

NURSING DIAGNOSIS

- Knowledge, Deficient
- Infection, Risk for
- Fluid volume, Risk for imbalanced
- Pain, Acute

Transplant, Liver

DEFINITION

- Liver transplantation involves transplanting all or part of liver and is performed when a patient has end-stage liver disease and meets certain criteria (see Box 4).

BOX 4

Conditions to Prioritize Organ Recipients

- Appropriate parameters are met regarding size of the liver, ABO (blood type) compatibility, and model end-stage liver disease (MELD) or pediatric end-stage liver disease (PELD) score.
- The amount of time spent on the waiting list.
- The degree of medical urgency.
  1. Candidates who have a life expectancy of less than seven days would include patients with fulminant liver failure.
  2. A person who has received a liver transplant in the last 7 days, but the transplant liver is nonfunctioning (defined as an AST greater than or equal to 5,000 *and* an INR greater than 2.5 or acidosis with pH less than 7.3 or lactate of 2 times the normal level).
  3. Hepatic artery thrombosis in the first seven days of liver implant.
  4. Decompensated Wilson's disease

Classifications

- Orthotopic liver transplant (OLT)—removes the diseased liver and implants a donated (live or cadaveric) liver or part of a liver.
- Auxiliary transplantation—leaves all or part of the patient's liver and grafts the donated (live or cadaveric) liver or part of a liver to the patient's liver.

Organ Sources

- Cadaveric organs come from patients who are brain dead. The whole liver may be transplanted, or the liver may be split to allowing transplantation to more patients.
- Live donor (living donor liver transplant) is usually donated by a family member. The ability of the liver to regenerate makes it possible for the donor and the recipient livers grow back to normal size.

KEY ASSESSMENTS

- Hemodynamic status
- Oxygenation status
- Bleeding
- Acute graft rejection (nausea, pain, fever, or jaundice)

- Level of consciousness (LOC)
- Urine output
- Hepatic artery thrombosis ([HAT], abdominal ultrasound)
- Bile production (drain)
- Infection

Diagnostics

- Liver biopsy may be formed if rejection is suspected.

Lab Tests

- Aspartate aminotransferase (AST), alanine aminotransferase (ALT), and Bilirubin
- Prothrombin time (PT), partial thromboplastin time (PTT), and international normalized ratio (INR)
- Electrolytes
- Arterial blood gases (ABGs)
- Blood urea nitrogen (BUN) and creatinine (Cr)

PLANNING AND IMPLEMENTATION

- Hourly vital signs
- Hourly urine output
- Encourage deep breathing
- Sterile wound care
- Treat incisional pain
- Strict hand washing
- Continuous cardiac monitoring
- Monitor labs
- Monitor for signs of rejection
- Monitor for signs of HAT (elevated AST, ALT, and thrombus noted on ultrasound)
- Monitor for signs of infection
- Administer immunosuppressive medications including corticosteroids, cyclosporine, FK-506, tacrolimus, sirolimus, imuran, and mycophenolate mofectil
- Monitor for side effects of immunosuppressive therapy

Discharge Planning

- Patients are at risk for infection and rejection for the rest of their lives. Patients must understand the medication therapy, the side effects, signs of infection, and signs of rejection and should not take any medication unless prescribed.

NURSING DIAGNOSIS

- Knowledge, Deficient
- Infection, Risk for
- Fluid volume, Risk for imbalanced
- Pain, Acute

Triage

DEFINITION

- Triage stems from the French word for "to sort" and is the process of rapidly assessing patients and assigning them a classification of priority of care.

The Objectives of a Triage System

- Identify patients requiring immediate care
- Use resources wisely
- Facilitate patient flow
- Provide assessment and reassessment of patients
- Initiate legal accountability

Classifications

Hospital triage

Care is rendered to the most critical patient first.

- Level I—critically ill or emergent (loss of limb or anaphylactic shock).
- Level II—intermediate or urgent (fractures or abdominal pain).
- Level III—low risk or stable (sprains or toothaches).

Mass casualty incident triage

Care is rendered to the patient likely to survive.

- Green—patients who will do well with minimal care (walking wounded).
- Yellow—patients who require moderate care but are fairly stable (fractures).
- Red—patients who require care but have good chances of survival (crushed limb requiring amputation).
- Black—patients who need most care and still may die (hemorrhagic shock due to large trauma).

Military triage

Care is based on the lives at stake, the resources available, and the capabilities of the medical personnel at the scene.

- Military tactical triage
  - Class I—minor injuries can be treated on an ouptpatient basis.
  - Class II—injuries require immediate attention, but require minimum amount of time, personnel, and resources.
  - Class III—treatment can be delayed without threat to life or limb.
  - Class IV—injuries are extensive and would require extensive time, highly trained personnel and a great deal of supplies. Caring for these patients would jeopardize the treatment of many others.
- Military nontactical triage
  - Priority I—patients with correctible life-threatening illness or injury.
  - Priority II—patients with serious but not life-threatening illness or injury.
  - Priority III—patients with minor injuries.
  - Priority IV—patients are dead or fatally injured.

Valve Repair

DEFINITION

- Valve repair is a procedure that restores the integrity of a heart valve. Postoperative care is described in Valve Replacement.

Three Main Types of Procedures

- Valvuloplasty is a procedure in which a balloon-tipped catheter is inserted via a peripheral artery into the heart, and the balloon is inflated in the valve and then removed. The inflation increases the valve diameter.
- Annuloplasty is a type of heart surgery in which a sternotomy incision is made, and the valve is repaired by either a ring procedure or a leaflet repair.
  - Ring procedure—a ring is placed at the junction of the valve leaflets and the heart muscle. This ensures the size of the valve opening preventing regurgitation.
  - Leaflet repair—the extra tissue causing stenosis of the valve is removed.

- Chordoplasty—the repair of the defect in the shape of the chordae tendineae of the mitral valve. The defect causes valvular regurgitation.

Valve Replacement

DEFINITION

- Valve replacement is a surgical procedure that replaces the defective valve with a mechanical or biological valve (bovine, porcine, or cadaver). The patient is cared for in the intensive care unit after surgery.

KEY ASSESSMENTS

- Heart rate and rhythm
- Sternal incision
- Vital signs
- Hemodynamic status
- Level of consciousness (LOC)
- Hemorrhage
- Oxygenation status
- Intake and output (I & O)

PLANNING AND IMPLEMENTATION

- Monitor hemodynamic status
- Monitor chest tube output
- Monitor urine output and call health are provider if less than 30 mL/hour
- Monitor for arrhythmias
- Treat arrhythmias as ordered
- Monitor LOC
- Monitor I & O
- Maintain a patent intravenous (IV) line
- Administer prophylactic antibiotics
- Administer anticoagulants (mechanical valve)
- Monitor wound for signs of infection
- Prophylactic antibiotics use
- Encourage deep breathing
- Treat incisional pain
- Monitor tissue perfusion

SPECIAL CONCERNS

Teaching Considerations

- Instruct patients about what to expect postoperatively in the intensive care unit, including expectations about monitors, lines, ventilator, pain, activity levels, and wound care.
- If patients receive a mechanical valve replacement, inform them that lifelong anticoagulation is necessary and discuss the risks.
- Discuss the possibility of banking the patient's blood because valve replacement surgery is usually planned in advance.

Wound Healing

DEFINITION

- Wound healing is the process in which skin, with a loss in integrity, becomes closed or healed. Wound closure occurs in three ways.
  - Primary intention—the wound heals using the normal wound repair process and occurs in clean wounds, such as a surgical wound.
  - Secondary intention—the wound heals by the spread of granulation tissue from the base of the wound, such as a venous leg ulcer.
  - Tertiary intention—the wound must be sutured through several layers of granulation tissue to close the wound surface, such as a complex decubitus ulcer.

Risks for Delayed Wound Healing

- Reduced blood flow to area
- Repetitive injury
- Altered nutritional status
- Presence of infection
- Older
- Smoking
- Diabetes mellitus

Phases of Wound Healing

- Inflammatory phase begins with presence of an injury site where chemicals are released and platelets are activated.
- Proliferative phase begins at three to four days when collagen is formed to seal off the wound.

- Remodeling phase collagen reforms into a scar tissue and may take up to years.

KEY ASSESSMENTS

- Wound size and appearance
- Presence of drainage, color, and quantity
- Skin color and temperature surrounding wound
- Signs of infection (fever or increased temperature)

PLANNING AND IMPLEMENTATION

- Document wound assessments every shift
- Wound care as prescribed by the health care provider
- Wound culture and sensitivity
- Anticipate antibiotic administration if an infection is present
- Collaborate with the skin care or ostomy nurse

SPECIAL CONCERNS

- Many wounds heal slowly. Encourage patients to become active in the wound care regime.

NURSING DIAGNOSIS

- Skin integrity, Impaired
- Infection, Risk for
- Knowledge, Deficient

Appendix A

Symbols and Abbreviations

SYMBOLS

~	similar	>	greater than
≅	approximately	<	less than
@	at	%	percent
√	check	+	positive
Δ	change	−	negative
↑	increased	♀	female
↓	decreased	♂	male
=	equals	△ △ △ (1, 2, 3)	trimester of pregnancy (one triangle for each trimester)
#	pounds		

ABBREVIATIONS

2,3-DPG	2,3-diphosphoglycerate
AACN	American Association of Colleges of Nursing
AAOHN	American Association of Occupational Health Nurses
AARP	American Association of Retired Persons
ABG	arterial blood gas
A/C	alternative/complementary
Acetyl-CoA	acetyl coenzyme A
ADA	Americans with Disabilities Act
ADAMHA	Alcohol, Drug Abuse, and Mental Health Administration
ADH	antidiuretic hormone
ADL	activities of daily living
ADP	adenosine diphosphate
ADR	adverse drug reactions
AEB	as evidenced by
AGF	angiogenesis factor
AHA	American Hospital Association
AHNA	American Holistic Nurses Association
AHRQ	Agency for Health Care Research and Policy
AIDS	acquired immunodeficiency syndrome
AJN	*American Journal of Nursing*
AMB	as manifested by
ANA	American Nurses Association
ANS	autonomic nervous system
AONE	Association of Nurse Executives
AORN	Association for Operating Room Nurses
APN	advanced practice nurse
APRN	advanced practice registered nurse
APTT	activated partial thromboplastin time
AST	aspartate aminotransferase
AT	axillary temperature
ATP	adenosine triphosphate
ATSDR	Agency for Toxic Substances and Disease Registry
BCR	bulbocavernous reflex
BMI	body mass index
BMR	basal metabolic rate
BN	bachelor's degree in nursing
BP	blood pressure
BScN	bachelor of science in nursing (in Canada)
BSE	breast self-examination
BSN	bachelor of science in nursing
BUN	blood urea nitrogen
C	Celsius; also called centigrade
CAT	computerized adaptive testing
CAUSN	Canadian Association of University Schools of Nursing
CBC	complete blood count
CBE	charting by exception
CDC	Centers for Disease Control and Prevention
CEUs	continuing education units
CHD	coronary heart disease
CLIA	Clinical Laboratory Improvement Act
cm	centimeter
CMS	Centers for Medicare & Medicaid Services
CNA	Canadian Nurses Association

continued

Symbols and Abbreviations—cont'd

ABBREVIATIONS—cont'd

CNATS	Canadian Nurses Association Testing Service
CNM	certified nurse midwife
CNO	community nursing organization
CNS	central nervous system
CNS	clinical nurse specialist
CO_2	carbon dioxide
COBRA	Consolidated Omnibus Budget Reconciliation Act
COPD	chronic obstructive pulmonary disease
CPK	creatine phosphokinase
CPM	continuous passive motion
CPN	central parenteral resuscitation
CPR	cardiopulmonary resuscitation
CPT	chest physiotherapy
CQT	continuous quality movement
CRNA	certified registered nurses anesthetist
CSF	cerebrospinal fluid
CST	computerized clinical stimulation testing
CT	computed tomography
CVA	cerebral vascular accident
DDS	doctor of dental science
DHHS	Department of Health and Human Services
dl	deciliter
DNR	do not resuscitate
DNSc	doctorate of nursing in science
DRGs	diagnosis-related groups
DSN	doctorate of science in nursing
DUS	Doppler ultrasound stethoscope
DVT	deep vein thrombosis
ECG	electrocardiogram (also known as EKG)
EEG	electroencephalogram
EN	enteral nutrition
EPA	Environmental Protection Agency
EPO	exclusive provider organization
ESR	erythrocyte sedimentation rate
ET	ear canal temperature
F	Fahrenheit
FAF	fibroblase activating factor
FAS	fetal alcohol syndrome
FDA	Food and Drug Administration
FiO_2	fraction of inspired oxygen
ft	feet
f	gram
GAS	general adaptation syndrome
GCS	Glasgow Coma Scale
gH	drop
GI	gastrointestinal tract
GNP	gross national product
HBD	alpha-hydroxybutyrate dehydrogenase
HBV	hepatitis B virus
HCFA	Health Care Financing Administration
Hct	hematocrit
HDL	high-density lipoprotein
HEPA	high-efficiency particulate air
Hgb	hemoglobin
HIS	hospital information system
HIV	human immunodeficiency virus
HMO	health maintenance organization
HPN	home parenteral nutrition
HQIA	Healthcare Quality Improvement Act
HRSA	Health Resources and Services Administration
HSV-2	herpes simplex virus 2
HT	healing touch
IHS	Indian Health Service
IM	intramuscular
in	inch
I & O	intake and output
IOM	Institute on Medicine
IPPB	intermittent positive-pressure breathing
IRA	individual retirement account
IV	intravenous
IVP	intravenous pyelogram
JCAHO	Joint Commission on Accreditation of Healthcare Organization
kcal	kilocalorie
kg	kilogram
LAS	localized adaptation syndrome
lb	pound
LDH	lactic dehydrogenase
LDL	low-density lipoprotein
LLQ	left lower quadrant
LOC	level of consciousness
LPN	licensed practical nurse
LUQ	left upper quadrant
LVN	licensed vocational nurse
m	meter
MA	master of arts degree
MAC	mid-upper-arm circumference
MAR	medication administration record

Symbols and Abbreviations—cont'd

ABBREVIATIONS—cont'd

MD	doctor of medicine
MDR	multi-drug-resistant
mEq	milliequivalent
mEq/L	milliequivalent per liter
mg	milligram
MH	malignant hyperthermia
MI	myocardial infarction
ml	milliliter; also abbreviated mL
mm	millimeter
mm Hg	millimeters of mercury
MN	master's degree in nursing
mOsm	milliosmole; also spelled milliosmol
mOsm/L	milliosmole per liter
MRI	magnetic resonance imaging
MRSA	methicillin-resistant *Staphylococcus aureus*
MSN	master of science in nursing
NACGN	National Association of Colored Graduate Nurses
NANDA	North American Nursing Diagnosis Association
NCEP	National Cholesterol Education Program
NCLEX	National Council Licensure Examination
NCLEX-PN	National Council Licensure Examination for Practical Nurses
NCNR	National Center for Nursing Research
NCSBM	National Council of State Boards of Nursing
NIC	Nursing Interventions Classification
NHI	National Institutes of Health
NINR	National Institute of Nursing Research
NLN	National League for Nursing
NP	nurse practitioner
NPO	*non per os* (nothing by mouth—to eat or drink)
NS	nutrition support
NST	nutritional support team
OAM	Office of Alternative Medicine
OBRA	Omnibus Budget Reconciliation Act
OR	operative room
OSHA	Occupational Safety and Health Administration
OT	occupational therapist
OTC	over-the-counter drugs

oz	ounce
P	pulse
PO_2	partial pressure of oxygen in a mixture of gases, or in solution
PA	physician's assistant
PaO_2 (PAO_2)	partial pressure of oxygen dissolved in arterial blood plasma
PAP	Papanicolaou test
PAT	pulmonary artery temperature
PC	potential complication
PCA	patient-controlled analgesia
PCO_2	partial pressure of carbon dioxide
PCP	primary care provider
PEG	percutaneous endoscopic gastrostomy
PERRLA	pupils equal, round, reactive to light, and accommodation
pH	hydrogen ion concentration of a solution
PID	pelvic inflammatory disease
PIE	problem, intervention, evaluation
PIEE	pulse irrigation enhanced evacuation
PKU	phenylketonuria
PMR	progressive muscle relaxation
PMS	premenstrual syndrome
PN	parenteral nutrition
PNI	psychoneuroimmunology
PNS	peripheral nervous system
PO	*per os* (by mouth)
POMR	problem-oriented medical record
POR	problem-oriented record
PPN	peripheral parenteral nutrition
PPO	preferred provider organization
PPS	prospective payment program
prn	*pro re nata* (as needed)
PRO	peer review organization
PSRO	Professional Standards Review Organization
PT	physical therapist
PT	prothrombin
PT	prothrombin time
PTSD	post-traumatic stress disorder
PTT	partial thromboplastin
PURT	prompted urge response toileting
q	every
QA	quality assurance
R	respiration
RAS	reticular activating system
RBC	red blood cell

continued

Symbols and Abbreviations—cont'd

ABBREVIATIONS—cont'd

RD	registered dietitian	SMI	sustained maximum inspiration
RDA	recommended dietary allowance	SO	source-oriented charting
RDDA	recommended daily dietary allowances	SOAPIE	Subjective data, Objective data, Assessment, Plan, Implementation, Evaluation
RHC	Rural Health Clinic		
RLQ	right lower quadrant	STD	sexually transmitted disease
RN	registered nurse	SUI	stress urinary incontinence
RNA	registered nurse's assistant	SW	social worker
ROM	range-of-motion	T	temperature
RPCH	rural primary care hospital	TEFRA	Tax Equity Fiscal Responsibility Act
RPh	registered pharmacist	TENS	transcutaneous electrical nerve stimulation
RT	rectal temperature		
RT	related to	TMJ	temporomandibular joint
RT	respiratory therapist	TNA	total nutrient admixture
RUQ	right upper quadrant	TPN	total parenteral nutrition
S-CDTN	Self-Care Deficit Theory of Nursing	TQM	total quality management
SA	sinoatrial node	TSE	testicular self-examination
SAECG	signal-averaged electrocardiography	TT	therapeutic touch
		UAP	unlicensed assistive personnel
SaO_2	percent saturation of arterial blood (hemoglobin) with oxygen	UHDDS	uniform hospital discharge data set
		USPHS	United States Public Health Service
SBC	school-based clinic	VA	Veterans Affairs
SI	*le Système International d'Unités* (the international system of units)	VLDL	very low-density lipoprotein
		V/Q	ventilation/perfusion mismatch
SL	sublingual	VRE	vancomycin-resistant enterococci
SLT	social learning theory	WBC	white blood cell
SMDA	Safe Medical Devices Act	WIC	Women, Infants, and Children

Appendix B

Body Mass Index (BMI)

	Healthy		Overweight					Obese				
BMI	19	24	25	26	27	28	29	30	35	40	45	50
Height	**Weight in Pounds**											
4′10″	91	115	119	124	129	134	138	143	167	191	215	239
4′11″	94	119	124	128	133	138	143	148	173	198	222	247
5′0″	97	123	128	133	138	143	148	153	179	204	230	255
5′1″	100	127	132	137	143	148	153	158	185	211	238	264
5′2″	104	131	136	142	147	153	158	164	191	318	246	273
5′3″	107	135	141	146	152	158	163	169	197	225	254	282
5′4″	110	140	145	151	157	163	169	174	204	232	262	291
5′5″	114	144	150	156	162	168	174	180	210	240	270	300
5′6″	118	148	155	161	167	173	179	186	216	247	278	309
5′7″	121	153	159	166	172	178	185	191	223	255	287	319
5′8″	125	158	164	171	177	184	190	197	230	262	295	328
5′9″	128	162	169	176	182	189	196	203	236	270	304	338
5′10″	132	167	174	181	188	195	202	209	243	278	313	348
5′11″	136	172	179	186	193	200	208	215	250	286	322	358
6′0″	140	177	184	191	199	206	213	221	258	294	331	368
6′1″	144	182	189	197	204	212	219	227	265	302	340	378
6′2″	148	186	194	202	210	218	225	233	272	311	350	389
6′3″	152	192	200	208	216	224	232	240	279	319	359	399
6′4″	156	197	205	213	221	230	238	246	287	328	369	410

To determine body mass index, find the patient's height in feet and inches. Follow the numbers across the page to the patient's weight in pounds. Then go to the top of the column for the BMI rating.

Common Intravenous (IV) Therapy Solutions

Common Intravenous Solution	Components	Clinical Use	Precautions	Nursing Actions
VOLUME EXPANDERS				
D_5W (Hypotonic) *Also listed isotonic* $D_{10}W$ (Hypertonic) $D_{20}W$ (Hypertonic) $D_{500}W$ (Hypertonic)	Carbohydrates in **water**	■ Provides calories for essential energy. ■ Provides breakdown of protein needs. ■ Prevents dehydration. ■ Improves hepatic function.	Do not administer with blood. Will cause hemolysis of red cells. Electrolyte-free solutions may result in hypokalemia.	Monitor intake and output (I & O). Monitor serum K+.
D_5 1/3 (Hypertonic) D_5 1/2 (Hypertonic)	Carbohydrates in **normal saline (NS)**	■ Hypertonic solutions useful to pull fluid from tissues into bloodstream, such as burns, increased intracranial pressure (ICP) and postoperatively to keep swelling from operative site. ■ Provides sodium chloride.	Do not administer to patients with cellular dehydration. Use cautiously in patients with cardiac disease, congestive heart failure (CHF), hypertension, and other fluid volume excesses or deficits because additional fluid will be moved into the bloodstream.	Monitor I & O. Monitor vital signs. Monitor for signs and symptoms of CHF.
D_5 NS (Hypertonic)	Carbohydrates in **NS**	■ Temporary treatment for excessive fluid loss. ■ Early treatment along with plasma or albumin for fluid loss due to burns. ■ Treatment for acute adrenocortical insufficiency.	Use with caution in patients with cardiac, renal, and hepatic disease. May result in acidosis and hypokalemia.	Monitor I & O. Monitor vital signs. Monitor patient for circulatory overload and shortness of breath. Monitor serum K+.

Common Intravenous (IV) Therapy Solutions—cont'd

Common Intravenous Solution	Components	Clinical Use	Precautions	Nursing Actions
VOLUME EXPANDERS—cont'd				
NaCl 0.9% (Isotonic; same tonicity as plasma)	Sodium chloride	▪ Restores circulatory volume. ▪ Treatment for hypovolemic hypotension. ▪ Treatment for metabolic acidosis. ▪ Replaces sodium chloride deficit. ▪ Initiation and termination of blood transfusions.	Use with caution in patients with cardiac, renal, and hepatic disease. May result in acidosis and hypokalemia.	Monitor I & O. Monitor vital signs. Monitor patient for circulatory overload and shortness of breath.
0.45% NS (Hypotonic) 0.33% NS (Hypotonic)	Sodium chloride	▪ Replaces sodium chloride deficits. ▪ Treatment of cellular dehydration.	Do not administer to patients with increased ICP, burns, or edema.	Monitor I & O. Monitor vital signs. Monitor extremities for edema.
Ringer's Lactate (Isotonic)	Sodium chloride, potassium, calcium, and lactate	▪ Replaces surgical and gastrointestinal losses. ▪ Treats dehydration. ▪ Fluid losses due to diarrhea and burns	Use with caution in patients with renal, cardiac, and liver diseases.	Monitor I & O. Monitor vital signs. Monitor blood gases.
Ringer's Injection (Isotonic)	Content approximates that of plasma and includes sodium, potassium, calcium, and chloride.	▪ Used to replace electrolytes. ▪ Provides water for hydration. ▪ Often used to replace extracellular fluid losses.	Do not use in severe metabolic acidosis or alkalosis. Does not contain calories. Use with caution in patients with renal, cardiac, and liver diseases. Can cause overhydration electrolyte excess, and caloric depletion.	Monitor I & O. Monitor serum electrolytes. Monitor blood gases.

continued

Common Intravenous (IV) Therapy Solutions—cont'd

Common Intravenous Solution	Components	Clinical Use	Precautions	Nursing Actions
PLASMA EXPANDERS				
Dextran 6% in NS Dextran 5% in sterile water	Dextran	▪ Increases blood volume temporarily. ▪ Restores excessive fluid loss to hypovolemic shock.	Do not use as sole replacement of blood.	Observe for allergic reactions such as wheezing, mild urticaria, nausea, and vomiting. Notify nurse manager and health care provider.
Hetastarch	Hetastarch	▪ Increases blood volume. ▪ Increase granulocyte yield during leukapheresis.	Can cause hypovolemia, electrolyte imbalances, tissue dehydration, anaphylactic reactions, and increased bleeding times. Preexisting conditions should be considered, such as renal or cardiac disease.	Monitor labs for serum protein and hematocrit.
Albumin	Albumin (natural plasma protein)	▪ Used for plasma volume expansion in treating shock or impending shock related to circulatory volume deficit. ▪ Albumin 5% solution generally used to treat hypovolemia. ▪ Albumin 5% solution reserved for treatment when there are fluid and sodium restrictions.	The potential for complications should be considered if cardiac, hepatic, or renal disease is present.	

Appendix D

Glasgow Coma Scale (GCS)

The Glasgow Coma Scale is used to measure eye response, motor response, and verbal response in patients. There are points assigned to each response, and the points are totaled for a best possible score of 15 or lowest score of 3. The scale is listed below.

EYE RESPONSE	
Spontaneously	4
To voice	3
To pain	2
No response	1
MOTOR RESPONSE	
Follows commands	6
Localizes to pain	5
Withdraws from pain	4
Decorticate	3
Decerebrate	2
No response	1
VERBAL RESPONSE	
Oriented and converses	5
Disoriented and converses	4
Inappropriate word use	3
Incomprehensible sounds	2
No response	1
Total score	

Appendix E

Nursing Management of Chest Drainage System

What to Check	Steps to Complete	Rationale
Observe patient condition	Assessment	▪ Observe for dyspnea. ▪ Assess pain using 10-point scale. ▪ Make sure chest tube dressing is secure and dry. ▪ Listen to breath sounds.
Verifying system operation	Placement of unit: ▪ Upright with floor stand open and perpendicular to the chest drainage device. ▪ Unit below level of patient's chest. ▪ Ensure patient clamp in the open position. ▪ Ensure all connections are secure.	▪ If the chest drainage device tips over, unrestricted atmospheric air may be infused back to the patient. ▪ If the drainage chamber tips over, you must change the entire system if the fluid collected moves into each of the three columns of fluid collection. ▪ If you place the unit above the level of the chest, you may accidentally infuse fluid or air into the pleural space.
Observe water seal for patient air leaks. Observe suction control chamber.	▪ Monitor bubbling in water seal leak monitor. ▪ Adequate water level.	▪ Continuous bubbling will confirm a persistent air leak. ▪ Intermittent bubbling confirms an alternating air leak. ▪ Absence of bubbling indicates no air leak is present. ▪ If needed, you may add water-to-water seal by syringe via the front face grommet. Fill only to 2 cm grommet line. ▪ Avoid vigorous bubbling because this can increase pressure and cause tissue damage. ▪ Add additional water to suction control by temporarily turning suction source off, add desired water, and slowly resume suction level.

Appendix F

Reference Laboratory Values

Laboratory Tests	Conventional Units	SI Units
Acid hemolysis	No hemolysis	No hemolysis
Alkaline phosphatase	14–100	14–100
Cell counts		
Erythrocytes		
Male	4.6–6.2 million/mm^3	4.6–6.2 × 10^{12}/L
Female	4.2–5.4 million/mm^3	4.2–5.4 × 10^{12}/L
Children (varies with age)	4.5–5.1 million/mm^3	4.5–5.1 × 10^{12}/L
Leukocytes, total	4,500–11,000/mm^3	
Leukocytes, differential counts		
Myelocytes	0%	0/L
Band neutrophils	3–5%	150–400 × 10^6/L
Segmented neutrophils	54–62%	3,000–5,800 × 10^6/L
Lymphocytes	25–33%	1,500–3,000 × 10^6/L
Monocytes	3–7%	300–500 × 10^6/L
Eosinophils	1–3%	50–250 × 10^6/L
Basophils	0–1%	15–50 × 10^6/L
Platelets	150,000–400,000/mm^3	150–400 × 10^9/L
Reticulocytes	25,000–75,000/mm^3	25–75 × 10^9/L

continued

Reference Laboratory Values—cont'd

Laboratory Tests	Conventional Units	SI Units
Coagulation tests		
Bleeding time	2.75–8 min	2.75–8 min
Coagulation time	5–15 min	5–15 min
D-dimer	less than 0.5 μg/mL	less than 0.5 μg/mL
Factor VIII and other coagulation factors	50–150 of normal	50–150 of normal
Fibrin split products	less than 10 μg/mL	less than 10 μg/mL
Fibrinogen	200–400 mg/dL	200–400 mg/dL
Partial thromboplastin time (PTT)	20–35 sec	20–35 sec
Prothrombin time (PT)	12–14 sec	12–14 sec
Coombs' test		
Direct	Negative	
Indirect	Negative	
Corpuscular values of erythrocytes		
Mean corpuscular hemoglobin	26–34 pg/cell	26–34 pg/cell
Mean corpuscular volume	80–96 μm^3	80–96 fL
Mean corpuscular hemoglobin concentration (MCHC)	32–36 g/dL	320–360 g/L
Haptoglobin	20–165 mg/dL	0.20–1.65 g/L
Hematocrit		
Male	40–54 mL/dL	0.40–0.54
Female	37–47 mL/dL	0.37–0.47
Newborn	49–54 mL/dL	0.49–0.54
Children (varies with age)	35–49 mL/dL	0.35–0.49

Reference Laboratory Values—cont'd

Laboratory Tests	Conventional Units	SI Units
Hemoglobin		
Male	13–18 g/dL	8.1–11.2 mmol/L
Female	12–16 g/dL	7.4–9.9 mmol/L
Newborn	16.5–19.5 g/dL	10.2–12.1 mmol/L
Children (varies with age)	11.2–16.5 g/dL	7–10.2 mmol/L
Hemoglobin, fetal	less than 1% of total	less than 0.01 of total
Hemoglobin A1C	3–5% of total	0.03–0.05 of total
Hemoglobin A2	1.5–3% of total	0.015–0.03 of total
Hemoglobin, plasma	0–5 mg/dL	0–3.2 μmol/L
Methemoglobin	30–130 mg/dL	19–80 μmol/L
Erythrocyte sedimentation rate (ESR)		
Wintrobe		
Male	0–5 mm/hr	0–5 mm/hr
Female	0–55 mm/hr	0–15 mm/hr
Westergren		
Male	0–15 mm/hr	0–15 mm/hr
Female	0–20 mm/hr	0–20 mm/hr

Appendix G

Electrocardiogram (ECG) Rhythm Wave Forms

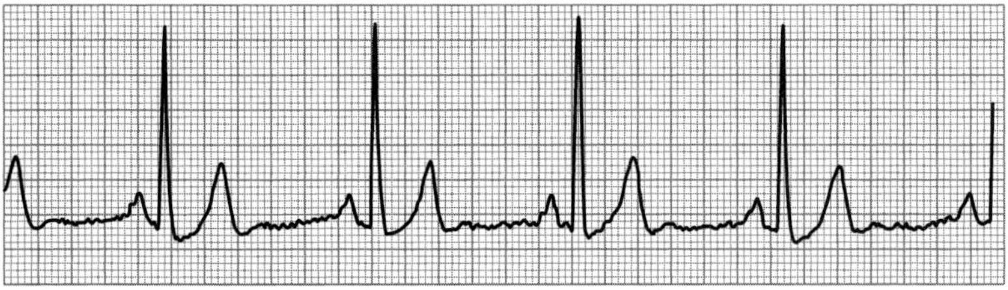

Figure 3 Sinus bradycardia. Ventricular rate 40, PR interval 0.20, QRS interval 0.12.

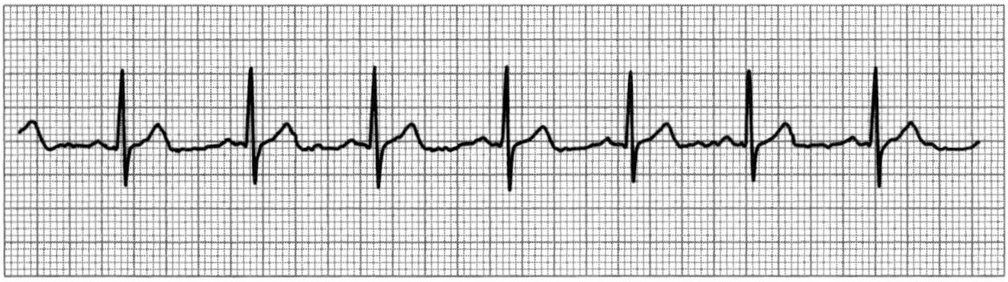

Figure 4 Normal sinus rhythm. Ventricular rate 70, PR interval 0.20, QRS interval 0.08.

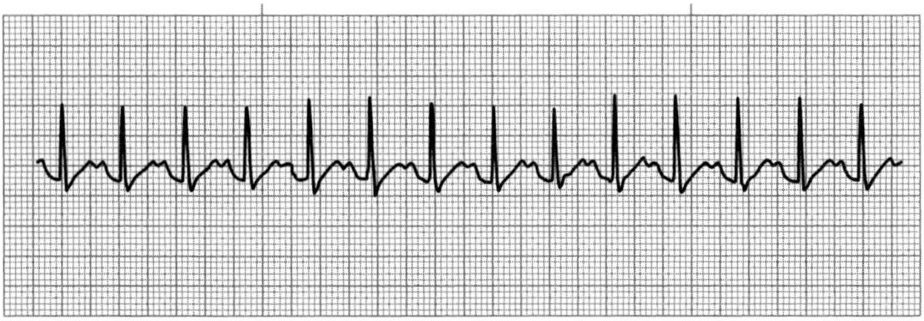

Figure 5 Sinus tachycardia. Ventricular rate 140, PR interval 0.16, QRS interval 0.06.

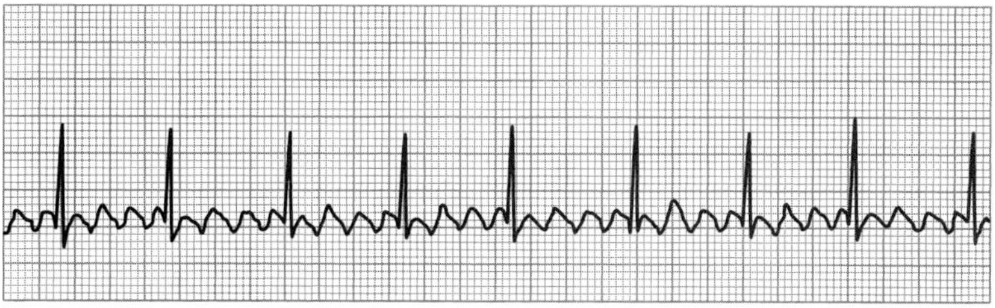

Figure 6 Atrial flutter. Ventricular rate 90, atrial rate 360, QRS interval 0.08. Note flutter waves; also called atrial flutter with 4:1 conduction.

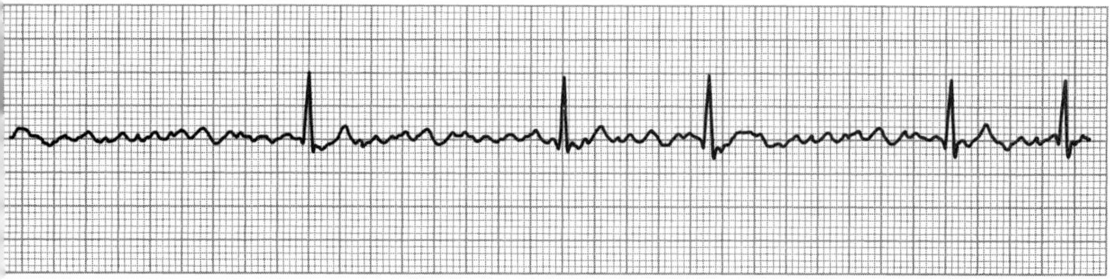

Figure 7 Atrial fibrillation. Ventricular rate 40, unable to measure PR interval because the atrium is fibrillating, QRS interval 0.10, and rhythm is irregular.

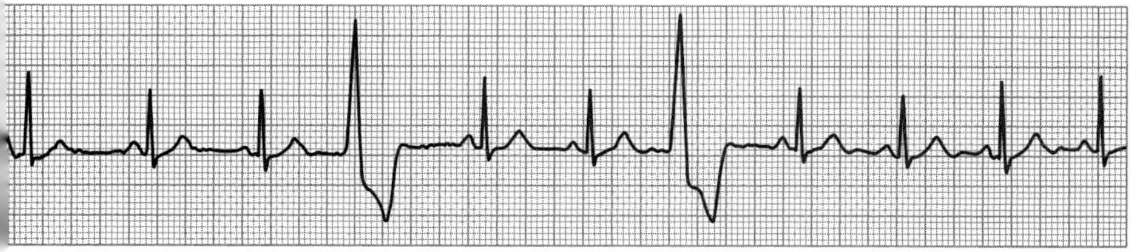

Figure 8 Normal sinus rhythm with premature ventricular contractions (PVCs). Underlying rhythm is normal sinus rhythm with two premature ventricular contractions. The PVCs arrive before the next expected beat (premature) and only have QRS complexes (ventricular contraction).

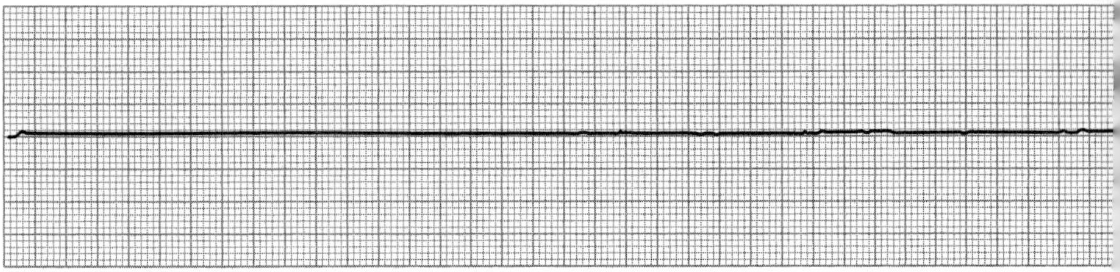

Figure 9 Asystole. No myocardial activity and is a medical emergency. To verify the rhythm, check leads to confirm they are intact and increase gain on ECG tracing.

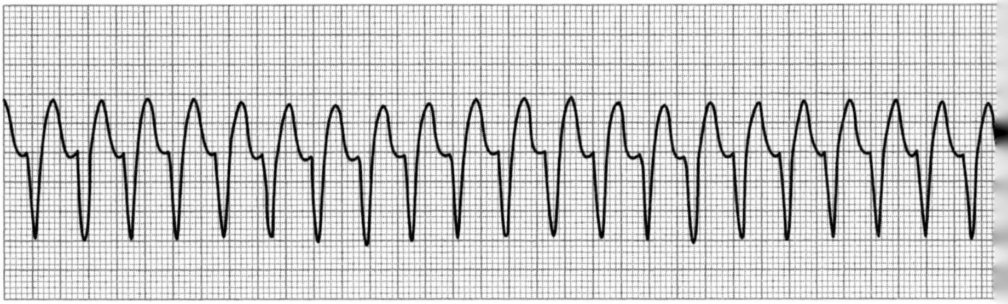

Figure 10 Ventricular tachycardia. The rhythm is regular, consists of wide QRS complexes, and is a medical emergency.

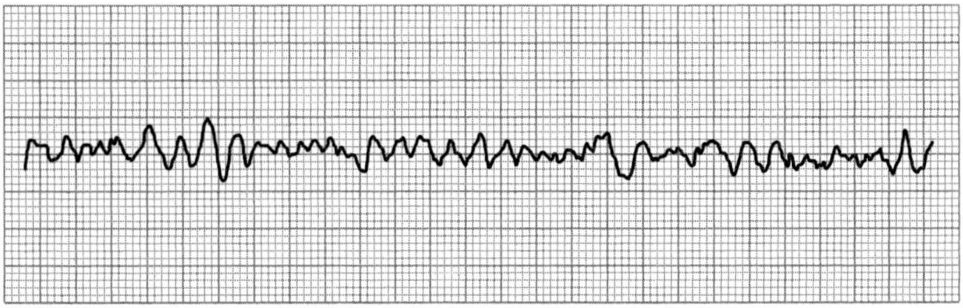

Figure 11 Ventricular fibrillation. The rhythm is erratic, represents the ventricles fibrillating, and is a medical emergency.

Appendix H

Spanish Words and Phrases

Being able to say a few words or phrases in the patient's language is one way to show that you care. It lets the patient know that you as a nurse are interested in the individual. There are three rules to keep in mind regarding the pronunciation of Spanish words.

- If a word ends in a vowel, or in n or s, the accent is on the next to the last syllable.
- If the word ends in a consonant other than n or s, the accent is on the last syllable.
- If the word does not follow these rules, it has a written accent over the vowel of the accented symbol.

Courtesy phrases, names of body parts, and expressions of time and numbers are included in this section for quick reference. The English version will appear first, followed by the Spanish translation and Spanish pronunciation.

COURTESY PHRASES

Please	Por favor	Por-fah-**vor**
Thank you	Gracias	**Grah**-the-as
Good morning	Buenos días	Boo-**ay**-nos **dee**-as
Good afternoon	Buenas tardes	Boo-**ay**-nos **tar**-days
Good evening	Buenas noches	Boo-**ay**-nos **no**-chays
Yes/No	Sí/No	See/No
Good	Bien	Be-en
Bad	Mal	Mahl
How many?	¿Cuántos?	Coo-**ahn**-tos?
Where?	¿Dónde?	**Don**-day?
When?	¿Cuándo?	Coo-**ahn**-do?

continued

Spanish Words and Phrases—cont'd

BODY PARTS

abdomen	el abdomen	el ab-doh-men
ankle	el tobillo	el to-**beel**-lyo
anus	el ano	el **ah**-no
anvil (incus)	el yunque	el **yoon**-kay
appendix	al apéndice	el ah-**pen**-de-thay
aqueous humor	el humor acuoso	el oo-**mor** ah-coo-**o**-so
bladder	la vejiga	la vah-**nee**-gah
brain	el cerebro	el thay-**ray**-bro
breast	el pecho	el **pay**-cho
buttock	la nalga	lah **nal**-gah
calf	la pantorrilla	lah pan-tor-**reel**-lyah
cervix	la cerviz	lah ther-**veth**
cheek	la mejilla	lah mah-**heel**-lyah
chin	la barbilla	lah bar-**beel**-lyah
choroid	la coroidea	lah co-ro-e-**day**-ah
ciliary body	el cuerpo ciliar	el coo-**err**-po the-le-**ar**
clitoris	el clitoris	el **clee**-to-ris
coccyx	el coxis	el **coc**-see
conjunctiva	la conjunctiva	la con-hoon-**tee**-vah
cornea	la córnea	lah **cor**-nay-ah
penis	el pene	el **pay**-nay
prostate gland	la próstata	lah **pros**-ta-tah
pupil	la pupila	lah poo-**pee**-lah
rectum	el recto	el **rec**-to
retina	la retina	lah ray-**tee**-nah

Spanish Words and Phrases—cont'd

BODY PARTS—cont'd

sclera	la esclerótica	lah es-clay-**ro**-te-cah
scrotum	el escroto	el ex-**cro**-to
seminal vesicle	la vesícula seminal	lah vay-**see**-coo-lah say-me-**nahl**
shoulder	el hombro	el **om**-bro
small intestine	el intestino delgado	el in-tes-**tee**-no del-**gah**-do
spinal cord	la médula espinal	lay **may**-doo-lah es-pe-**nahl**
spleen	el bazo	el **bah**-tho
stirrup (stapes)	el estribo	el es-**tree**-bo
stomach	el estómago	el es-**toh**-mah-go
temple	la sien	lah se-**ayn**
testis	el testículo	el tes-**tee**-coo-lo
thigh	el muslo	el **moos**-lo
thorax	el tórax	el **to**-rax
tongue	la lengua	lah **len**-goo-ah
trachea	la tráquea	lah **tray**-kay-ah
upper extremities	las extremidades superiores	las ex-tray-me-**dahd**-es soo-pay-re-**or**-es
ureter	el uréter	el oo-**ray**-ter
uterus	el útero	el **oo**-tay-o
vagina	el vagina	lah vah-**hee**-nah
vitreous humor	el humor vítreo	el oo-**more vee**-tray-o
wrist	la muñeca	lah moo-**nyah**-cah

EXPRESSIONS OF TIME, CALENDAR, AND NUMBERS

after meals	después de comer	des-poo-**es** day co-**merr**
at bedtime	al acostarse	al ah-cos-**tar**-say

continued

Spanish Words and Phrases—cont'd

EXPRESSIONS OF TIME, CALENDAR, AND NUMBERS—cont'd

before meals	antes de comer	**ahn**-tes day co-**merr**
daily	el diario	el de-**ah**-re-o
date	la fecha	lay **fay**-chah
day	el día	el **dee**-ah
every hour	a cada hora	ah **cah**-dah **o**-rah
hour (time)	la hora	lah **o**-rah
how often	cada cuánto tiempo	**cah**-dah coo-**ahn**-to te-**em**-po
noon	el mediodía	el may-de-o-**dee**-ah
now	ahora	ah-**o**-rah
once	una vez	**oo**-nah veth
today	hoy	**oh**-e
tomorrow	mañana	man-**nyah**-nah
tonight	esta noche	**es**-tach **no**-chay
week	la semana	lah say-**mah**-nah
year	año	**a**-nyo
Sunday	el domingo	el do-**meen**-go
Monday	el lunes	el **loo**-nes
Tuesday	el martes	el **mar**-tes
Wednesday	el miércoles	el me-**err**-co-les
Thursday	el jueves	el hoo-**ay**-ves
Friday	el viernes	el ve-**err**-nes
Saturday	el sábado	el **sah**-bah-do
zero	cero	**thay**-ro
one	uno	**oo**-no
two	dos	dose

Spanish Words and Phrases—cont'd

EXPRESSIONS OF TIME, CALENDAR, AND NUMBERS—cont'd

three	tres	trays
four	cuatro	coo-**ah**-tro
five	cinco	**theen**-co
six	seis	**say**-ees
seven	siete	se-**ay**-tay
eight	ocho	**o**-cho
nine	nueve	noo-**ay**-vay
ten	diez	de-**eth**

NURSING CARE SENTENCES AND QUESTIONS

What is your name?
¿Cómo se llama usted?
¿Co-mo say **lyah**-mah oos-**ted**?

I am a student nurse.
Soy estudiante enfermero(a).
Soy es-too-de-**ahn**-tay en-fer-**may**-ro(a).

My name is. . .
Mi nombre es. . .
Me **nom**-bray es. . .

Do you need a wheelchair?
¿Necesita usted una silla de rueda?
¿Nay-thay-**se**-ta oos-**ted oo**-nah **seel**-lyah day roo-**ay**-dah?

How do you feel?
¿Cómo se siente?
¿Co-mo say se-**ayn**-tah?

When is your family coming?
¿Cuándo viene su familia?
¿Coo-**ahn**-do vee-**en**-nah soo fah-**mee**-le-ah?

This is the call light.
Esta es la luz para llamar a la enferemera.
Es-tah es la looth **pah**-ra lyah-**mar** a lah en-fer-**may**-ra.

If you need anything, press the button.
Si usted necesita algo, oprima el botón.
See oos-**ted** nay-thay-**se**-ta **ahl**go o-pre-**ma** el bo-**tone.**

continued

Spanish Words and Phrases—cont'd

NURSING CARE SENTENCES AND QUESTIONS—cont'd

Do not turn without calling the nurse.
No se voltee sin llamar a la enferemera.
No say vol-tay seen lyah-**mar** a lah en-fer-**may**-ra.

The side rails on your bed are for your protection.
Los rieles del costado están para su protección.
Los re-**el**-es del cos-**tah**-do es-**tahn pah**-ra so pro-tec-the-**on.**

Please do not try to lower or climb over the side rail.
Por favor no pretenda bajarlos (barjarlas) o treparse sobre ellos.
Pr-fah-**vor** no pray-**ten**-dah ba-**har**-los o tray-**par**-say **so**-bray **ayl**-los.

The head nurse is. . .
La jefa de enfermera es. . .
La **hay**-fay day en-fer-**may**-ras es. . .

Do you need more blankets or another pillow?
¿Necesita usted más frazadas u otra almohada?
¿Nay-thay-**si**-ta oos-**ted** mahs frall-**thad**-dabs oo **o**-trah al-mo-**ah**-dah?

You may not smoke in the room.
No se puede fumar en el cuarto.
No say poo-**ay**-day foo-**mar** en el coo-**ar**-to.

Do you want me to turn on (turn off) the lights?
¿Quiere usted que encienda (apague) la luz?
¿Ke-**ay**-ray oos-**ted** day en-the-**en**-dah (a-**pah**-gay) lah looth?

Are you thirsty?
¿Tiene usted sed?
¿Tee-**en**-nah oos-**ted** sayd?

Are you allergic to any medication?
¿Es usted alérgico(a) a alguna medicina?
¿Es oos-**ted** ah-**lehr**-hee-co(a) ah ah-**goo**-nah nay-de-**thee**-nah?

You may take a bath.
Usted puede bañarse.
Oos-**ted** poo-**ay**-day bah-**nyar**-say.

Do not lock the door, please.
No cierre usted la puerta con llave, por favor.
No the-**err**-ray oos-**ted** lah poo-**err**-tah con **lyah**-vay por-fah-**vor.**

Call if you feel faint or in need of help.
Llame si usted se siente débil o si necesita ayuda.
Lyah-mah see oos-**ted** say se-**ayn**-tah **day**-bil o see nay-thay-**se**-ta ah-**yoo**-dah.

Spanish Words and Phrases—cont'd

NURSING CARE SENTENCES AND QUESTIONS—cont'd

Call when you have to go to the toilet.
Llame cuando tenga que ir al inodoro.
Lyah-mah coo-**ahn**-do **ten**-gah kay eer al in-o-**do**-ro.

I will give you an enema.
Le pondra una enema.
Lay pon-**dray oo**-nah ay-**nay**-mah.

Turn on your left (right) side.
Voltese a su lado izquierdo (derecho).
Vol-**tay**-say ah soo **lah**-do ith-ke-**er**-do(dah) (day-**ray**-cho[cha]).

Here is an appointment card.
Aqui tiene usted una tarjeta con la información escrito.
Ah-**kee** tee-**en**-nah oos-**ted oo**-nah tar-**hay**-tah con lah in-for-mah-the-**on** es-**cree**-to.

You are going to be discharged (released) today.
A usted le van a dar de alta hoy.
Ah oos-**ted** lay vahn ah dar day **ahl**-tah **oh**-e.

How did this illness begin?
¿Cómo empezó esta enfermedad?
¿Co-mo em-pa-**tho es**-tah en-fer-may-**dahd**?

Is the pain better after the medicine?
¿Siente usted alivio depués de tomar la medicina?
¿Se-**ayn**-tah oos-**ted** al-**lee**-ve-o des-poo-**es** day to-**mar** lah may-de-**thee**-nah?

Where is the pain?
¿Qué la duele? (or) ¿Dónde le duele?
¿Kay lah doo-**ay**-le? (or) ¿**Don**-day lay doo-**ay**-le?

Do you have pains in your chest?
¿Tiene usted dolores in el pecho?
¿Tee-**en**-nah oos-**ted** do-**lor**-es en el **pay**-cho?

Are you in pain now?
¿Tiene usted dolores ahora?
¿Tee-**en**-nah oos-**ted** do-**lor**-es ah-**o**-rah?

Is it constant pain or does it come and go?
¿Es un dolor constante or va y vuelve?
¿Es oon do-**lor** cons-**tahn**-tay o vah ee voo-**el**-vah?

¿Is there anything that makes the pain better?
¿Hay algo que lo alivie?
¿Ah-ee **ahl**-go kay lo al-**le**-ve?

continued

Spanish Words and Phrases—cont'd

NURSING CARE SENTENCES AND QUESTIONS—cont'd

Is there anything that makes the pain worse?
¿Hay algo que lo aumente?
¿Ah-ee **ahl**-go kay lo ah-oo-**men**-tay?

Where do you feel the pain?
¿Dónde siente usted el dolor?
¿Don-day se-**ayn**-tah oos-**ted** el do-**lor?**

Point to where it hurts.
Apunte usted por favor, adonde le duele.
Ah-**poon**-tay oos-**ted** por fah-**vor** ah-**don**-day lay doo-**ay**-le.

Show me where it hurts.
Enaéñeme usted donde le duele.
En-**say**-nah-may oos-**ted** don-**day** lay doo-**ay**-le.

Is the pain sharp or dull?
¿Es agudo o sardo el dolor?
¿Es ah-**goo**-do o **sor**-do el do-**lor?**

Do you know where you are?
¿Sabe usted donde está?
¿Sah-**bay** oos-**ted** don-**day** es-**tah?**

You are in a hospital.
Usted está en el hospital.
Oos-**ted** es-**tah** en el os-pee-**tahl.**

You will be okay.
Usted va a estar bien.
Oos-**ted** vah a es-**tar** **be**-en.

Do you have any drug reactions?
¿Tiene usted alguna sensibilidad a productos químicos?
¿Te-**en**-nah oos-**ted** al-**goo**-nah sen-se-be-le-**dahd** a pro-**dooc**-tos **kee**-me-cos?

Have you seen another doctor or native healer for this problem?
¿Ha vista usted a otro médico a curandero tocante a este problema?
¿Ah **vees**-to oos-**ted** a **o**-tro **may**-de-co o coo-ran-**day**-ro to-**cahn**-tay a **es**-ah pro-**blay**-mah?

Have you vomited?
¿Ha vomitado usted?
¿Ah vo-me-**tah**-do oos-**ted?**

Do you have any difficulty in breathing?
¿Tiene usted alguna dificultad para respirar?
¿Te-**en**-nah oos-**ted** ah-**goo**-nah de-fe-cool-**tahd** **pah**-ra res-pe-**rar?**

Spanish Words and Phrases—cont'd

NURSING CARE SENTENCES AND QUESTIONS—cont'd

Do you smoke?
¿Fuma usted?
¿Foo-**mar** oos-**ted?**

How many per day?
¿Cuántos al día?
¿Coo-**ahn**-tos al **dee**-ah?

For how many years?
¿Par cuántos años?
¿Por coo-**ahn**-tos **a**-nos?

Do you awaken in the night because of shortness of breath?
¿Se despiena usted por la noche par falta de respiración?
¿Say des-pee-**err**-tah oos-**ted** por lah **no**-chay por **fahl**-tah day res-pe-rah-the-**on?**

Is any part of your body swollen?
¿Tiene usted alguna parte del cuerpo hinchada?
¿Te-**en**-nah oos-**ted** ah-**goo**-nah **par**-tay del coo-**err**-po in-**chah**-da?

How much water do you drink daily?
¿Cuántos vasos de agua bebe usted diariamente?
¿Coo-**ahn**-tos **vah**-sos day **ah**-goo-ah **bay**-be oos-**ted** de-ah-re-ah-**men**-tay?

Are you nauseated?
¿Tiene náusea?
¿Te-**en**-nah **nah**-oo-say-ah?

Are you going to vomit?
¿Va a vomitar?
¿Vah a vo-me-**tar?**

When was your last bowel movement?
¿Cuánto tiempo hace que evacúa usted?
¿Coo-**ahn**-to te-**em**-po **ah**-the kay ay-vah-**coo**-ah oos-**ted?**

Do you have diarrhea?
¿Tiene usted diarrea?
¿Te-**en**-nah oos-**ted** der-ar-**ray**-ah?

How much do you urinate?
¿Cuánto orina usted?
¿Coo-**ahn**-to o-**re**-nah oos-**ted?**

Did you urinate?
¿Orino usted?
¿O-re-**no** oos-**ted?**

continued

Spanish Words and Phrases—cont'd

NURSING CARE SENTENCES AND QUESTIONS—cont'd

What color is your urine?
¿De qué color es la orina?
¿Day kay co-**lor** es lah o-**re**-nah?

Call when you have to go to the toilet.
Llame usted cuando tenga que ir al inodoro.
Lyah-mah oos-**ted** coo-**ahn**-do **ten**-gah kay eer al in-o-**do**-ro.

I need a urine specimen from you.
Necesito una muestra de orina de usted.
Nay-thay-**se**-to **oo**-nah moo-**ays**-trah day o-**re**-nah day oos-**ted.**

We will put a tube in your bladder so that you can urinate.
Le pondremos un tubo en la vejiga para que puede orinar.
Lay pon-**dray**-mos un **too**-be en lah vay-**hee**-gah **pah**-rah kay poo-**ay**-day o-re-**nar.**

When was your last menstrual period?
¿Cuándo fue se última menstruación?
¿Coo-**ahn**-do foo-**ay** soo **ool**-te-mah mens-troo-ah-rhe-**on?**

Are you bleeding heavily?
¿Está sangrando mucho?
¿Es-tah san-**grahn**-do moo-cho?

Take off your clothes, please.
Desvístase usted, por favor.
Des-**ves**-tah-say oos-**ted** por-**fah**-vor.

Just relax.
Relaje usted el cuerpo.
Ray-**lah**-he oos-**ted** el coo-**err**-po.

I am going to listen to your chest.
Voy a escucharle el pecha.
Voye a es-coo-**char**-lay el **pay**-cho.

Let me feel your pulse.
Déjeme tomarle el pulso.
Day-ha-me to-**mar**-lay el **pool**-so.

I am going to take your temperature.
Voy a tomarle la tempetarura.
Voye a to-**mar**-lay lah tem-pay-rah-**too**-rah.

Lie down, please.
Acuéstese, por favor.
Ah-coo-**es**-tah-say por fah-**vor.**

Spanish Words and Phrases—cont'd

NURSING CARE SENTENCES AND QUESTIONS—cont'd

Do you understand?
¿Me comprende usted?
¿May com-**pren**-day oos-**ted?**

That's right.
Así. Bien.
Ah-**see. Be**-en.

You are doing very well.
Usted va muy bien.
Oos-**ted** vah **moo**-e **be**-en.

Do not take any medicine from home.
No tome usted ninguna medicina traída de su casa.
No **to**-may oos-**ted** nin-**goon**-ay may-de-**thee**-nah trah-**ee**-dah day soo **cah**-sah.

I am going to give you an injection.
Voy a ponerle una inyección.
Voye a po-**nerr**-lay **oo**-nah in-yec-the-**on.**

Take a sip of water.
Tome usted un traguito de agua.
To-may oos-**ted** un trah-**gee**-to day **ah**-goo-ah.

Very good. That was fine.
Muy bien. Excelente.
Moo-e **be**-en. Ex-thay-**len**-tay.

Don't be nervous.
No se ponga nervioso(a).
No say **pon**-gah ner-ve-**o**-so(ah).

Do you feel dizzy?
¿Se siente vertigo?
¿Say see-**ayn**-tah **verr**-to-go?

Please lie still.
Quédese inmóvil, por favor.
Kay-day-say in-**mo**-veel por-fah-**vor.**

You must drink lots of liquids.
Usted debe tomar muchos liquidos.
Oos-**ted day**-bay to-**mar moo**-chos **lee**-ke-dos.

continued

Spanish Words and Phrases—cont'd

REFERENCES

Kelz, R. K. (1997). *Conversational Spanish for health professionals* (3rd ed.). Clifton Park, NY: Delmar Learning.

Velazquez de la Cadena, M., Gray, E., & Iribas, J. (1985). *New revised Velazquez Spanish and English dictionary*. Clinton, NJ: New Win Publishing, Inc., 1985.

Index

Page references followed by *t*, *f*, and *b* refer to tables, figures, and boxes.

Notes

Notes

Notes

Notes

Notes

Notes

Notes

Notes

Notes

Notes